DOCTORS
and
DISEASES

in the Roman Empire

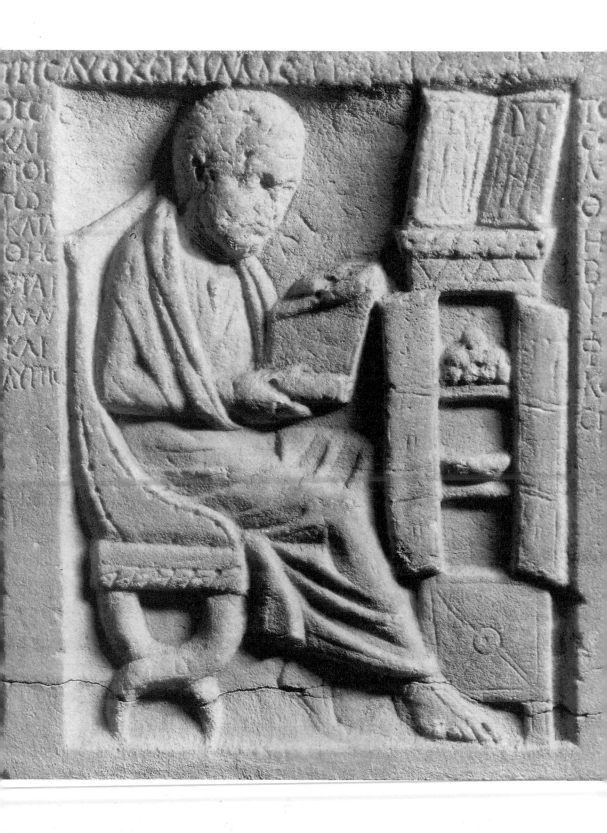

DOCTORS
and
DISEASES
in the Roman Empire

Ralph Jackson

BRITISH MUSEUM ⬚ PRESS

For Liz, Huw, Tom, Lindsay and Owen

Cover Drawing of a sard sealstone, showing a
seated physician, perhaps intended to represent
the great Hippocrates. He examines his young
patient watched over by Asklepios, god of
healing and patron of doctors. The god is dressed
in characteristic garb and leans on the serpent-
entwined staff, symbol of his miraculous powers.
1st–2nd century AD.

Frontispiece A physician reading from a scroll
before a cabinet which holds his surgical
instruments. From a marble sarcophagus, 4th
century AD.

Published by British Museum Press
A division of The British Museum Company Ltd
46 Bloomsbury Street, London WC1B 3QQ

First published 1988
First published in paperback 1991
Reprinted 1993, 1995, 2000 with corrections

British Library Cataloguing in Publication Data

Jackson, Ralph
    Doctors and diseases in the Roman Empire.
    1. Ancient Roman medicine
    I. Title
    610'.937
    ISBN 0-7141-1398-0

Design by Noelle Derrett
Cover design by Martin Richards

Typeset in Plantin and printed in Great Britain by
The Bath Press, Bath

Contents

Photographic acknowledgements

The author and publishers gratefully acknowledge the following for providing illustrations:

Bath Archaeological Trust 47
Susan Bird 13, cover illustration
The Trustees of the British Museum 2 (Dept of Coins and Medals); 4 (Dept of Egyptian Antiquities); 5, 11, 15, 22, 27, 32, 36, 40, 41, 42, 50 (Dept of Greek and Roman Antiquities); 20, 26, 44 (Dept of Prehistoric and Romano-British Antiquities)
Henry Buglass 39
Cirencester Excavation Committee 48
Philip Compton 43
Deutsches Archäologisches Institut, Athens 28, 38
Deutsches Archäologisches Institut, Rome 34
Metropolitan Museum of Art, New York (Gift of Earnest and Beata Brummer, 1948, in memory of Joseph Brummer) 17
Musée Barrois, Bar-le-Duc, photo Musée d'Histoire et d'Archéologie, Antibes 31
Musées de Metz 21
Musée du Louvre, Paris 3, 14
Museo Civico, Piacenza (photo Manzotti) 1
Museo Archeologico Nazionale, Naples (photo Soprintendenza Archeologica delle Province di Napoli e Caserta) 33
Museo Ostiense, Ostia (photo Fototeca Unione) 24
National Museums and Galleries on Merseyside 30, 46
Österreichische Nationalbibliothek, Vienna 19
T. W. Potter 9
Rheinisches Bildarchiv, Cologne 25b
Rheinisches Landesmuseum, Bonn 35
Römisch-Germanisches Museum, Cologne (photos Ralph Jackson) 18, 25a, 37
Römisch-Germanisches Zentralmuseum, Mainz 16, 23, 29
Society of Antiquaries of London 45
Dr Calvin Wells, and the Calvin Wells Laboratory for Burial Archaeology, School of Archaeological Sciences, University of Bradford 49
York Archaeological Trust and Derek Phillips 10

All other photographs are the copyright of the author.

Preface

Graeco-Roman medicine is a wonderfully challenging field of study with a prodigious range and volume of source material. The results of detailed research are to be found in the specialist literature of medical and classical historians and archaeologists, and there are general summaries in wider-ranging histories of medicine, but there have been few attempts to present the whole subject to a wide readership. In 1969, when John Scarborough published his *Roman medicine*, he noted that there had been 'no work putting Roman medicine and its development before the modern reader' since Sir Clifford Allbutt's *Greek medicine in Rome* had appeared in 1921. Equally, there has been no work to replace Scarborough's book which, despite some notable omissions, has remained the single most useful survey in English for almost twenty years. Not surprisingly, there have been many new and interesting developments in that time.

In this book, therefore, I have tried to give a broad but concise account of classical medicine as it culminated in the Roman Empire, for the interested but non-specialist reader, incorporating the results of recent discoveries and research. In doing so I have particularly sought to reveal the intriguing mixture of striking similarities and fundamental differences between the concepts, techniques, instruments and drugs of classical and modern medicine, and the equally fascinating relationship between rational and non-rational elements, the healing profession and the healing deities. I cannot hope to have covered every aspect in equal depth for, like any author, I have my own particular biases and preferences: the imprint of archaeologist and museum curator will be apparent. Nevertheless, I have tried to achieve a balanced view by marshalling the evidence from every possible source: from the treatises of Greek and Roman medical authors, our principal evidence for medical theory and practice; extracts from the works of lay writers, including geographers, historians, poets, social commentators, satirists and men of letters, which often give the patient's side of the story in fascinating, amusing and grisly anecdotes or wry and ironical asides; papyrus documents and letters, and inscribed tombstones, which shed light on the personal, social and legal aspects of medicine; carved stone reliefs, mosaics, gems, vase-paintings and wall-paintings, which provide us with 'snapshots' of doctors, midwives and healing deities at work; finely made surgical instruments and medical apparatus, which highlight the Roman technical achievement; the excavated remains of hospitals and healing sanctuaries, which demonstrate the complex arrangements devoted to the treatment of the sick in two very different branches of healing; traces of drugs and medicines, which amplify the written evidence of the classical pharmacopoeias; and plant remains, animal bones, micro-organisms and human skeletal remains, the ever more sophisticated study of which has begun to provide exciting and fundamentally important information on diet and disease.

In the gathering of material from such diverse sources I have benefited from the work and ideas of many people, both through their publications and through formal and informal discussion. In particular I am indebted to Dr Vivian Nutton of the Wellcome Institute for the History of Medicine, who read a draft of this book and offered invaluable advice. I am grateful, too, to Dr Ernst Künzl of the Römisch-Germanisches Zentralmuseum, Mainz, to Peter Jones, Fellow and librarian of King's College Cambridge, to Paul Swain, Surgical Unit, School of Medicine, University College London, to Mr John R. Kirkup, to my colleagues at the British Museum, especially Don Bailey, Lucilla Burn, Brian Cook, Ian Jenkins (Department of Greek and Roman Antiquities), Catherine Johns and Tim Potter (Department of Prehistoric and Romano-British Antiquities), and to the curators and staffs of many museums and institutions who have kindly assisted me. I would also like to record my debt to the late Roy Davies, who died, tragically, in 1977. His excellent publications on Roman military medicine fuelled my early interest in the subject and served to encourage me in my own research. Finally, my thanks go to Jenny Chattington of British Museum Publications, who has been a kind and encouraging editor; and to my wife and children who have shown remarkable forbearance during the prolonged and sometimes difficult 'gestation' of this book.

Chapter 1

Origins

> When the [bladder] stone has been extracted, if the patient is strong and
> has not suffered excessively, it is well to let the bleeding go on, so that
> less inflammation may follow. Besides it is not unfitting for him to move
> about a little in order that any blood clot still inside may drop out. But
> if again the bleeding does not cease of its own accord, it must be stopped
> lest all his strength be used up. (Celsus, *De Medicina* VII, 26, 5; trans.
> W. G. Spencer)

> The best of all safeguards against serpents is the saliva of a fasting human
> being, but our daily experience may teach us yet other values of its use.
> We spit on epileptics in a fit, that is, we throw back infection. In a similar
> way we ward off witchcraft and the bad luck that follows meeting a person
> lame in the right leg. (Pliny, *Natural History* XXVIII, vii, 35; trans. H.
> Rackham *et al.*)

These extracts, and many others like them, illustrate the startling mixture of sound
scientific procedures and bizarre practices that comprised classical medicine. Today
this commingling of opposites seems almost incomprehensible, but in Greek and
Roman society it occurred as a direct response to real and pressing needs, both physical
and spiritual.

Celsus and Pliny the Elder were near contemporaries in Roman Italy of the
first century AD and came from the same upper tier of society. Neither was a doctor,
and their writings are therefore those of intelligent laymen with an interest in medicine.
Celsus' work *De Medicina*, 'On Medicine', is the principal surviving part of his general
encyclopaedia, which also included books on agriculture, military art, rhetoric, philosophy and jurisprudence. It is a fine survey, in eight books, of medicine at his time,
compiled from selected written sources – mainly Greek – and personal observations.
Systematically arranged and written in a clear style for Latin lay readers, it includes
sections on dietetics and preventive medicine, diseases and their treatment, pharmacology and surgery. Some of the surgical procedures, like the measures to avoid inflammation after lithotomy quoted above, have been highly praised, while many of the
methods advocated in dietetics and preventive medicine are similar to those of today.

The counterpart to Celsus' synthesis of Graeco-Roman medicine, Pliny's medical
writings are as diffuse as Celsus' work is precise. They are part of his wide-ranging
Historia Naturalis, 'Natural History' in thirty-seven books, a unique compilation which
culled material from well over a hundred authors. The strength of the work, its
comprehensiveness, is also its weakness, for Pliny refused to select from his sources.
The result is that absurd theories rub shoulders with sensible measures, and many
of his medical remedies, including that above, we would regard as little more than
superstitious nonsense. However, the use of loathsome ingredients and bizarre rituals,

though repellent today, is strikingly similar to medieval magical cures and to those recorded by modern anthropologists. This brand of folk medicine rooted in ignorance and fear is one of the earliest instinctive stages in the struggle against disease, and can be identified in the evolution of most societies.

Both Celsus and Pliny were wealthy Roman landowners. They exemplify the Roman intellectual ideal of the self-sufficient *pater familias*, a man of wide learning and practical outlook. Part of medicine they regarded as a craft, the realm of those who worked with their hands, the remainder they believed to be the preserve of their own class. By observation, experience and reading they felt they could master the art of medicine without recourse to any kind of formal study or training, just as they mastered the techniques of agriculture or the methods of military or civilian administration, and with a large estate work-force there were sound practical reasons to be well versed in medicine. The concept of a professional physician was at odds with these traditional Roman values and might result in suspicion of others who claimed to be expert in a particular field. It is within this context that Pliny's sometimes scathing comments on doctors should be viewed: 'It is at the expense of our perils that they learn, and by conducting experiments they put us to death; a physician is the only man that can kill a man with sovereign impunity ... I shall not even attempt to denounce their avarice, the rapacious haggling while their patients' fate hangs in the balance.'[1]

By Pliny's day, however, Romans had become at least accustomed, if not agreeable, to the existence of trained physicians. Some three centuries earlier Greek physicians making their first contact with Rome encountered open hostility: 'The Greeks ... are a quite worthless people, and an intractable one ... When that race gives us its literature it will corrupt all things, and even the more if it sends hither its physicians. They have conspired together to murder all foreigners with their physic.'[2] Pliny quoted this hysterical outburst from Cato (234–149 BC), who saw increasing Greek influence as a threat to Roman traditions. Cato was no doctor, but he prided himself on his ability to supervise the health and well-being of his household, both family and slave alike. This was not altruism but hard-headed materialism: sick slaves cannot work efficiently, so to ensure profit they must be kept in health. The slave was a possession, part of the wealth-making equipment of the farm, and Cato, like any other Roman of his day, would have seen no distinction between the upkeep of slave, oxen or plough. Certainly, the brand of medicine he dispensed to the human work-force was little different to that of the livestock, while an unhealthy slave fared no better than damaged stock: 'Sell worn-out oxen, blemished cattle, blemished sheep, wool, hides, an old wagon, old tools, an old slave, a sickly slave, and whatever else is superfluous.'[3]

Cato's medicine, a mixture of magical incantations and animal and vegetable remedies – cabbage administered both internally and externally was his favourite 'cure-all' – was the heritage of Italic folk medicine. Another part of this heritage was the veneration of ancient gods, principally those of agriculture and fertility but also numerous spirits whose function was to safeguard the individual. For example, for childbirth Alemona guarded the foetus, Partula presided over the birth, Vagitanus ensured the first cry, Cunina watched over the cradle and Rumina was the spirit of breast-feeding, while the aid of many other spirits was invoked at subsequent transitional stages in life. These gods and spirits were the personified but mysterious forces of nature which both caused and alleviated disease. Thus early Italic medicine involved primarily the treatment of symptoms, because it was believed that prevention, diagnosis and prognosis – the forecast of the course of an illness – were controlled by gods and were beyond the realm of human action. Occasionally an illness or disease, especially those which were remittent, may have cleared or improved at the time a remedy was administered. This would have prolonged belief in archaic treatments, which often combined a simple food or drug therapy with the forces of magic liberated by obscure rituals or rhythmic chants.[4] Doctors had no part in this system of healing. The cure was believed to arise entirely from the remedy, which was paramount, and no special expertise was required of the person who administered it. Within the family control was vested in the *pater familias*, who either dispensed the remedy himself or ensured that his nominee employed the correct ingredients, words and rituals.

There was also an attempt to ward off disease at a higher level. With Etruscan influence Roman state religion had developed the practices of augury and divination, by which the priests were believed to be able to discern the will of the gods. The liver of a sacrificed animal was regarded as a particularly sensitive indicator. An elaborate ritual of slaughter and inspection by the specialist priest, the *haruspex*, combined with the consultation of related tables and texts, gave direction to important affairs of state or guidance in the case of serious outbreaks of disease.

1 Etruscan bronze model of a sheep's liver. The divisions probably related sections of the liver to regions of the sky and would have helped the priest to interpret as good or bad omens the signs he observed in the liver of a freshly sacrificed animal. From Piacenza, 3rd century BC.

The practice of divination, coupled with Etruscan contact with the Greek settlements of southern Italy, may be connected with the apparently early development of surgery by the Etruscans. Dentistry, too, was well advanced, at least in the provision of crowns and bridges (30). Nevertheless, Roman medicine remained generally unsophisticated, and in 295 BC, when Rome was held in the grip of plague, outside assistance had to be sought. Significantly it was not Greek physicians but the Greek

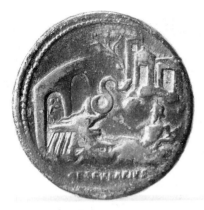

2 Asklepios comes to Rome. A sacred snake from Epidauros disembarks from the prow of a ship onto the island in the River Tiber to stem the plague of 295 BC and establish the first temple of Asklepios at Rome. Reverse of a medallion of Antoninus Pius.

healing god Asklepios whose help was enlisted. A temple was dedicated to him at Rome, though with characteristic suspicion it was erected outside the city on an island in the River Tiber. The plague subsided, and with this slender foothold the resistance to Greek doctors gradually decreased.

From this first contact began the process of amalgamation of Greek and Roman medicine that was ultimately to bring Rome to pre-eminence over the medical centres of Greek lands. However, although the diffuse lore of Italic folk remedies was absorbed into the framework of Greek and Hellenistic medicine, it was a comparatively minor influence. Rome borrowed heavily from Greece and an understanding of Roman medicine requires an examination of the origins and development of Greek medicine.

Evidence for the earliest stages of Greek medicine is sparse. While it might be assumed that the brilliant civilisation of the Greek Bronze Age – the Minoan culture of Crete and the Mycenaean culture of mainland Greece – had medical concepts as advanced as the artistic achievements, there is in fact little evidence to sustain such an assumption. Although excavations have shown there was an awareness of the importance of public health, with a well-designed drainage system at Knossos and other palace sites, these were adequate rather than highly sophisticated sanitary installations. Equally, evidence for the supply of water suggests a simple approach, utilising wells, springs and cisterns rather than any more elaborate system.

Further, indirect evidence is available in the form of Homer's *Odyssey* and *Iliad*, composed in the eighth century BC but depicting life in the Greek Bronze Age. The Homeric references to physicians and disease form a small but valuable body of information. In the *Odyssey*, for example, the physician is classed together with prophet, shipwright and minstrel as a 'worker for the public good',[5] which sheds a little light on his social standing. He was clearly of some importance, but as an itinerant worker he would not have been a landowner and therefore did not belong to the highest level of society. From earliest times these peripatetic doctors would have been patronised by aristocratic households, especially in times of war, when 'a healer is worth many other men for extracting arrows and spreading gentle remedies upon the wound'.[6]

In the *Iliad* is the earliest account of disease, the plague cast by Apollo upon the Greek army before Troy, while in both books there are descriptions of fearful injuries suffered in battle:

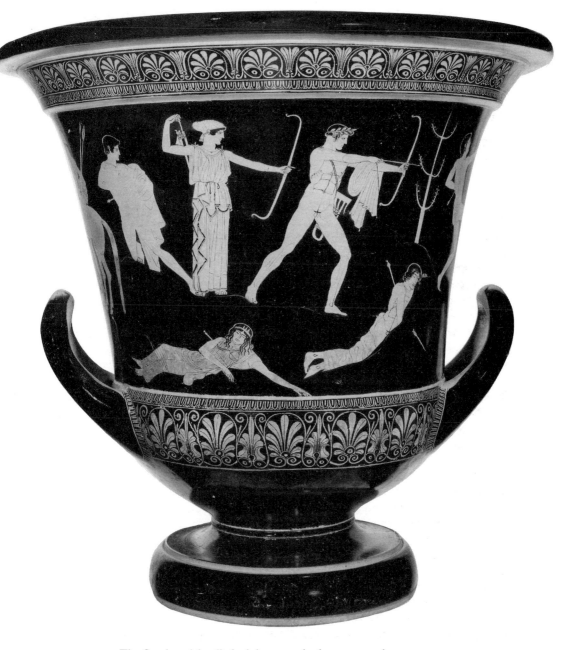

3 The Greek god Apollo had the power both to avert and to cause
mortal suffering. Here, with his sister Artemis, he looses his 'arrows
of death' on the children of Niobe. *Calyx-crater*, *c*. 455–450 BC, from
Orvieto.

> Then Idomeneus smote Erymas upon the mouth with a thrust of the pitiless bronze, and clean through passed the spear of bronze beneath the brain, and clave asunder the white bones; and his teeth were shaken out, and both his eyes were filled with blood; and up through mouth and nostrils he spurted blood as he gaped, and a black cloud of death enfolded him. (*Iliad* XVI, 345–50; trans. A. T. Murray)

Such wounds revealed interior structure and organs, albeit often damaged or dislodged, and allowed some rudimentary perception of anatomy, apparent in the descriptions themselves. How far such observations advanced the state of surgery it is not possible to say, for the treatment described was seldom other than missile extraction, washing and bandaging carried out either by a physician or a fellow warrior. Superstition played a large part, and sung incantations were used to stop the bleeding from one of Odysseus' wounds. Drugs, primarily powders or ointments concocted from dried herbs, were also frequently applied.[7]

In medicine, as in other spheres, the Minoans and Mycenaeans were in contact with Egypt, whence some of the more exotic herbs were obtained in trade, 'for the fertile soil of Egypt is most rich in herbs', Homer records, and, he continues; 'in medical knowledge the Egyptian leaves the rest of the world behind'.[8] An aid to the furthering of medical knowledge in Egypt, over and above the natural abundance of plants with medicinal properties, was the form of burial rite, embalming. This process, which involved the removal of the viscera, allowed regular observation of the interior organs and at least laid the basis for a partial understanding of human anatomy, though no clear link can be demonstrated between embalmers and physicians. In fact, progress was minimal, probably as a direct result of religious restrictions on human dissection, and it was to be many centuries before the study of anatomy received its great stimulus under the Ptolemies in Hellenistic Alexandria.

If anatomy and physiology were only rudimentarily understood, other aspects of early Egyptian medicine were well advanced. Both mummified bodies and a number of papyrus documents have preserved evidence of sound surgical techniques. Splinting of fractures was practised as early as the 5th Dynasty (2750–2625 BC), the use of palm fibre splints yielding particularly good results.[9] Also beneficial would have been the mouldy bread, rich in antibiotics, which some Egyptian doctors prescribed for wounds, while through embalming the antiseptic qualities of saltpetre and common salt were discovered, knowledge which may well have been put to good use in the treatment of wounds.

The Edwin Smith papyrus,[10] the remains of a great Egyptian surgical treatise of the seventeenth century BC, lists forty-eight cases of clinical surgery, mainly covering injuries and wounds to the head, chest and spine. Many interesting symptoms are noted: paralysis in limbs and sphincter following dislocation of cervical vertebrae; deafness resulting from fracture of the temporal bone; and the feeble pulse and fever observed in patients with mortal injuries to the head. Each case history is set down in a logical and methodical manner: the descriptive title, which is in the form of a provisional diagnosis, examination, listing of symptoms, diagnosis, prognosis, and treatment. As will be seen, this approach foreshadows the achievements of the great Hippocrates some twelve centuries later.

Another fascinating medical document, written about a century after the Edwin

4 Disorders of the anus and rectum are described on this Egyptian papyrus of the
19th Dynasty (*c.* 1200 BC). The remedies include four-hourly doses of carob beans,
fresh dates, castor oil, honey and water.

Smith papyrus, is the Ebers papyrus,[11] which came to light in Thebes in 1872. It
is an encyclopaedic compilation which includes a lengthy and detailed list of diseases.
Those of the ear and eye are prominent, and include a description of trachoma,
a contagious inflammation of the eye and a frequent cause of blindness in the past,
for which one of the remedies was a copper-based application similar to some still
in use today. As examination of mummies has made abundantly clear, intestinal and
other parasites were widespread, and the writer of the Ebers papyrus lists many,
including ancylostoma, schistosoma, filaria, taenia and ascaris. The prescriptions for
'hardening in the limbs' – arthritis – also echo the evidence from mummies and
skeletons: the nature of the climate and the unremitting toil of hard physical work
seem to have spared few in their later years from the pain and disability of osteoarthritis.

The therapeutics of the Ebers papyrus is extensive, though not necessarily sophisticated, and amongst some sound medical remedies there are also magical incantations.
However, the section on tumours is remarkable. Here, as in the Edwin Smith papyrus,
there is an attempt at accurate clinical description. Embryonic versions of some of
the ethical precepts expressed in the Hippocratic works have also been discerned
in these and other early Egyptian medical papyri.

Despite such promising beginnings progress in Egyptian medicine was not sustained, and there was little development of early ideas. Physicians remained largely
bound by religious restrictions which, combined with a natural conservatism, seem
to have had a stultifying effect, and the early systems became fossilised into magico-
religious formulae jealously guarded by the priests. Furthermore, by the fifth century
BC, as Herodotus reveals, spurious specialisation was rife: 'The art of medicine is
thus divided among them: Each physician applies himself to one disease only, and
not more. All places abound in physicians; some physicians are for the eyes, others
for the head, others for the teeth, others for the intestines and others for internal
disorders.'[12] Impressive as this sounds, such narrow specialisation without a broad
basis was rather a barrier than an aid to progress. Dental specialists, for instance,
spent much of their energy and ingenuity in seeking remedies to drive out the 'worms'

believed to be the source of decay and disease in teeth. Similarly, the proliferation of drugs, resulting in a vast and intricate pharmacopoeia, does not necessarily indicate an advancement of the art of healing. More probably it represents a stagnation, masses of drugs being prescribed in ignorance rather than a few well-chosen ones being used with skill and discrimination.

Egyptian medicine did not become entirely moribund, however, and speculation on disease, if not accompanied by active investigation, certainly took place. One theory in particular, that of 'corrupt residues', was to influence Greek medical writers. It was thought that gases given off by putrefying food residues in the bowel filtered through the body, causing ill health and disease. The Greek historian Herodotus noted the preventive measures that were taken in his day: 'They purge themselves every month, three days in succession, seeking to conserve health by emetics and clysters; for they suppose that all diseases to which men are subject proceed from the food they use.'[13] Nevertheless, it was not the theoretical but the practical side of Egyptian medicine – pharmacy, surgery and gynaecology – that was to have the most profound effect on early Greek physicians.[14] By the sixth century BC the impetus to medical progress no longer came from Egypt, and although the great Persian king Darius (reigned 521–486 BC) still employed Egyptians as his court physicians, it was a Greek doctor who successfully treated him after a hunting accident. The episode is related by Herodotus in his account of the life of Democedes of Croton, whom he described as 'the most skilful physician of his time'.[15] The account is of great value for the light it sheds on the dangers and rewards faced by early Greek doctors.

Democedes' father, Calliphon, had been a priest of Asklepios at Cnidus (on the south-west coast of Asia Minor) before moving to Croton in southern Italy. The two fell out and Democedes left home to set up in medical practice on the Greek island of Aegina. Within a year, as Herodotus relates, 'he excelled all the other physicians, although he had no equipment nor any of the implements of his calling. In his second year the Aeginetans paid him a talent to be their public physician; in the next the Athenians hired him for an hundred minae, and Polycrates in the next again for two talents.' His post as personal physician to Polycrates, tyrant of Samos, was short-lived, for Polycrates was 'foully murdered' by Oroetes, satrap of Sardis, and Democedes was enslaved. Before long Oroetes himself was put to death by order of Darius. Then, sometime later, suffering from a badly dislocated ankle, the king heard that one of his slaves was rumoured to have been a famous physician, and he sent for him. Democedes had been reluctant to reveal his knowledge of medicine for fear that it would hinder his return to Greek lands, a clear illustration of how sought-after skilled doctors were at this time. However, threats of torture brought the truth, and he successfully cured the king, taking the opportunity to criticise the rough and outmoded methods of the Egyptian doctors. Democedes, now in high favour, was rewarded with gold and a magnificent house, although these did not diminish his wish to return home, and when he was asked by the king's wife to treat a breast tumour, he did so on the understanding that she would help him reach Greece.

After her cure the queen persuaded Darius to send Democedes with a group of Persian envoys who were to carry out a reconnaissance of a number of Greek settlements. They journeyed via Phoenicia to Greece and thence to the Greek colonies in southern Italy, where Democedes was at last able to escape to Croton. Here he settled and married a daughter of the famous wrestler Milon, but his travels were not yet ended, for later, with the aristocratic Pythagoreans, he was driven out of Croton by the democrats and fled to Plataea.

Democedes was the most famous physician of his day and was clearly a skilled practitioner. His trials and tribulations, and the considerable distances he traversed may not have been typical, but evidence from other sources does indicate that doctors of this period were frequently well travelled. Quite apart from the need to seek patrons (and, in Democedes' case, to escape them), travel enabled the observation of regional diseases and the effect of different climates on health, part of the active investigation and analysis of observed phenomena which were to become the hallmark of early Greek medicine. The appearance, from the sixth century BC onwards, of literary and archaeological evidence for medical thought and practice coincides with the great burst of activity in all fields at that time which culminated in the remarkable achievements of the full Greek Classical period that followed. Medicine grew up alongside philosophy; indeed, in the early stages aspects of the two were closely linked, a development of profound importance, for Greek medicine early acquired the complex theoretical framework which marked it out from that of other cultures.

Although Democedes had prospered at the court of Polycrates, others were less fortunate, and at about the time that Democedes arrived Pythagoras emigrated in the reverse direction – from Samos to Croton – probably to escape Polycrates' tyranny. Under Pythagoras' influence Croton became the foremost of all the Greek towns in Italy. He believed that the soul was a fallen divinity, trapped in the body and condemned to a cycle of reincarnation from which it could only escape by means of physical and spiritual purity. An important element in this purity was study, and he established in Croton a form of religious order whose adherents sought to abide by strict ethical precepts and whose basis was the investigation of nature.

Pythagoras had considerable influence on and through his followers. Another influential author was Alcmaeon of Croton (fl. *c.* 450 BC), a man of wide interests, both a physician and a natural scientist. In the surviving fragments of his writings are some of the earliest records of true anatomical observations: amongst other things he discerned the optic nerves and the tubes between the nose and ear cavities; and he identified the brain as the source of intelligence to which all the sensory channels were connected. In addition, using the theory of the interaction of opposites as an explanation both of human affairs and of bodily conditions, Alcmaeon formulated one of the most fundamental and enduring theories of Greek and Roman medicine: the concept of health as a harmony of the bodily powers, its constituent fluids. Good health was an equilibrium of these fluids, while illness and disease occurred when the dominance of one caused an imbalance. The fluids were imbued with specific qualities and causal properties – heat, cold, wetness, dryness, sweetness, bitterness, and so on. They formed the basis of the Hippocratic humours and reached their ultimate expression some seven centuries later in the humoral pathology of Galen.

Several other far-reaching theories belong to this period, when pre-Socratic nature philosophers contemplated and speculated on the most fundamental principles of creation and existence. Akin to the doctrine of humours was the doctrine of elements, one of whose earliest and most forceful advocates was Empedocles (fl. *c.* 445 BC), who lived in Acragas, modern Agrigento, in south-west Sicily. He was a famous polymath whose biological theories were adapted by Plato and Aristotle, and whom Galen called the founder of the Sicilian medical 'school'. Empedocles taught that all things in the Universe, inanimate and animate, were formed from the mingling, in different proportions, of four 'roots' or basic elements – fire, air, earth and water. Each element had a corresponding characteristic – hot, cold, dry, wet – and the health of living organisms was determined by their balance. Together, the concepts of humours and elements, as agents of health and disease, permeated medical thought for the next two thousand years.

Anaxagoras (*c.* 500–*c.* 428 BC), who lived in Clazomenae, on the south shore of the Gulf of Smyrna, further refined the doctrine of elements, proposing that each element was composed of a mixture of tiny invisible 'seeds'. His main contribution to medicine was in physiology, most notably in nutrition, and his 'seeds' theory would have helped to explain how bodily tissues grew from, and were nourished by, foods to which they bore no resemblance. The invisible 'seeds' were supposed to be released from food in the process of digestion and then reconstituted into different parts of the body. In a further development in the later fifth century Democritus and Leucippus postulated 'atoms' as the basic building-blocks of matter. These invisible, indestructible particles were in perpetual motion, and it was through collisions and combinations of atoms that creation was believed to have occurred. In living creatures the differing dimensions and positions of atoms determined their physiology and health. Despite rejection by some, notably by Plato, Aristotle and the Stoics, atomism was an influential doctrine. It was utilised by the great physiologist Erasistratus in the third century BC and, some two centuries later, by his 'disciple' Asclepiades; and, modified to a concept of particles and pores, it was subsequently incorporated into the doctrine of the Methodist sect of medicine.

Another concept current among the nature philosophers was that *pneuma* (roughly equivalent to 'air') was the source of all things. Its life-giving properties would have been evident enough from earliest times, but Diogenes of Apollonia (fl. *c.* 440 BC), reviving earlier ideas, went so far as to endow *pneuma* itself with life, intelligence and divinity. It was additionally soul and mind in living creatures who breathed it, and its quantity and quality, varying from one species to another, dictated the physical condition of man or animal. The weakness of the doctrine was apparent even at the time, and was satirised by Aristophanes. Nevertheless, its influence may be found in several of the Hippocratic treatises, and the idea of *pneuma* as a life force was retained by many subsequent medical theorists. Indeed, it later became the central doctrine of the medical sect known as the Pneumatists.

In these early attempts at explaining the cosmos and the essence of life a stock of ideas was gradually built up, the pattern of which was constantly changing as new theories were added, existing ones modified or adapted and outmoded ones cast aside. The interest lies not only in the theories, some of which were remarkably long-lived, but in the processes of observation, hypothesis and evaluation that were evolved. For the practising physician the doctrines themselves may have been of use in impressing a client, but they would seldom have had any practical application, and even the results of anatomical and physiological investigations were limited in scope. The natural progression was for medicine to 'fly the nest' of philosophy and emerge as a separate discipline no longer constrained by the need for its doctrines to conform with wider philosophical speculation. In his brief account of the development of medicine Celsus attributes this separation to Hippocrates:

> At first the science of healing was held to be part of philosophy, so that treatment of disease and contemplation of the nature of things began through the same authorities ... Hence we find that many who professed philosophy became expert in medicine ... But it was Hippocrates of Cos, a man first and foremost worthy to be remembered, notable both for professional skill and for eloquence, who separated this branch of learning from the study of philosophy. (*De Medicina* Prooemium, 6–8; trans. W. G. Spencer)

In fact, Hippocrates' influence was but one stage in a process, albeit a significant one, and it was not the case that there was a complete break with what had gone before. Side by side with the nature philosophers, physicians like Democedes and others less eminent had continued to attempt cures largely through use of the knife and drugs. Their contribution to the store of medical knowledge would have been obtained through empirical observation of patient, disease and environment, and passed on by word of mouth if not by the written word. Most of the works of the Hippocratic Corpus reflect these two main strands of enquiry. There is a fusion of ideas, both general theories and practical details, which in some places demonstrates a truly scientific approach.

Of Hippocrates the man woefully little is known with any degree of certainty, other than that he lived in the latter half of the fifth century BC, a contemporary of Socrates, and that his fame as a physician was established already by the time of Plato. According to a biography written several hundred years after his death, he was born in 460 BC on Cos, a Greek island, near Rhodes, off the south-west coast of Asia Minor. His father was a member of the 'family of Asclepiads', a close-knit group which traced its origins back to the god Asklepios, and amongst whom the practice of medicine passed from one generation to the next. Through intermarriage the 'family' expanded and became a sort of guild of physicians. Two main centres arose, one on Cos and the other in the town of Cnidus on the facing mainland. Hippocrates became the leader of the Coan 'guild' or 'school' after studying with his father and other teachers, but later left to work as a physician in Thessaly. As with Democedes, success was followed by fame, and he was invited to set up practice in many different places, including Athens and the court of the Persian king Artaxerxes. But it was to Thessaly that he returned towards the end of his life, and he is supposed to have died in old age at Larissa in 380 BC.

Even this much is doubtful and most of the descriptions of his activities and achievements were invented to suit the times in which they were written. The same process may be seen at work in the depictions of Hippocrates.[16] No contemporary statue or bust has survived, if indeed one was ever made in his lifetime. Sculpture, in any case, did not always portray individuals as they actually appeared, tending instead towards certain 'ideals' or 'types'. Thus the most famous bust of Hippocrates is a Roman marble copy of a Hellenistic original which depicts the 'Father of Medicine' as an elderly bearded man with thinning hair, a portrait type used particularly for philosophers. Nevertheless, this is probably one of the best surviving likenesses and is similar to the portrait on a coin issue of Cos. Appropriately, the bust was found in a doctor's tomb in Ostia, together with a stone inscription which begins with the famous opening words of the *Aphorisms* of the Hippocratic Corpus: 'Life is short, the Art long' (Lat. *ars longa vita brevis*).

This and other statues, as well as a wealth of literature, demonstrate Hippocrates' pre-eminent position in the field of medicine from the Hellenistic period onwards. Unfortunately, by an irony of fate, the reverence which has preserved his name has obscured his beliefs and doctrine. There are two main causes of this obscurity. First, there has always been a tendency by medical writers to select and adapt material from the Corpus to assist in the projection of their own views, often at the expense of the original overall meaning. Such misuse, not necessarily intentional, has continued right up to the present day and is a hazard of any study or commentary on early works. Galen's was perhaps the most celebrated and insidious 'adaptation' of Hippocrates, and although he set himself up as Hippocrates' champion it was often his own theories that he was propagating or defending under the mantle of Hippocratic respectability.[17]

But what were the Hippocratic writings that were suffering in this way? Not all modern medical historians would now claim that any work in the Hippocratic Corpus was certainly written by Hippocrates, though almost every book has been suggested at some time over the last two thousand years. Thus the second main impediment to an understanding of Hippocrates' own views is the failure of any known written work of his to survive, whether as an original or a copy. The tendency to use Hippocrates as a 'mirror of the times' has been shown to have started in the Hellenistic period, and the most reliable glimpses of his doctrine come from references in pre-Hellenistic authors, notably Plato, and Aristotle's pupil Meno, who wrote a history of medicine. From Plato's writings it has been deduced that Hippocrates regarded the body as an organism, claiming that its nature cannot be understood without an understanding of 'the nature of the whole'. Plato's interpretation of this was that having established whether the body is simple or complex, it is then necessary to determine its power of acting on or being acted upon by other things. This was viewed as the key to scientific knowledge.

From Meno comes a brief account of his understanding of Hippocrates' views on the origin of disease. This Hippocrates attributed to gases (*physai*) emanating from the residues (*perissomata*) of undigested food, which rose through the body and displaced health-giving breath (*pneuma*). Although details may have differed, this was not a totally new concept, for, as we have seen, the Egyptians had formulated a similar theory of putrefactive residues which seems to have passed into Greek medical thought in the sixth century BC. However, the source of Meno's account, a fragmentary second-century AD papyrus known as *Anonymus Londinensis*,[18] is a very incomplete copy of what was probably a series of lecture notes, written by a medical student at several removes from Meno's history. It appears to have incorporated several separate though related compilations, and the summary of Hippocratic doctrine attributed to Meno is disappointingly brief. This prevents any unequivocal assessment of Meno's interpretation which, in any case, may itself have misrepresented Hippocrates' own doctrine.

If, then, the Hippocratic Corpus is not the work of Hippocrates, what is it? The generally accepted view today is that it is a collection of medical treatises brought together from many sources and reflecting a range of medical traditions. There are many different literary styles, differing approaches, internal inconsistencies and actually conflicting theories. The sort of process that led to its formation is illustrated in an intriguing passage in Galen (his commentary on the Hippocratic book *Epidemics III*). It concerns the great Library of Alexandria and the acquisitiveness of Ptolemy III Euergetes (r. 246–221 BC): 'And, they say, the Ptolemy who was the King of Egypt became so greedy for books, that he ordered that the books of everyone who arrived by ship be brought to him. After he had them copied on new paper, he gave the copies to the owners of the books ... and deposited the confiscated books themselves in the library'.[19] Many of these confiscated books would themselves have been copies, made for the use of owners who sometimes may have chosen to have had texts from more than one original source transcribed together in a single 'volume'. Thus the emergence of the Hippocratic Corpus in Alexandria probably resulted not from a deliberate collection of the works of one 'school' of medicine or the acquisition of a complete medical library, but from a haphazard and piecemeal agglomeration of unsigned texts and extracts, most of which, however, had their origin in the medical literature of the fifth and fourth centuries BC.

The three major medical centres of this period were those of Cos, Cnidus, and southern Italy, and ideas attributed to both the Coan and the Cnidian 'schools' have been traced in the Corpus. According to Galen, the Cnidians took pleasure in classification, listing the number of diseases for each organ of the body, while the Coans sought understanding through a general description of each illness and a forecast of its likely course. However, the recognition of distinct Coan and Cnidian doctrines is a vexed question. Galen wrote at a time when there had long been a tradition of opposing sects of medicine, but there is no evidence that this was the case as early as Hippocrates. In fact, a certain unity of ideas underlies the Hippocratic Corpus, in particular the theory of humours, suggesting that Cos and Cnidus, as also the lesser Greek medical centres, shared fundamentally the same medicine. Galen himself did not specify opposing sects at Cos and Cnidus, and it is much more likely that the two centres shared in the gradual amalgamation of a store of common knowledge, exchanging and debating new ideas in a spirit of friendly rivalry. Divisions, if they existed at all, were probably between those who held on to traditional views and those who espoused new theories, irrespective of the medical centre at which they were based.[20]

How much of the Corpus reflects the doctrine of Hippocrates, or even that of different 'schools', is therefore impossible to tell, and seems to have been so since before the time of Galen. Why it became known as the Hippocratic Corpus is equally unanswerable, but by a complicated historical process Hippocrates himself became immortalised as the ideal physician, and the writings that came to bear his name acquired an equivalent respect. Whether a source of ammunition for its proponents or fodder for its critics, the Corpus became the basis of Western medicine and exercised a profound influence on subsequent medical thought. Though it lacks a logical arrangement, it nonetheless contains sections on most aspects of medicine which include, in today's terminology, anatomy and physiology, regimen, therapy, clinical description and pathology, surgery, gynaecology and obstetrics, and other more general matters including medical ethics and etiquette. While the sections on regimen are often striking for their modern-sounding approach, those books that deal with anatomy and physiology reveal most clearly the great gulf between Hippocratic and modern medicine.

Anatomy, on which depend physiology, pathology and surgery, is the cornerstone of modern medicine, and the key to its understanding is dissection. In fifth-century Greece, however, human dissection almost never took place, partly because it was socially unacceptable, but also because there was little concept of its crucial role in medicine. Consequently, none of the internal organs was properly understood, and, although there was some notion of the vascular system and pulse, the function of the heart as a pump and the circulation of blood were completely unknown, as was, too, the mechanism of breathing. It was the need to fill this gaping hole in anatomical and physiological knowledge that gave full rein to the two bodies of doctrine most characteristic of Greek medicine: the theory of *humours* and the theory of *pneuma*. Both had evolved through the nature philosophers and were already current by the time of Hippocrates, but in the Corpus they became securely established.

The mixture of humours in the body determined constitution, temperament and health, while *pneuma* was seen as the source of consciousness in thought, perception and sensation. In many places in the Corpus the classical four humour doctrine was adopted: blood, phlegm, yellow bile and black bile, which have been identified respectively as blood, mucus (especially that of the nose), bile and excreted or vomited blood from internal haemorrhage, though the latter identification is uncertain. Another view was of bile and phlegm alone as the critical bodily fluids. In both schemes it was the excess or deficiency of one or more of the fluids, which might be attributed to such factors as climate, weather or diet, that caused illness. To regain a balanced state – health – steps had to be taken to create 'coction', a mixing of the humours, which usually involved purging and blood-letting as well as the use of emetics and dietary controls.

It is in the last of these, diet, and the wider sphere of regimen that the most advanced and enduring aspects of Greek medicine are to be found. In an age with so little control over disease once it had struck, considerable endeavour was channelled into preventive medicine based on a concept of positive health. There was a detailed classification of food and drink according to their perceived properties – strong, weak, drying, moistening, cooling, heating, binding, laxative, and so on. For example, beef was strong and binding, beans were astringent and laxative, seafood dry and light, and cheese strong and nourishing. The type and quantity of food would be adjusted for each individual to maintain a balance between the elemental fire and water of which all living creatures were thought to be composed. Water, cold and moist, equated with nourishment and a calm temperament, fire, hot and dry, with movement and an energetic temperament.

For the sick and for invalids barley water or gruel was normally administered, and the author of *Regimen in Acute Diseases* extols the virtue of a wide range of recipes and describes their application. As the thinnest strained juice it could be given to the very ill, more solid forms being substituted as the patient gained in strength. Certain wines had a place in the sick diet, but more often hydromel, a mixture of honey and water, or oxymel, a mixture of honey and vinegar, would be administered. However, other things also affected the body, and baths, exercise and sleep were imbued with the same range of properties as those attributed to foods and had to be tempered accordingly.

Much space is devoted to the regimen for fever patients, and the generally sound procedures advocated were followed almost unchanged until recent times. Fever, although divided into different types, was regarded and treated as a disease in itself rather than a reaction of the body. The descriptions given are seldom precise enough to permit a retrospective diagnosis, but many of the fever cases were probably a result of remittent or intermittent malaria. Infectious diseases appear to have been rare, there being no sure descriptions of measles, chicken-pox, smallpox, scarlet fever or even influenza in the Hippocratic Corpus. There is, however, an intriguing account of the outbreak of an epidemic disease among the population of the island of Thasos in the late fifth century BC:

> Many people suffered from swellings near the ears, in some cases on one side only, in others both sides were involved. Usually there was no fever and the patient was not confined to bed. In a few cases there was slight fever. In all cases the swellings subsided without harm and none suppurated as do swellings caused by other disorders. The swellings were soft, large and spread widely; they were unaccompanied by inflammation or pain and they disappeared leaving no trace. Boys, young men and male adults in the prime of life were chiefly affected and of these, those given to wrestling and gymnastics were specially liable. Few women took it. Many patients had dry, unproductive coughs and hoarse voices. Soon after the onset of the disease, but sometimes after an interval, one or both testicles became inflamed and painful. Some had fever, but not all. These cases were serious enough to warrant attention, but for the rest, there were no illnesses requiring care. (*Epidemics* I, i; trans. Chadwick and Mann)

The disease has been diagnosed as mumps. Its unfamiliarity to the author, who had no name for it, leaves little doubt as to its rarity, and, indeed, there is no other reference to the disease in Greek medical literature. An important, probably critical limiting influence on the occurrence of acute contagious diseases must have been their dependence on large, densely populated communities, which were never common in antiquity. Nevertheless, it has been observed that as the majority of cases at Thasos were young men it is improbable that this was the first outbreak of mumps there.[21]

Unlike the acute contagious diseases, chest troubles, in particular pneumonia, pleurisy and pulmonary tuberculosis, are very frequently referred to by Greek writers. There are many references in the Corpus to draining empyema from the lungs in pneumonia patients, showing that physicians had a sound understanding of the disease and knew both how and when to operate. Though regularly performed, it was nonetheless a serious operation, one of the few surgical procedures attempted on interior organs and soft parts. The draining agent was usually a heated cautery, the commonest use of this feared instrument in Greek medicine. Normally termed 'fire' or 'iron', its use was considered the most extreme therapeutic measure: 'What drugs will not cure, the knife will; what the knife will not cure, the cautery will; what the cautery will not cure must be considered incurable.'[22]

Hippocratic surgery focused particularly on bones and their accompanying tissues, the one aspect of anatomy that was well understood. Much of what was written in *Fractures* and *Joints* has been generally admired and was practised almost unaltered up to recent times. The Roman author Celsus borrowed heavily from Hippocrates, including the techniques for setting fractures, traction, bandaging, amputation and trephination. Considerable skill and ingenuity went into the development of apparatus for the extension and counter-extension of fractures and dislocated limbs, and the famous 'Hippocratic Bench' with its range of adjustable fittings – levers, cross-bars, windlasses, straps and cords – is another of the positive aspects of the Corpus.[23]

The coverage of gynaecology and obstetrics is patchy, and there is no account of the procedures involved in a normal delivery. Instead there are scattered references to unusual presentations and other obstetrical difficulties, although there is no hint that caesarean section was performed. A range of women's diseases is described but the lack of even a rudimentary knowledge of the upper part of the reproductive tract is very evident. Thus although menstrual problems feature prominently, the fact that neither the ovaries nor the Fallopian tubes were known meant that there was no understanding of the causes and mechanism of menstruation. That abortion was sometimes practised, whether or not with approval, is made clear in the specific provision forbidding it in *The Oath*: 'I will use my power to help the sick to the best of my ability and judgement; I will abstain from harming or wronging any man by it. I will not give a fatal draught to anyone if I am asked, nor will I suggest any such thing. Neither will I give a woman means to procure an abortion.[24]

Women faced considerable dangers in childbirth, and many, like the wife of Dromeades, must have perished from uterine haemorrhage or infection. The onset and course of her illness, terminating in death a week after childbirth, is carefully, if briefly, recorded in one of the forty-two clinical histories in the First and Third Books of *Epidemics*, a pathetic memorial to the frailty of life in the pre-antisepsis era:

The wife of Dromeades, having given birth to a daughter and progressing in all other respects normally, was seized by rigors on the second day, accompanied with high fever.

A pain started on the subsequent day in the hypochondrium; nausea and shivering supervened. She did not sleep on succeeding days and was distraught. Breathing deep and slow, each breath immediately drawn back again.

On the second day after the rigors, her stools were normal; the urine thick, white and cloudy, of the appearance of urine with sediment which has been stirred up after standing a long while. But in her case no sediment was formed. She did not sleep at night.

Third day: about noon rigors, a high fever, urine as before, pain in the hypochondrium, nausea. A restless night with insomnia. Generalized cold sweats, but soon followed by warmth again.

Fourth day: slight relief of the pain in the hypochondrium, a heavy headache. Fell into a stupor; a slight epistaxis occurred. Tongue dry, thirst. Urine little, thin and oily. Slept a little.

Fifth day: thirst, nausea; character of urine unchanged, constipated.

About noon much delirium followed quickly by a lucid phase. On going to stool she became comatose and chilled, slept during the night but was delirious.

Early on the sixth day she suffered from rigors followed quickly by fever and generalized sweating; the extremities were cold and she was delirious with a slow rate of breathing. After a little while convulsions supervened starting in the head and death soon followed.' (*Epidemics* I, xi; trans. Chadwick and Mann)

On the positive side is the ordered approach and remarkable attention to detail in these case-histories which, if practised widely, must have led to a rapid accumulation of knowledge permitting the identification of recurrent symptoms in particular illnesses. However, because illness was regarded as a struggle between the body's constitution and a disturbance in the balance of the humours, a large part of the physician's role was to ensure, by diet and regimen, both that the patient's constitution was as well equipped as possible for the struggle, and that nothing impeded the natural course of the disease. He monitored its progress by making careful observation of the various stages reached, gauging these from such indicators as the condition and form of urine, stools and sputum. There were critical days and normally a major crisis, after which, if the patient survived, excess residues would be evacuated and a recovery would take place following a restoration of the equilibrium.

These case-histories were probably written up from notes made by both the visiting physician and one of his assistants. For there was no system of trained nurses, and where skilled care was required it seems to have devolved upon young trainee physicians, who thereby acquired much of their experience. In the less serious cases slaves or relatives might fulfil the role, but this does not seem to have been encouraged:

Let one of your pupils be left in charge, to carry out instructions without unpleasantness, and to administer the treatment. Choose out those who have already been admitted into the mysteries of the art, so as to add anything necessary, and to give treatment with safety. He is there also to prevent those things escaping notice that happen in the intervals between visits. Never put a layman in charge of anything, otherwise if a mischance occur the blame will fall on you. (*Decorum* XVII; trans. Jones and Withington)

This extract is from one of several books devoted to medical ethics and etiquette. They are of equal importance to the truly medical books for the insight they give both into the ideals that were striven after and the kinds of malpractice that must often have occurred. The stress was not just on high moral standards for their own sake, but on a concerted attempt to safeguard medicine from its critics, distance it from the mumbo-jumbo of magic and sorcery and raise it above the charlatanry of drug-peddlers. To gain the confidence of the patient and the approval of the community at large, young physicians were encouraged to offer constructive advice to fellow doctors instead of quarrelling or jeering, and they were advised to provide their services free of charge occasionally. Furthermore, they were to avoid flamboyance in public lectures and were never to trouble a sick patient with a discussion of fees during the illness.

The apprenticeship system, in which a master physician might take on one or more trainees, tended to result in a continuity of doctrine. Unfortunately, such respect for earlier medical thought often became exaggerated and rather than assisting in the advancement of Greek medicine actually restrained its progress. For this conservatism might result in inflexibility, a reluctance to accept fresh views if they could not be accommodated within existing doctrine, and suspicion or downright disbelief of totally new theories.

However, although this affected the fundamental theories of disease and medicine, it did not impede the development of many individual aspects. Thus Diocles, whom Pliny[25] ranked second only to Hippocrates, broke new ground in physiology, pharmacology and dietetics, whilst synthesising, adjusting and elaborating the earlier theories of Empedocles, Hippocrates and others. Diocles came from Carystos, a town on the island of Euboea, and lived at Athens in the fourth century BC. His botanical book *Rhizotomika* was the first in which plants were listed alongside a description of their effects on the human body, and this created the pattern which was followed for centuries after. Most of our information on his work has been transmitted through the writings of Pliny and Galen, but one possible surviving fragment is an intriguing document in the form of a letter to the Macedonian king Antigonus (382–301 BC).[26] It comprises a brief survey of the causes and symptoms of diseases and the measures to be taken against them. The purpose of the letter may well have been to seek royal patronage, for it is couched in terms intended to flatter the king, as well as advertising the advanced medical thinking of its author. The survey is in four main sections according to regions of the body – head, thorax, intestines and bladder – an interesting division which we may presume to reflect the areas most commonly afflicted by disease. Unfortunately, doubt has been cast on the status of this letter.

We do not know whether Diocles' letter resulted in his appointment at the Macedonian court, but we do know that he was a contemporary of Aristotle (384–322 BC) and a member of his Peripatetic school in Athens, the most important Greek centre of scientific study at this time. Aristotle's interests were wide and included medicine, but it was in biology and comparative anatomy that he was to have a lasting and profound influence. There he combined shrewd observation and acute reasoning with a passion for order to produce his best work. His interest in zoology was shared by Diocles, and both carried out dissection of animals. Diocles wrote the first book devoted entirely to anatomy, and was one of the first to recognise a difference between arteries and other vessels. Aristotle provided good descriptions of some of the internal organs, but his researches do not seem to have extended far into human anatomy and physiology. Instead, he appears to have been a major influence in this field through his philosophical views. Before him Plato had differentiated the body from the immortal soul, and Aristotle, though he did not accept that the soul was immortal, reiterated its pre-eminence and the subservient role of the body. As the teaching of Plato and Aristotle became more widespread amongst the learned, so the consequent reduction in the sanctity of the human corpse – an empty shell without soul – would have weakened the barrier to active investigation of its structure: dissection.

Within fifty years of the death of Aristotle the systematic dissection of human cadavers in the pursuit of anatomical information became briefly established in the Greek city of Alexandria. The Hellenistic period was ushered in with the military expansionism of Aristotle's most famous pupil, Alexander the Great (356–323 BC). He left Egypt in the hands of the Ptolemies, a line of Macedonian kings, and under their influence Alexandria became one of the foremost cities of the ancient world and the greatest Greek centre of learning. Largely for their own prestige they sought to attract the most eminent scholars from both arts and sciences, and used as bait the unrivalled facilities of their Library and Museum. Through an active, sometimes ruthless collecting policy, as already seen, the Ptolemies acquired a vast and important collection of written works. In their heyday the Library and Museum together formed a sort of institute of study and research, and in the third century BC conditions were right for free thought and experimentation. There was a brilliant period of scientific progress during which medical science, in particular anatomy, received a massive impetus that was to stand it in good stead for centuries to come.

The two most important medical scientists of this phase were Herophilus and Erasistratus.[27] Herophilus, who came from Chalcedon, a Greek city on the Asiatic side of the Bosphorus, received his medical training from the eminent Praxagoras, on the island of Cos. In the early third century BC he went to Alexandria, where he wrote at least eleven treatises, none of which, unfortunately, survives. From later writers, most notably Galen, however, we know that he was not only a great medical scholar but also a physician and surgeon whose crucial contribution to medicine arose in large part from his awareness of the equal importance of reason and experience. Theories were necessary but were dependent upon or had to be modified by the experience of practical work. The other determining factor in the success of his enquiries was the freedom to apply these qualities. In Ptolemaic Alexandria this meant the unrestricted use of human cadavers for dissection.

Applying logical method to direct investigation, Herophilus made anatomical discoveries of profound importance, most notably in his investigations of the eye, liver, brain, genital organs, vascular and nervous systems. He identified both sensory and motor nerves, though still regarding them as channels for the *pneuma*, traced the origin and course of nerves from the fourth ventricle of the brain and the spinal cord, and isolated the brain as the seat of the intellect, believing it to be the centre of the nervous system. He discovered the Fallopian tubes and the ovaries, whose structure and function he compared with the male testes, while his work on the pulse, which modified that of his former teacher, Praxagoras,[28] although faulty in the basic tenets, brought a rationale to its use in diagnosis. Furthermore, according to Galen, Herophilus attempted to integrate the results of his anatomical studies with a range of exercises and dietary requirements aimed at restoring and maintaining health.

The second of the two great Hellenistic medical writers, Erasistratus of Ceos, was a younger contemporary of Herophilus. Just as Galen believed Herophilus to be the outstanding pioneer of human anatomy, Erasistratus is often called 'the Father of Physiology'. The son of a doctor himself, he left his home on the Greek island of Ceos to study at Aristotle's Peripatetic school in Athens, whence he is believed to have travelled to Cos before going to Alexandria. None of his writings has survived, but his achievements and theories are better known than those of Herophilus because

Galen took a greater exception to his physiological doctrines and spent longer refuting them. Erasistratus continued Herophilus' studies of the nervous system, giving a more accurate description of the human brain and distinguishing the cerebrum from the cerebellum. Through experimentation with live brains he noted that damage to the outer membrane, the *dura mater*, upset the functioning of the motor nerves. He contrasted the size of the human brain with that of other animals and attributed man's superior intelligence not just to the greater size of his brain but to the marked convolutions of its surface.

Rejecting the prevalent ideas of occult or hidden forces as an explanation of movement in the body fluids, Erasistratus subscribed to Strato's theory of *horror vacui*, the natural tendency of a vacuum to become refilled. He retained the notion of *pneuma* and regarded the arteries as vessels for *pneuma* alone. His observation, therefore, that blood flowed from severed arteries involved a mental contortion: he believed the *pneuma* rushed out, unseen, causing blood from neighbouring veins to enter the arteries through their walls due to *horror vacui*. He distinguished two kinds of *pneuma*, vital *pneuma* which sustained life and was drawn from outside by way of the lungs to the heart's left ventricle for distribution, and psychic *pneuma* which had its seat in the brain and was distributed through the nerves.

Erasistratus came closer than anyone to William Harvey's discovery of the circulation of blood, for he correctly defined the heart as a distributor of blood. In his system blood was sucked into the right ventricle and was driven into the veins via the lungs, but his belief in the *pneuma* theory required that the left ventricle, aorta and arteries be interpreted as the means of distribution of *pneuma*. In the process of this work he nevertheless identified the action of the bicuspid, tricuspid and semi-lunar valves and acquired a good knowledge of the route of the major vessels. He also described a 'three-fold network' of veins, arteries and nerves that accompanied each organ and part of the intestines, and he proposed that their infinitesimally small terminals, impossible to perceive but predictable according to reason, bound together the tissues.

The work of Herophilus and Erasistratus was a great step forward which had far-reaching consequences, and we might expect others to have continued the series of major discoveries that they initiated. Yet after their time the impetus seems to have disappeared from Alexandrian medical research. The cause is not entirely clear and probably depended upon a number of factors. As is often the case, a period of rapid progress and innovation was followed by one of consolidation, as existing schemes were modified by or adapted to the wealth of new ideas and information. Different views were taken over the interpretation of the new data, and argument over the theory of medicine seems to have largely taken the place of practical research. In addition, the Greek anti-dissection lobby gradually reasserted itself, and while the earlier Ptolemies had not just protected medical researchers from these pressures but had positively encouraged them, the later kings, who were politically weaker, perhaps found it expedient to avoid a confrontation over dissection. A deciding factor may have been the more emotive issue of human vivisection at Alexandria, which Celsus describes alongside dissection. If the clear division between the two became somewhat obscured, the positive revulsion and hostility engendered by vivisection may have contributed to the demise of dissection:

Moreover, as pains, and also various kinds of diseases, arise in the more internal parts, they hold that no one can apply remedies for these who is ignorant about the parts themselves; hence it becomes necessary to lay open the bodies of the dead and to scrutinise their viscera and intestines. They hold that Herophilus and Erasistratus did this in the best way by far, when they laid open men whilst alive – criminals received out of prison from the kings – and whilst these were still breathing, observed parts which beforehand nature had concealed ... Nor is it, as most people say, cruel that in the execution of criminals, and but a few of them, we should seek remedies for innocent people of all future ages. (*De Medicina* Prooemium, 23–6; trans. W. G. Spencer)

Thus Celsus reports the views of the Dogmatic 'school' of medicine, that the good of vivisection outweighed the evil. However, he balances this with a summary of the opposing view, that of the Empiric sect:

... but what remains, cruel as well, to cut into the belly and chest of men whilst still alive, and to impose upon the Art [of medicine] which presides over human safety someone's death and that too in the most atrocious way ... it is only when the man is dead that the chest and any of the viscera come into the view of the medical murderer, and they are necessarily those of a dead, not of a living man. It follows, therefore, that the medical man just plays the cut-throat, not that he learns what our viscera are like when we are alive ... That for these reasons, since most things are altered in the dead, some hold that even the dissection of the dead is unnecessary; although not cruel, it is nonetheless nasty. (*De Medicina* Prooemium, 40–4; trans. W. G. Spencer)

Celsus' own thoughts on the matter are stated at the end of his preface: 'to lay open the bodies of men whilst still alive is as cruel as it is needless; that of the dead is a necessity for learners, who should know positions and relations, which the dead body exhibits better than does a living and wounded man'.[29] He takes the middle path, approving dissection but opposing vivisection. The Christian author Tertullian, writing around AD 200 but drawing on sources of the first century AD, also voiced abhorrence at vivisection, calling Herophilus a butcher who cut up people to investigate nature.[30] Neither Celsus nor Tertullian were physicians and they probably had little to lose by such pronouncements. However, if attitudes did harden, it would have become increasingly difficult, whether in Alexandria or elsewhere, for physicians who practised or merely approved dissection to avoid censure, and this probably explains the silence on the matter by most medical writers.

Whether or not human dissection continued at Alexandria, progress there was not completely eclipsed. For the introduction of systematic instruction made Alexandria the first true medical teaching centre, raising the status of doctors and maintaining the importance of the city. It was at this period also, the second and first centuries BC, that surgery became a specialism within medicine at Alexandria, a development which must have owed much to the sheer size of the city. Erasistratus had been a competent surgeon whose operations included the opening of the abdomen to treat the liver directly, and catheterisation for the relief of strangury (slow and painful urination). His example was followed by others, and Celsus noted the growth of surgery in Alexandria: 'This branch, although very ancient, was more practised by Hippocrates ... than by his forerunners. Later it was separated from the rest of medicine, and began to have its own professors; in Egypt it grew especially by the influence of Philoxenus, who wrote a careful and comprehensive work on it in several volumes.'[31] Philoxenus (fl. *c.* 75–50 BC) was not only a fine surgeon but an expert on tumours, especially cancers of the womb and intestines. Another surgeon, Ammonius, developed a technique for the crushing of bladder stone.

Thus part of the heritage of Herophilus and Erasistratus was the formal distinction of surgery, which also led to the evolution of other specialisms. This separation, together with the very practicality of surgery, probably ensured its progress by safeguarding it from the doctrinaire disputes of opposing sects or schools of medicine. The process that led to a division into sects had already begun in the time of Erasistratus and was paralleled by a similar development in philosophy.[32] Instead of working within a common framework of medical knowledge, theories polarised and became a hindrance to progress as medical men devoted more time and energy to discrediting the doctrine of others than to advancing the knowledge of medicine.

We have already encountered the differing views on dissection of the Empiric and Dogmatic sects. The Dogmatists approved dissection, for knowledge of anatomy assisted in the development of logical theories concerning both evident and hidden causes of disease. The need to understand disease was the core of their doctrine, but the explanations, as recorded by Celsus, all logical in their own terms, were many and varied: an imbalance of the four elements, of the humours, or of the *pneuma*; a migration of the blood into the vessels which carried *pneuma*; or a blockage of the bodily passages by 'atoms'. Dogmatic medicine was essentially theoretical and its proponents were attacked for being 'talkers not doers', who hardly knew one end of a patient from the other.

Their main opponents were the Empirics, who were opposed to the study of anatomy, through either vivisection or dissection, because they rejected all search into the causes of health and disease. They held that immediate causes were obvious and hidden ones incapable of discovery. Thus the channelling of energy into attempts at comprehending such things as pulse, digestion or breathing was pointless. Theirs was a very practical medicine, in which experience was valued above logical argument. Observation was the key to understanding, and their approach to illness was to note the patient's symptoms and to treat them using remedies that had been found to be effective against similar symptoms in the past.

Both Dogmatists and Empirics found confirmation of their theories in the Hippocratic Corpus, and the doctrine of another later sect, that of the Methodists, also drew on aspects of the Corpus. The Methodists rejected humoral pathology and all complicated theories, stressing instead the fundamental importance of regimen. Their other basic tenet was the belief that a few general conditions were common to many different diseases, and it was the *methodos* that they developed to treat these conditions that gave the sect its name. Methodism was especially important among Greek physicians in the Roman Empire, where their practical approach apparently held considerable appeal.

The fourth medical sect, that of the Pneumatists, was a splinter group of the

Dogmatic sect which reverted to the theories of *pneuma* and the four humours. *Pneuma* was regarded as the primordial matter from which life sprang, and its disturbance in the body, triggered by an imbalance of the humours, was the cause of disease.

These four 'schools' were most prominent in medical thought in the century before and after the birth of Christ, and they therefore span the main period when Greek medicine came to Rome. Although earlier contact had been made, and by tradition Archagathus of Sparta in 219 BC was the first Greek doctor to settle in Rome, the most significant event was the arrival of Asclepiades of Bithynia in the later second century BC.[33] He was a rhetorician, but while in Rome he saw better prospects in medicine and became a self-taught physician. Aware of the strong resistance to Greek theories of medicine, he aligned himself with Roman thought and tempered reasoning with a sound practical approach. Furthermore, he turned his back on extreme treatments and replaced the exotic or disgusting drugs prevalent at that time with simple therapeutic measures, hence his nicknames 'wine-giver' and 'cold water-giver'.[34] He was criticised by other medical writers, above all by Galen, for his rejection of the humours in favour of the then outmoded 'atomist' theory of medicine. However, Celsus viewed him as one who broke with tradition and 'changed in large measure the way of curing',[35] and it was his moderation of Greek medical thought combined with the empathy he had with his Roman patients that ultimately ensured not just his own success but also the acceptance of Greek doctors and medicine in the Roman Empire.

Chapter 2

Fitness, food and hygiene

Dietetics, pharmacology and surgery, according to Celsus, were the three branches into which medicine became divided after the time of Hippocrates.[1] Though the divisions were not hard and fast, this tri-partite system had a long history through Greek and into Roman medicine. Dietetics had a far broader meaning then than today, and involved regimens which covered not only the regulation of food and drink, but also exercise, bathing, relaxation and medicines. Originally it had developed in Greece as a response to the needs of athletes training for games, but soon it became established as an important method of treating the sick and then, applied to the healthy, as a means of avoiding illness.

Preventive medicine was always an important aspect of the physician's work, not least because of the unreliability of the therapeutic measures at his disposal. However, some wealthy hypochondriacs took dietetics to the extreme and put themselves under the constant supervision of a doctor, whose dietetic rules might be so time-consuming that they prevented any kind of normal life. Only the rich could afford to indulge in that sort of regimen, but even among the poorer classes dietetics took a firm hold. It was especially prominent in the mechanistic medicine advocated and practised by Asclepiades in Rome in the early first century BC. According to Pliny, Asclepiades 'recognised especially five principles of general application: fasting from food, in other cases abstinence from wine, massage, walking, and the various kinds of carriage-rides'.[2] These principles were in accord with his physical theory of the organism. Reviving and adapting earlier theories, he regarded the body as an aggregate of 'atoms' in constant motion, permeated by invisible pores through which passed *pneuma* and the body fluids. Health, which depended on the condition and number of these constituents, could be controlled through dietetics. Pliny was scathing of Asclepiades' medicine and only grudgingly observed that he 'brought round to his view almost all the human race, just as if he had been sent as an apostle from heaven'.[3] Celsus, however, seems to have approved of Asclepiades' methods, and he included many in his own medical books, though not without some modification.

Celsus epitomised the Roman pragmatic approach to dietetics: while recognising its importance for the weak, notably scholars and city-dwellers, he believed that most people could regulate their own health and need have recourse to physicians only if they became ill: 'A man in health, who is both vigorous and his own master, should be under no obligatory rules, and have no need, either for a medical attendant, or for a rubber and anointer. His kind of life should afford him variety; he should be now in the country, now in town, and more often about the farm; he should sail, hunt, rest sometimes, but more often take exercise.'[4] He should also show moderation in eating, drinking, exercise and sexual intercourse.

Greater care still should be taken by the weak, 'among whom are a large portion of townspeople, and almost all of those fond of letters . . . he who has not digested should lie up altogether, and neither work nor take exercise nor attend to business . . . He should also reside in a house that is light, airy in summer, sunny in winter; avoid the midday sun, the morning and evening chill, also exhalations from rivers and marshes.'[5] In the morning, after waking, he should lie still in bed for a while before rising. Then he should wash his face in cold water, except in winter, and next observe the colour of his urine to check whether his body is healthy. Later: 'He who has been engaged in the day, whether in domestic or on public affairs, ought to keep some portion of the day for the care of the body. The primary care in this respect is exercise, which should always precede the taking of food . . . and . . . ought to come to an end with sweating, or at any rate lassitude.'[6] Baths and a short rest should follow before eating, in which, again, restraint should be shown.

Celsus advised against a surfeit or an excessive abstinence of food, remarking, however, that if intemperance occurred, over-drinking was less harmful than over-eating. Savouries or salads preceded the main course, which should be boiled or roasted meat, and, for those whose constitution allowed it, a dessert of dates or apples might round off the meal. If taken at all, especial moderation was to be shown with preserved (honeyed) fruits, which were indigestible but also a temptation, 'because more is taken owing to their sweetness'.[7]

Wealth, leisure and self-discipline were the major prerequisites of Celsus' regimen, which was written primarily for people of his own social class, and may well indeed reflect the pattern of his own life. Thus his list of exercises is geared towards the literate rich with a country residence.[8] They should read aloud, march, run, even play hand-ball, but mostly Celsus favoured walking exercises, more or less strenuous according to the constitution of the individual. Certainly these exercises are far from the demanding schedules of the gymnasium where dietetics originated. Doctors had long held the view that the regimen for athletes was not at all conducive to good health. 'The condition of the athlete is not natural. A healthy state is superior in all', said the author of the Hippocratic treatise *Nutriment*, while Celsus observed that 'bodies thus fed up . . . age very quickly and become infirm'.[9] Although some trainers claimed expertise in medicine, these two branches of dietetics continued to diverge. Galen more than once took issue with trainers and left no doubt as to the derision he felt for them and their trade:

The healthy city hates and despises this activity which perverts all one's force for living, and turns it into an unworthy condition of the body. I have often found myself stronger than highly respected athletes. They were useless when it came to traveling or military activity, and more so in political life and farming. And if it is necessary to stay with a sick friend, they are totally worthless for consolation, consultation, or assistance – just like pigs. Nevertheless the most unsuccessful of them, who have never won a prize, of a sudden set themselves up as trainers, and cry their wares loudly as swine in their barbarian voices. Some even try writing, about massage or conditioning, or hygiene, or exercise, and dare to take on and contradict people they don't understand at all. (*Thrasybulus*, (*Whether Hygiene is a Part of Medicine or Gymnastics*), trans. in Smith 1979, 107–8).

Galen saw health as a mean between two extremes and believed that regimens should be developed to avoid excesses of heat, cold, moisture and dryness. Although he deplored the extremes of athletic training and the ignorance of the trainers, he did not reject the techniques themselves. Like Celsus, he commended the use of appropriate levels of exercise, diet, baths and massage, not just for those in the prime of life but for old and young, strong and weak alike. He even wrote a short treatise on the benefits to health from playing ball games.[10] Massage in particular had long been practised as a means of toning the body, and both Celsus and Galen cited Hippocrates as the authority on 'rubbing', as it was known: 'Hippocrates... said that rubbing, if strenuous, hardens the body, if gentle, relaxes; if much, it diminishes, if moderate, fills out. It follows, therefore, that in the following cases rubbing should be employed, when either a feeble body has to be toned up, or one indurated has to be softened, or a harmful superfluity is to be dispersed, or a thin and infirm body has to be nourished.'[11] The wealthy would be massaged in their own home, by their personal physician or his assistant, but many others received treatment at public baths, where both trainers and doctors plied their trade. The pummelling and slapping of hand on flesh was one of the many distracting noises complained of by Seneca, who had an apartment over a town baths.[12]

Massage also had a recuperative role for convalescents, especially those recovering from fever, and was used to bring relief to those suffering from prolonged headaches or a partially paralysed limb. Rocking, among which was included Asclepiades' 'carriage-rides', is a less familiar technique today, but a form of therapy that was widely practised in Roman medicine. An essentially passive form of exercise, Celsus thought it suitable for those recovering from chronic maladies, especially for those patients weakened by a bout of fever. The slightly more energetic 'rocking' attained by horse-riding was prescribed for convalescents and those who suffered from 'looseness of the bowels'.[13]

A common aim of most ancient regimens was to diminish or remove various substances from the body. Thus Celsus included as methods of 'depletion' blood-letting, purging, vomiting, exercise, rubbing and rocking. 'Nourishment' was the natural concomitant, and food and drink were 'of general assistance not only in diseases of all kinds but in preserving health as well; and an acquaintance with the properties of all is of importance, in the first place that those in health may know how to make use of them'.[14] By 'properties' Celsus meant the degree of nourishment that different types of food or drink would supply, and he divided them into three classes accordingly. To the strongest class of foods, 'that which has most nourishment', belonged bread, pulses, the meat from large game and large domesticated animals, large birds, 'sea monsters' (including whale), honey and cheese; to the middle class smaller game, birds, fish and pot herbs whose roots or bulbs were eaten; and to the weakest class vegetables, fruit, olives, snails and shellfish.

Strength was further determined by the size and age of food animals, the particular cut of meat, the type of soil on which crops were grown, the quality of the water in which fish were caught, the freshness of the food and its means of cooking, and several other factors. Such subdivisions and subtle distinctions would have provided the physician with a complex framework, with which he could demonstrate his knowledge and skill by selecting a diet appropriate to the needs of every individual, sick or healthy. 'Thus', as Celsus observed, 'the quality of the food administered should be in accordance with the patient's strength, and the quantity in accordance with its quality. For weak patients, therefore, there is needed the lightest food; food of the middle class best sustains those moderately strong, and for the robust the strongest is the fittest.'[15]

Even Roman cookery books, like that of Apicius, included dietetic and medical recipes. In Apicius several were described as *ad ventrem*, 'to be used as a laxative', or *digestibile*, 'to promote the digestion'.[16] These must often have been needed as a tonic to the rich and indigestible dishes so prominent in descriptions of the more elaborate Roman meals. A cook in Plautus' *Pseudolus* complains of the Roman fondness for over-seasoning. 'Other cooks', he said, 'thrust herbs at you then proceed to season those herbs with other herbs.'

> They put in coriander, fennel, garlic and horse parsley, they serve up sorrel, cabbage, beet and spinach, pouring into this a pound of asafoetida and pounding up wicked mustard which makes the pounders' eyes water before they've finished. When they season their dinners they don't use condiments but screech owls, which eat out the intestines of the guests alive. That is why life is so short for men in this world, since they stuff their bellies with suchlike herbs, fearful to speak of, not just to eat. (*Pseudolus* I, 810; trans. in Renfrew 1985, 23)

Most people ate only once or twice a day. Breakfast, if taken at all, was a very simple affair, Galen, for instance, eating only a little bread.[17] Lunch, too, was

5 In the gymnasium. An umpire prepares to strike one of the contestants in a *pankration* bout – a form of all-in wrestling – for gouging the eyes of his opponent. To the left two boxers spar. Red-figured *kylix* made in Athens *c.* 490–480 BC.

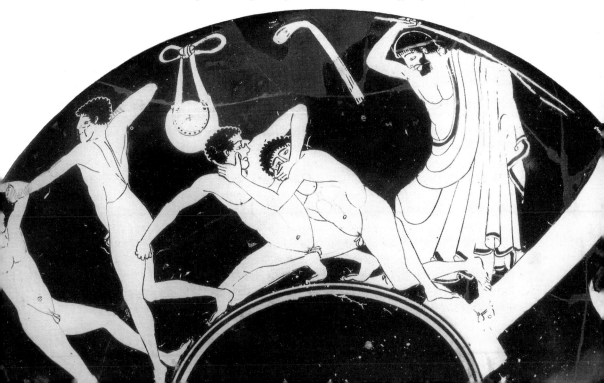

usually at most a light buffet or snack, and the main Roman meal was *cena*, eaten in the evening. For the moderately wealthy *cena* normally comprised three courses. The first, *gustatio*, was our hors-d'oeuvre or entrée and took many forms, usually comparatively simple preparations of vegetables, mushrooms, eggs or shellfish. The main course, *primae mensae*, consisted of boiled and roast meat dishes, beef, lamb, pork and ham, as well as poultry and many different kinds of sausage, usually stuffed or covered with spicy and piquant sauces. Sweet and sour sauces were popular, but the favourite was *garum*, also known as *liquamen*, a sort of anchovy essence made by leaving the salted entrails of small fish in a pan in the sun for several weeks before straining away the residue to extract the sauce. Always sharp and sometimes postively vicious, *garum*, together with oysters and exotic shellfish was often singled out by Roman writers both as a symbol of gluttony and over-indulgence and as a cause of ill health and disease.[18] Seneca, for example, praised the austerity of his predecessors, while the Younger Pliny favoured a simple, but hardly meagre diet, which was, however, not always to the liking of his guests: 'Who are you, to accept my invitation to dinner and never come?... It was all laid out, one lettuce each, three snails, two eggs, barley-cake, and wine with honey chilled with snow ... besides olives, beetroots, gherkins, onions, and any number of similar delicacies. You would have heard a comic play, a reader or singer, or all three if I felt generous. Instead you chose to go where you could have oysters, sow's innards, sea-urchins, and Spanish dancing-girls.'[19]

As we have seen in Celsus' warning over honeyed fruits, the third course was usually, like ours, a sweet. Whether orchard fruit or pastries were eaten, honey was a common ingredient for it was the almost universal sweetener. Wine diluted with water might accompany the second course, but usually serious drinking did not begin until the meal had ended. Like food, drinks were also imbued with different 'strengths', and Celsus placed vintage wine, sweet wine, wine concentrate (must), mead and beer in his strongest class, while water was the weakest and plain wines were 'intermediate in quality'. *Acetum* was also an important Roman beverage. Basically a cheap, low-quality wine similar to vinegar, when mixed with water it made a refreshing drink known as *posca*, which was drunk by the poorer classes and serving soldiers. Soldiers also drank beer, *cervesia*, especially in the provinces of Gaul, Britain and Germany, where the best and strongest varieties were made by the grain-malting process. The consumption of alcohol seems to have been of importance in early Celtic society, especially amongst the warrior and chieftain class, and their habit of quaffing large quantities of undiluted imported wine surprised and shocked early Greek and Roman travellers.

Perhaps the Celts were right to drink their wine quickly, for few wines could be improved by laying down, and most were best drunk within a couple of years. Even then a wide variety of additives were required to preserve wine or improve the flavour of that which had soured. They included honey, spices, resin, herbs, brine and must (*defrutum* or *sapa*). Galen's father added sulphur, a preservative that is still used in wines today.[20] Must, also used extensively in cooking, was a wine concentrate, reduced by boiling down wine to a third or half of its volume. For this process it was specified that pans of lead should be used. If this was indeed the case it is difficult to imagine that serious lead-poisoning could have been avoided, and many illnesses and premature deaths attributed to other causes may well have occurred through the long-term consumption of wine or food contaminated with lead.[21]

There were other problems of food contamination also linked to the difficulty of preservation, for without refrigeration meat and fish were particularly vulnerable. Whenever possible, as in pre-industrial communities today, fish and shellfish would have been transported alive in tanks and food animals 'on the hoof', to be killed immediately before cooking. But for the many occasions when this was not appropriate preservatives had to be used. For fish, especially sea-fish, the answer was normally close at hand in the form of brine, obtained by evaporation from sea water. By heating the brine it could be converted to salt crystals, and coastal saltings were widespread. Many probably doubled as *garum*-making sites.

Meat was also salted, and Apicius devoted a recipe to removing the salt flavour from meat preserved in this way. He also recommended the use of vinegar to help preserve fried fish and to pickle oysters, but 'to keep meat fresh as long as you like

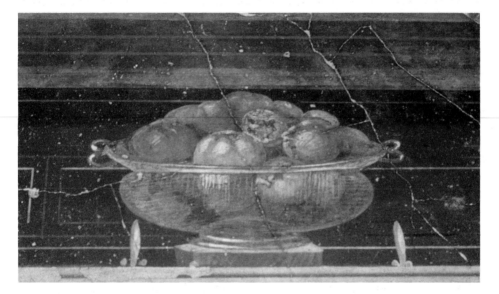

6 An apple a day . . . Vivid detail from a Roman fresco of the 1st century AD showing fresh fruit, probably plums and pomegranates, in a glass bowl. Oplontis, Villa of Poppaea, Room 23.

without pickling' he advised: 'Cover meat that you wish to keep fresh with honey, but suspend the receptacle, and use when required. This is better in winter; in summer it will keep in this manner only a few days.'[22]

Both meat and fish were also cured by drying and smoking,[23] but often, through accident or necessity, bad food must have been eaten. Food poisoning caused by fish is recorded in the literature, while the bowel parasites found in Roman sewage deposits are just as likely to have had their source in contaminated meat as in poor hygiene.[24] Indeed, as more analyses are carried out, it is becoming increasingly clear that in many places certain intestinal parasites were endemic. It is only too easy to understand why stomach-ache is the complaint most frequently mentioned in the medical sections of Pliny's *Natural History*.

Despite such hazards, meat was an important part of the diet in most areas of the Roman Empire, as the large quantities of animal bone found on excavated sites reveal. Analysis of bone assemblages has shown how wide a variety of animals and fish were eaten, as well as demonstrating regional or social preferences.[25] For the majority the meat diet would normally have been dictated by the species of wild or domesticated animals that were available locally, and there may well have been seasonal shortages. This would also have applied to the vegetable and fruit component of the diet, and vitamin deficiencies cannot have been uncommon. Hippocrates and Galen were apparently acquainted with 'night blindness', a vitamin A deficiency condition usually due to a lack of animal fats and oils in the diet, while the effects of scurvy, caused by an insufficient consumption of vitamin C in fresh fruit and vegetables, were described by Hippocrates and Pliny.[26] It seems likely, too, that rickets and osteomalacia, diseases arising from a low intake of vitamin D in dairy foods and fish-liver oils, must have taken their toll among the poor in some parts of the Empire. Soranus, an eminent physician of the first century AD, seems to allude to rickets in the paediatric section of his *Gynaecology* when he describes a bow-legged condition of infants that was especially common in Rome.[27] However, there are difficulties both in recognising and in interpreting the skeletal changes consistent with chronic or acute food shortages, and there are few instances of skeletons which show such diseases as scurvy or rickets.[28]

Although supplemented by meat, fish, vegetables and fruit, the staple diet throughout most of the Greek and Roman world was food grains processed into porridge, bread and, occasionally, pasta. The earlier forms of wheat were mainly husked varieties (emmer) known as *far*, which, like barley, were converted into gruels or porridge (*puls*). However, they were not suitable for baking, and as leavened breads began to take the place of porridges in the diet, the naked species of wheat became more intensively cultivated. Naked wheat, *frumentum* as it became known, required fewer processing stages than barley or emmer. The grain was simply sieved, ground between mill-stones and either boiled into porridge or kneaded and baked into bread. The size and type of mill varied widely from small 'family' hand-mills to the man- or animal-powered donkey-mills that operated in bakeries like those at Pompeii. Larger, and technologically still more important, were the water-mills, such as those which helped to supply the garrisons attached to Hadrian's Wall. Although the harnessing of water power permitted a larger scale of production, water-mills were restricted to those regions with watercourses of a fairly constant annual flow. Hand- and donkey-mills required comparatively little power output and both remained popular manufacturing techniques.[29]

The product from all these techniques was a coarse meal. Partially ground grains and the larger bran fragments might be removed by sieving, but the resulting flour must still have contained many impurities, and Horace's complaint that the bread at Canosa was '*lapidosus*' may suggest that it was 'full of grit' from the milling process rather than 'rock-hard'.[30] Certainly, both grits and unground grains in bread must have contributed to the marked attrition of teeth often observed in skeletons. Although the coarseness of some mixed cereal breads may have prevented the complete absorption of their nutritional component, bread was normally a vital part of the diet. Celsus placed it in his most nourishing category of foods, while Habinnas, at the banquet of Trimalchio, praised brown bread above white because it was nourishing and also prevented constipation.[31] Several different types were available, including wholemeal bread, the *panis militaris* eaten by soldiers,[32] which would have been both palatable and rich in vitamins, notably B_1.

The importance of bread may be seen in the considerable lengths to which Rome went to ensure a constant corn supply, the Annona.[33] Egypt and Africa were especially jealously guarded as 'Rome's granaries', while a carefully organised supply network was established to provision the army wherever it went. The poorest urban classes were at particular risk in times of food shortage, and at the time of Julius Caesar 150,000 poor households qualified for the free daily corn dole in Rome, a figure that rose to 175,000 by the end of the second century AD.[34] Elsewhere many other cities and provinces had special officials who organised food supplies along similar lines. Private philanthropy also played a part, as in the arrangement known as *alimenta*, in which an allowance was given for the sustenance of poor children.[35] To ensure continuity this often took the form of an endowment of land, like that made by the Younger Pliny to his native town of Comum, the rent charge from which was administered by a town or state official to feed a fixed number of children.[36]

Despite such measures, life for the majority must often have been a struggle for survival and hunger a common companion. There was an obscene disparity between their humble fare and the gross over-indulgence of a few immensely wealthy families. At the infamous banquet of Trimalchio, extravagant even in Imperial Rome, the many dishes offered to guests included such things as dormice in honey, hare served with sows' udders, and imitation pea-fowl eggs made of pastry stuffed with spiced garden warblers. Some, at least, felt their conscience pricked when their life of luxury was scrutinised:

> when I used to hear Attalus denouncing sin, error and the evils of life, I often felt sorry for mankind and ... often desired to leave his lecture room a poor man. Whenever he castigated our pleasure-seeking lives ... the desire came upon me to limit my food and drink ... That is why I have forsaken oysters and mushrooms for ever: since they are not really food, but are relishes to bully the sated stomach into further eating, as is the fancy of gourmands and those who stuff themselves beyond their powers of digestion: down with it quickly, and up with it quickly! (Seneca, *Epistulae Morales* CVIII, 13–15; trans. R. M. Gummere).

Seneca yearned for the days when a simple diet kept the body healthy, and he blamed the excesses of some of the rich, in particular their gluttony, for the rise of a whole range of new ills. According to Plutarch, the Roman world no longer suffered from the diseases of want and deprivation but was now beset with diseases of luxury.[37] However, the dietary complaints of the poor majority would still have been malnutrition, vitamin deficiencies and food-poisoning,[38] and only the rich could afford to inflict upon themselves such afflictions as:

> paleness, and a trembling of wine-sodden muscles, and a repulsive thinness, due rather to indigestion than to hunger. Thence weak tottering steps,

and a reeling gait just like that of drunkenness. Thence dropsy, spreading under the entire skin, and the belly growing to a paunch through an ill habit of taking more than it can hold. Thence yellow jaundice, discoloured countenances, and bodies that rot inwardly, and fingers that grow knotty when the joints stiffen, and muscles that are numbed and without power of feeling, and palpitation of the heart with its ceaseless pounding. Why need I mention dizziness? Or speak of pain in the eye and in the ear, itching and aching in the fevered brain, and internal ulcers throughout the digestive system? Besides these, there are countless kinds of fever, some acute in their malignity, others creeping upon us with subtle damage, and still others which approach us with chills and severe ague. Why should I mention the other innumerable diseases, the tortures that result from high living? (Seneca, *Epistulae Morales* XCV, 16–18; trans. R. M. Gummere).

Seneca deplored the fact that women, too, indulged the same vices as men and suffered the consequences: 'nowadays they run short of hair and are afflicted with gout'. The Elder Pliny also noted the appearance of new diseases in Rome, disfiguring skin complaints which, though not painful or dangerous, were so distressing that 'any kind of death would be preferable'.[39] Certainly, Rome was a centre of immense wealth in the first century AD, with luxury commodities imported from all corners of the ancient world, but the new diseases must have been as much a result of the increasing pressures of urbanisation as a result of gluttony. In addition, the mobility throughout the Empire of groups and individuals, both military and civilian alike, would have facilitated and increased the spread of regional diseases. The plague that gripped Rome in AD 166 was one of many epidemics brought back from the east by the army, while Pliny recorded that one of the new skin diseases, *mentagra*, had its origin in Asia Minor and was introduced to Rome by a returning government official. Pliny was intrigued by the fact that, unlike most epidemic diseases, *mentagra* at first struck almost exclusively aristocratic males. One of these, the legate of the province of Aquitania, paid 200,000 sesterces for treatment, though the benefits of this were dubious: 'The scar left on many who had been hardy enough to endure the treatment was more unsightly than the disease, for caustics were the method employed, and the loathsome complaint broke out afresh unless the flesh was burnt through right to the bones.'[40] The outbreak led to the arrival from Egypt of physicians who 'devoted all their attention to this complaint only, to their very great profit'.

Such hazards of city life, where diseases were more readily contracted, encouraged many who could do so to reside in the country. There they could follow healthy pursuits and more easily adopt a regimen like that recommended by Celsus. In his letters the Younger Pliny often yearned for the tranquillity of rural life. To a poet friend from his native town he wrote: 'Are you reading, fishing, or hunting or doing all three? You can do all together on the shores of Como, for there is plenty of fish in the lake, game to hunt in the woods around, and every opportunity to study in the depths of your retreat. Whether it is everything or only one thing I can't say I begrudge you your pleasures; I am only vexed at being denied them myself, for I hanker after them as a sick man does for wine, baths, and cool springs.'[41] Pliny's own properties included a villa at Tifernum (Umbria), 'at the very foot of

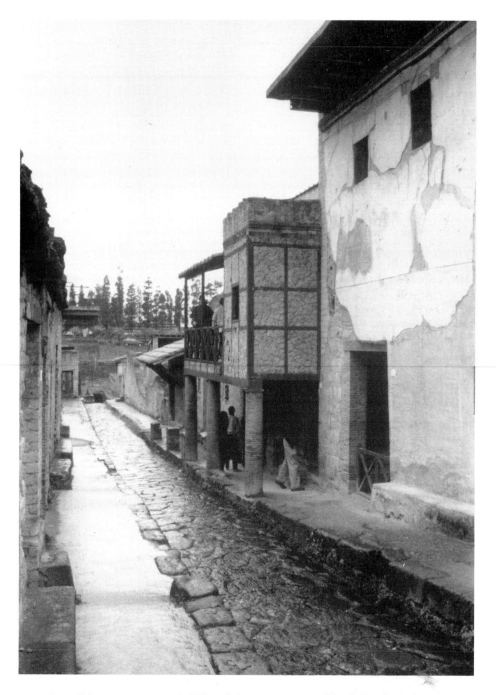

7 A small Roman apartment building of the 1st century AD. The timber-framed construction was light and economic but a fire hazard, while the projection of the upper floor over the pavement was a practice not normally tolerated. Herculaneum, Casa a graticcio.

the Apennines, which are considered the healthiest of mountains', and another near Ostia, from which he commuted to Rome: 'It is seventeen miles from Rome, so that it is possible to spend the night there after necessary business is done, without having cut short or hurried the day's work.'[42]

Pliny's descriptions highlight those aspects that the Romans considered most desirable in a villa. The region should preferably have a temperate climate, avoiding all extremes. There should be breeze rather than wind, streams but not marshland, sunshine without excessive heat, and so on. The building itself should be large and dignified though not pretentious, and the rooms orientated and arranged to take best advantage of the elements. Pliny rated warmth, sunlight and peace especially highly, as well as rural and sea vistas, and he reserved his highest praise for those rooms in which he could enjoy all or several of these pleasures. Essential to any villa were the colonnaded courtyards and gardens, which provided areas of warmth and sunshine as well as cool and shaded spots. At Tifernum Pliny's gardens combined formal arrangements with carefully nurtured 'wild' areas, and an integral part of their character came from oranamental pools and the play of water in fountains and rivulets, the *sine qua non* of any self-respecting villa-owner. Thus the country villas of the rich were dedicated to the enjoyment of nature, but a nature that was regulated by artifice. Pliny had no doubt as to the benefits: 'everywhere there is peace and quiet, which adds as much to the healthiness of the place as the clear sky and pure air. There I enjoy the best of health, both mental and physical, for I keep my mind in training with work and my body with hunting. My servants too are healthier here than anywhere else.'[43]

Those among the wealthy who found it necessary to live in towns often attempted to create a rural ambience in their houses. The hubbub of commerce could be shut out by arranging the rooms around internal courtyards, while *trompe l'oeil* frescos and the clever use of garden space, in particular utilising fountains and ingenious water installations, gave some semblance of life in the country. Houses of this design have been recognised in towns throughout the Roman Empire, just as rich villas have been discovered in every province, but most people, whether in town or country, dwelt in less spacious and less salubrious premises. In towns artisans and their family usually lived in one or two rooms behind or above their workshop, while agricultural workers occupied similarly basic quarters on villa estates or in villages. At Pompeii and Herculaneum the owners of many of the larger houses let out rooms, usually with a separate access from the street, while in especially densely occupied towns, as at Rome and Ostia, apartment blocks several stories high were common. Building techniques, usually sound, varied according to locally available materials and traditions, and timber houses could be as substantial as those of brick or stone. However, unscrupulous property magnates, especially in Rome, built flimsy multi-storey structures which not infrequently collapsed or burnt down.[44]

A more universal health hazard was the low standard or complete absence of basic facilities, notably arrangements for cooking, heating and sanitation. Only the rich could afford separate kitchens, underfloor heating, piped water, private baths and private latrines, and most people managed with considerably less. Cooking was usually done by boiling or spit-roasting over open fires. The more sophisticated households would have had raised hearths with charcoal fires and gridirons, like that in

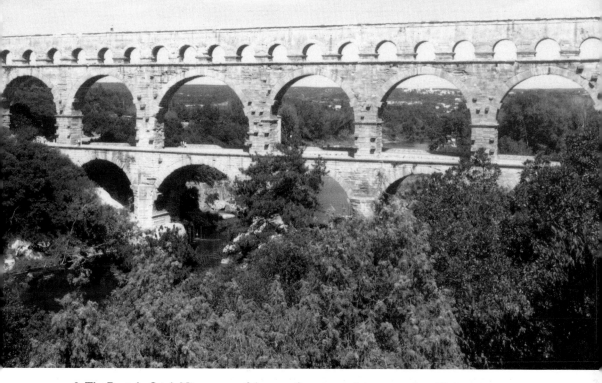

8 The Pont du Gard, Nîmes, one of the most famous surviving examples of Roman aqueduct construction. The aqueduct itself, a simple channel, was here carried across the valley of the River Gard on a magnificent triple-tiered bridge (height 49 m), built in the late 1st century BC.

the House of the Vettii at Pompeii, while in the British and Gallic provinces large cauldrons were still occasionally used, suspended from the roof beams over central open fires. Heating, too, was normally provided by an open hearth or a brazier, and artificial lighting depended on olive-oil lamps or, more commonly in north-west Europe, fish-oil lamps and wax candles. In consequence even in summer when ventilation was more straightforward most homes would have been frequently pervaded by smoke and fumes. Quite apart from the considerable risk of fire, like those that destroyed Rome in AD 64 and a large part of Verulamium (Roman St Albans) in the mid-150s AD, the coughing and sneezing provoked by irritant smoke would have caused and spread respiratory infections. In cold and damp climates especially sinusitis must often have developed into bronchitis.

Arrangements for the provision of water were extremely varied, and although there is a tendency to regard aqueducts as quintessentially the Roman water source, many other supply systems were employed. The first aqueduct brought water to Rome in 312 BC, but it was not until the Aqua Traiana was completed on 24 June AD 109 that the part of the city on the right of the Tiber received a ducted supply. At about that time Rome consumed daily many millions of gallons of water brought to the city in eight aqueducts.[45] The desire to have a copious supply of fresh spring water coupled with a pride in large civic enterprises prompted many other municipal authorities to initiate aqueduct construction projects. The aqueduct bridges alone at Pont du Gard near Nîmes in France and at Segovia, in Spain, and the arched masonry substructures at Rome itself are eloquent testimony to the expertise of Roman engineers. Less visible but no less impressive are the underground channels which were the normal form taken by aqueducts for most of their course. With a sound understanding of basic techniques, for instance inverted siphonage, sophisticated and carefully levelled watercourses were constructed, some of which continued to function effectively up to recent times.

A successful outcome did not always result, however, and there are examples of ill-conceived or foundered projects, like that at Nicomedia in the province of Bithynia, described by the Younger Pliny in a letter to the emperor Trajan. There, it seems, the skill of the engineers did not match the aspirations of the city fathers:

> The citizens of Nicomedia, Sir, have spent 3,318,000 sesterces on an aqueduct which they abandoned before it was finished and finally demolished. Then they made a grant of 200,000 sesterces towards another one, but this too was abandoned, so that even after squandering such enormous sums they must still spend more money if they are to have a water supply.
>
> I have been myself to look at the spring which could supply pure water to be brought along an aqueduct, as originally intended . . .
>
> The first essential is for you to send out an engineer or an architect to prevent a third failure. I will add only that the finished work will combine utility with beauty, and will be well worthy of your reign. (*Letters* 10, 37; trans. B. Radice)

The importance attached to the supply of water is clear in the provision at Rome of a water commissioner, *curator aquorum*. This was one of the most prestigious imperial appointments, and we are fortunate to have a full description of the duties and guiding principles of one of these men in the *De Aquis Urbis Romae*, 'On the Aqueducts of Rome', of Sextus Iulius Frontinus, who held the office in AD 97. He worked zealously to increase the efficiency of the aqueduct network and to put an end to corrupt practices: 'a considerable amount of this [water], however, is lost by leaks in the conduit . . . But we also detected some illicit pipes within the City'. Water had been appropriated not just by town-dwellers, 'who were taking water without grant from the sovereign', but by 'a large number of landed proprietors also, past whose fields the aqueducts run', and even by water officials and maintenance workers, 'whom we have detected diverting water from the public conduits for private use'. After the necessary reforming measures Frontinus claimed: 'But now . . . whatever was unlawfully drawn by the water-men, or was wasted as the result of negligence, has been added to our supply; just as though new sources had been discovered. And in fact the supply has been almost doubled, and has been distributed with such careful allotment that wards which were previously supplied by only one aqueduct now receive the water of several.'[46]

Frontinus was keenly aware of the 'health and safety' aspect of water and saw his role as much in ridding Rome of its unhealthy atmosphere as in beautifying the city with fountains. Thus, apart from securing a reliable public supply, he believed his new distribution would be 'felt still more in the improved health of the city, as a result of the increase in the number of the works, reservoirs, fountains, and water-basins. Not even the waste water is lost; the appearance of the City is clean and altered; the air is purer; and the causes of the unwholesome atmosphere, which gave the air of the City so bad a name with the ancients, are now removed.' His pride bubbled over as he contemplated the Roman technical achievement and, above all, the utility of the aqueducts in his care: 'With such an array of indispensable structures carrying so many waters, compare, if you will, the idle Pyramids or the useless, though famous, works of the Greeks!'[47]

Although few people benefited from public water systems in the form of a piped supply to private houses, the opportunity to fetch uncontaminated water from street fountains and basins would have helped to keep disease and infection at bay. Considerable care was taken in the location of an aqueduct water source, normally a spring, but occasionally a river, that was pure, palatable, and of fairly constant flow. Rome's aqueducts tapped many different sources, a few of which were particularly prized as drinking water. Whatever the purity of the source, however, the water might deteriorate on its journey to the consumer. In order to remove the coarsest impurities and clarify the water it passed through settling tanks at or outside the city boundary, where, 'taking fresh breath, so to speak, after the run, they deposit their sediment'.[48] In addition, although unknown at the time, its temporary storage in the relatively quiet state of the settling tanks would have effectively eradicated much of any harmful bacteria present in the water.[49] After having travelled some considerable distance in a closed channel the water was often flat and poor-tasting, but its sparkle and palatability could be restored by aeration either within special chambers or by the simple expedient of allowing the water to cascade from one tank to another at or near the final point of delivery.

Almost a century before Frontinus, the Roman architect Vitruvius described the basic method of water distribution adopted by towns supplied by aqueduct. Once the water reached the town it entered a collecting reservoir from which it debouched into the distribution tank, a triple receptacle, the outer two parts of which received water only if there was an overflow from the middle one: 'From the middle receptacle pipes will be taken to all pools and fountains; from the second receptacle to the baths, in order to furnish a public revenue; to avoid a deficiency in the public supply, private houses are to be supplied from the third'. Piped water was regarded very much as a public benefit and Vitruvius included his third division not so much as a service, but 'in order that those who take private supplies into their houses may contribute by the water rate to the maintenance of the aqueducts'.[50]

Distribution was by means of conduits, or of pipes made of lead, earthenware or hollowed timber. Vitruvius favoured those of earthenware as being both cheaper than lead and providing better quality water:

> ... water is much more wholesome from earthenware pipes than from lead pipes. For it seems to be made injurious by lead, because white lead is produced by it; and this is said to be harmful to the human body ...
>
> We can take example by the workers in lead who have complexions affected by pallor. For when, in casting, the lead receives the current of air, the fumes from it occupy the members of the body, and burning them thereupon, rob the limbs of the virtues of the blood. Therefore it seems that water should not be brought in lead pipes if we desire to have it wholesome. (*De Architectura* VIII, vi, 10–11; trans. F. Grainger)

The harmful effect of certain industrial processes was well enough known, if not the precise reason, and steps might be taken to avoid them or to counter them. Pliny the Elder, for instance, noted the use of protective masks to combat the toxicity of cinnabar dust: 'Persons polishing cinnabar in workshops tie on their face loose masks of bladder-skin, to prevent their inhaling the dust in breathing, which is very pernicious.'[51] However, the degree of contamination of cold water running through lead pipes was probably low and almost insignificant in comparison to the many other health hazards that assailed the Roman town-dweller. Indeed, the common and rapid deposition of calcium carbonate from hard water would quickly have formed a protective coating on the inside of lead pipes. Certainly, archaeology confirms that they were widely used, not only for private housing, as at Pompeii and Herculaneum, but extensively in public baths and military bases, as at Bath and Chester.

Under the 'health and safety' umbrella we might also view Vitruvius' instructions on well-digging, in which he warns of the dangers of 'mighty currents of air':

> When these are heavy and come through the porous intervals of the soil to the wells which are being dug, they affect the excavators, in so far as the nature of the exhalation chokes the animal spirits in their nostrils. Hence those who fail to escape at once, die there.
>
> The precautions against this are to be carried out as follows. Let a lighted lamp be lowered. If it remains alight, the descent will be accomplished without danger. If, however, the light is extinguished by the power of the exhalation, then air-shafts are to be dug right and left adjoining the well. In this way the vapours from the air will be dissipated. (*De Architectura* VIII, vi, 12–13; trans. F. Grainger)

Despite such occasional dangers in their construction, wells were always an important means of supply, especially for domestic purposes. Pliny noted that they were 'generally used in towns' and, indeed, wells have been found on most Roman sites, either as an alternative or a supplement to streams or aqueducts. They could normally be sunk precisely where required, thus avoiding either the cumbersome task of carrying water or a reliance on the intermittent supply of aqueduct water which, even when available, and when a licence had been obtained, could only be tapped at certain hours. This convenience seems to have outweighed considerations of hygiene, for wells are commonly found adjacent to pits filled with cess and other household rubbish. In fact, there often appears to have been little concept of human waste matter as an agent of disease and therefore no real appreciation of its danger to health by ground water contamination. Where advice was given on the choice of a spring source, for instance, it concentrated mainly on palatability and the avoidance of natural, not human, hazards. Water from hilly or mountainous regions was the best, while that which was stagnant, slimy and fetid was to be avoided: 'if the water itself in the spring is limpid and transparent and if wherever it comes or passes, neither moss nor reeds grow nor is the place defiled by any filth, but maintains a clear appearance, the water is indicated by these signs to be light and most wholesome.'[52]

Nevertheless, Pliny warned that 'well water should issue from the bottom, not the sides', and Vitruvius, too, recognised the process, whether harmful or beneficial, of seepage into water sources from their surrounding soil: 'There are also some acid springs... which have this property that, when they are drunk, they dissolve the stones which form in the human bladder. This seems to happen by nature, because a sharp and acid juice is present in the soil, and when currents of water pass out of it, they are tinctured with acridity.'[53]

Such phenomena held a special fascination for both Vitruvius and Pliny, who avidly collected details of those springs which were famous for their mineral waters.[54] These often became the centre of healing shrines or sanctuaries, but springs with less exceptional properties were equally important as good-quality water sources. They sometimes supplied towns by means of long-distance aqueducts, but more commonly they served the needs of the local rural communities. The site of a farm or villa was often carefully chosen with regard to a convenient water supply, and many were built on sloping ground at or near the spring line.

On the quality of rain-water there was some disagreement. Vitruvius stated that 'rain-water has more wholesome qualities, because it comes from the lightest and most finely tenuous of all sources'.[55] Pliny, however, believed that wells yielded 'the most commendable water', and he took issue with those physicians and medical authors who recommended rain-water as the most beneficial for drinking. Celsus was one such author. Like Vitruvius, he regarded rain as the lightest form of water and placed it in his weakest category of food and drink, that most appropriate to the needs of convalescents.[56] Because of its purity, physicians also favoured rain-water as a medical ingredient, as, for example, in the mixing of eye-salves, or in a treatment for diarrhoea.[57] But Pliny was convinced neither of its 'lightness' nor of its purity, observing that 'as it falls it is infected with exhalations from the earth', that 'rain-water is found to be full of dirt', and that it 'becomes putrid very quickly'.[58] Once again Pliny's comments relate rather to taste than health, but the physicians with whom he differed may have observed that those who drank rain-water were less likely to suffer from certain classes of diseases and more likely to recover if once they became ill. In the absence of the microscope, micro-organisms like those that caused typhoid and other water-borne diseases could never be detected, but physicians may occasionally have arrived at some sort of empiric knowledge of suspect water sources.

Nevertheless, apart from specific medical uses, rain-water appears to have been seldom used as a prime water source. Rather surprisingly, there is little evidence for its regular large-scale collection as run-off from the roofs of buildings, even in those parts of the Empire where precipitation was significant and fairly consistent. In drier regions it was often collected in a cistern set below the cool atrium of Roman houses, though usually as a standby to augment another source. Pliny, at least, did not relish the idea of drinking stale rain-water: 'cistern water even physicians admit is harmful to the bowels and throat because of its hardness, and no other water contains more slime or disgusting insects'.[59] Occasionally though, when neither lake, river, spring nor well could be tapped, cisterns were essential, as at Tiberius' magnificent palace retreat, the so-called Villa Iovis, set on a rugged cliff promontory of the island of Capri. There, as recommended by Vitruvius, a series of four huge semi-subterranean vaulted cement chambers was constructed, each divided into three or four compartments: 'If the cisterns are double or treble, so that they can be changed by percolation, they will make the supply of water much more wholesome. For when the sediment has a place to settle in, the water will be more limpid and will keep a flavour unaccompanied by smell.'[60]

Water suitable for drinking was vital, but another and usually greater draw on the supply was the quota for baths, for which water of lesser quality was acceptable.[61] A town of any pretension normally had at least one bathing establishment, whose construction and upkeep, like other public buildings, was largely funded by benefactors. As a result the entrance fee was nominal – one *quadrans*, the smallest copper coin[62] – while children, soldiers and occasionally slaves entered free of charge. Hence admission was not restricted and the public baths commonly combined a social role with their primary hygienic function. Mixed bathing was not unknown, but by the second century AD there were usually either separate male and female facilities or periods of the day, announced by the ringing of a bell, reserved for each sex. Many exercised or played ball games in a colonnaded courtyard, an integral part of most baths, while others availed themselves of the services of a masseur, but there was also a host of other activities and a flourishing 'service industry' that centred on the town baths. Seneca vividly described the resulting din:

> I have lodgings right over a bathing establishment. So picture to yourself the assortment of sounds, which are strong enough to make me hate my very powers of hearing! When your strenuous gentleman, for example, is exercising himself by flourishing leaden weights; when he is working hard, or else pretends to be working hard, I can hear him grunt; and whenever he releases his imprisoned breath, I can hear him panting in wheezy and high-pitched tones. Or perhaps I notice some lazy fellow, content with a cheap rub-down, and hear the crack of the pummelling hand on his shoulder, varying in sound according as the hand is laid on flat or hollow. Then, perhaps, a professional comes along, shouting out the score; that is the finishing touch. Add to this the arresting of an occasional roysterer or pickpocket, the racket of the man who always likes to hear his own voice in the bathroom, or the enthusiast who plunges into the swimming-tank with unconscionable noise and splashing. Besides all those whose voices, if nothing else, are good, imagine the hair-plucker with his penetrating, shrill voice – for purposes of advertisement – continually giving it vent and never holding his tongue except when he is plucking the armpits and making his victim yell instead. Then the cake-seller with his varied cries, the sausageman, the confectioner, and all the vendors of food hawking their wares, each with his own distinctive intonation. (*Epistulae Morales* LVI, 1–2; trans. R. M. Gummere)

People went to baths to cleanse themselves, take exercise, meet friends, chat and hear the latest news. In addition, they might have a massage or a manicure, even have unwanted hair removed, or take advice on dietetics from one of the trainers whom Galen so despised. Occasionally they may have gone for medical treatment to a doctor in one of the small booth-like shops that often flanked the street entrance of town baths, and a small set of surgical instruments found in a room at the Roman baths at Xanten[63] probably belonged to such a man. For baths were regarded not just as places for cleansing and social intercourse but also as centres of treatment. This is hardly surprising, as from earliest times, and especially under Asclepiades, doctors prescribed bathing as a means of curing illness as well as maintaining health. No less than blood-letting, baths were the Roman doctor's panacea. To treat 'diseases of sinews' or a humoral imbalance, for example, Celsus recommended sweating, elicited either in a hot-water bath or in the *laconicum*, a small sweating-room utilising dry heat, sometimes added to the normal suite of rooms at a baths. Amongst the many other conditions for which baths were considered appropriate were 'wasting disease', fever and convalescence: 'Now the bath is of double service: for at one time after fevers have been dissipated, it forms for a convalescent the preliminary to a fuller diet and stronger wine; at another time it actually takes off the fever; and it is generally adopted, when it is expedient to relax the skin and draw out corrupt humor and change the bodily habit. The ancients used it rather timidly, Asclepiades more boldly. There is indeed nothing to be apprehended from its use, if it be timely.'[64]

By the late Republican period Roman baths were usually of the modern Turkish type with rooms of graded temperature and humidity, and immersion was only a part of the process. By progressing through the cool and warm rooms to the hot room and returning in the reverse order the body was well cleansed and there was little risk of catching a chill. In the heated rooms grime and sweat were scraped from the skin with metal strigils, and there were basins with hot or cold water for washing and refreshing. The final stage normally involved the application of oils and sweet-smelling unguents. There has been justifiable admiration for such hygienic arrangements, which would have done much to maintain personal health. More important still, perhaps, was the effect on community health, for, despite the presence of the sick and ailing, regular visits to baths would have reduced the frequency and transmission of those epidemic diseases whose vectors were insects, like fleas, lice and ticks, which thrive on unclean human bodies.

Baths, unlike some other Roman institutions, were enthusiastically adopted throughout the Roman Empire, and they were to be found in small as well as large towns, in forts, in villas and in villages. They were available to the majority of the population, from senators in Rome to humble artisans in the peripheral province of Britain. To avoid the rabble the rich had private bath suites in their town houses and in their country villas, though the less extravagant, like the Young Pliny, might sometimes choose to take advantage of public baths and hired baths: 'There is... a village, just beyond the next house, which can satisfy anyone's modest needs, and here there are three baths for hire, a great convenience if a sudden arrival or too short a stay makes us reluctant to heat up the bath at home.'[65]

Although baths were common and widespread, the level of hygiene at different establishments must have varied tremendously, depending to a great extent on the water source. Even at those baths supplied by an aqueduct or an open leet, pumps, like the double-action force-pump found at Silchester,[66] would frequently have been required to raise the water to the level of the hot-water boilers. Moreover, baths were not invariably served with a running supply, and where water had to be carried or raised it would inevitably have been used rather more sparingly. By changing the water in the pools and cold plunges less often than that in the basins, for instance, baths could be operated with comparatively small quantities of water, but the result would have been less conducive to good health, especially if the clientele included

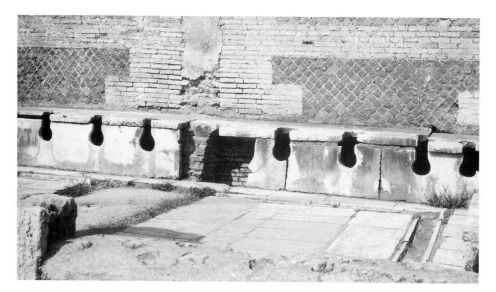

9 Public latrine opposite the Forum Baths at Ostia. This spacious establishment appears to have been installed when the baths were refurbished in the late 4th century AD.

those with habits like Thais, of whom Martial paints a particularly sordid picture: 'In order craftily to substitute for such a reek another odour, whenever she strips and enters the bath she is green with depilatory, or is hidden behind a plaster of chalk and vinegar, or is covered with three or four layers of sticky bean-flour.'[67]

We may assume that Martial, as so often, was exaggerating the atypical to satirise a small section of Roman society. In some places at least, if not all, rules were laid down to maintain standards at public baths, and self-interest would probably have further ensured that 'man's greedy love of baths', as the Elder Pliny put it, was not spoiled.[68]

Baths normally incorporated another important sanitary facility, the latrine. This was a natural adjunct, as baths were not only well visited but also yielded large quantities of waste water. Indeed, the counterpart to water supply was waste-water disposal, and the baths, as one of the biggest consumers of water, required a soundly constructed drainage system. With little extra effort a flushed latrine could be incorporated in this system, and examples have been found throughout the Roman Empire. The usual arrangement was to divert a branch drain beneath the floor of the latrine so that the water in the drain, whether it flowed intermittently or continuously, washed the effluent away from the latrine into a main sewer. The design was simple but effective and remained unsurpassed until recent times.

Public latrines independent of baths were also to be found in the busier regions of towns, notably near the forum and at main street intersections, where, with only a small entry charge they could still be profitable enterprises.[69] Although they would normally have afforded separate provision for the sexes, they were not divided into individual cubicles and so were public in a fuller sense than modern conveniences. Hardly less than the baths they were regarded as meeting places and no embarrassment was felt in conversing there with a friend, even exchanging dinner invitations.[70] Normally some ten to twenty people could be accommodated on wooden or stone seating around three sides of the room. Sometimes there were ornately carved marble seats and statues in ornamental niches, while in a latrine at Ostia, appropriately enough, an altar to Fortune, goddess of health and happiness, was discovered.[71] In place of toilet paper a small sponge tied to the end of a stick was commonly used, and this could be rinsed in the water in a small channel which ran around the room at floor level in front of the seating before descending into the sewer. Finally, handwashing water was often provided in marble or stone basins.

At their best latrines of this kind could have helped to reduce the spread of disease, although the sponges would have been breeding grounds for bacteria and, if communally used, would probably have negated all of the other sound provisions. Previously known from literary references, toilet sponges have recently been identified archaeologically in a Roman sewer at York. However, they were doubtless often replaced by other substances as, for example, the moss detected in sewage deposits from the fort latrine at Bearsden, Scotland. If indeed it served such a function it would have been less satisfactory than sponge in certain respects but would at least have had the virtue of single usage.[72]

While, too, some Roman sewers provoke admiration by their size and careful

10 Part of a Roman sewer system beneath the legionary fortress at York. For cleaning and maintenance a series of manholes gave access to the channel which is about 1 m high and 0.45 m wide. Constructed at the beginning of the 2nd century AD, the sewer appears to have continued to function until at least the late 4th century.

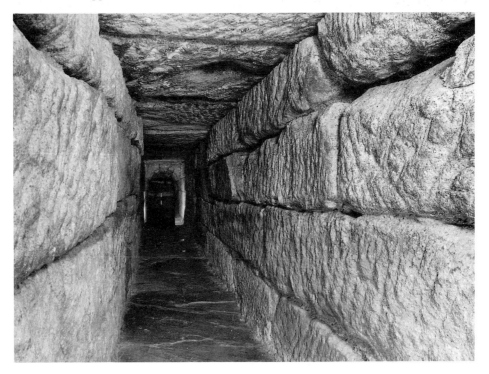

construction – as, for example, the famous Cloaca Maxima at Rome, the elaborate system beneath the imperial baths at Trier, or the network under the legionary fortress at York (10) – sewage disposal was never on a sound hygienic footing. The Younger Pliny, who had earlier held the post of *curator* of the bed and banks of the Tiber and sewers of Rome, wrote to the emperor Trajan from his province of Bithynia: 'Amongst the chief features of Amastris, Sir, (a city which is well built and laid out) is a long street of great beauty. Throughout the length of this however, there runs what is called a stream, but is in fact a filthy sewer, a disgusting eyesore which gives off a noxious stench. The health and appearance alike of the city will benefit if it is covered in, and with your permission this shall be done.'[73] We would question Pliny's assertion that the city was 'well built and laid out' when it clearly lacked a properly functioning system of purpose-built sewers. Furthermore, Pliny's solution, subsequently ratified by the emperor, was only to hide the offending stream from view and smell, not to prevent the contamination or construct a sewer *de novo*.

Another glimpse of the official attitude appears in an edict quoted by Frontinus on the use of surplus aqueduct water: 'there must necessarily be some overflow from the reservoirs, this being proper not only for the health of our City, but also for use in the flushing of the sewers.'[74] It is noteworthy that 'the flushing of the sewers' was not considered as part of 'the health of our City'. The primary intent was to shift waste because it smelt foul, not because it transmitted disease. Thus main drains and sewers seldom extended far beyond the limits of the occupied area, and they were often channelled into the town ditch or into the nearest river, which might constitute a water source for communities further downstream. At Rome Galen observed the marked difference in quality between fish caught in the relatively pure water upstream of the city and those caught in the filthy water downstream. He further noted that the effects of the pollution extended some distance seaward of the mouth of the Tiber.[75] In many instances the sewers themselves would have posed a considerable health risk, either because they were laid too close to the surface or because they were not connected to a continuous supply of running water. Some were constructed of rough coursed stone which would have trapped noxious debris; blockages, causing seepage and flooding, must have been a common occurrence if sewers were not regularly inspected and maintained.

Flushed latrines, usually with one or two seats, have also been found in the grander Roman houses, and sometimes a system of chutes permitted the provision of a latrine at first-floor level. Much more commonly, however, domestic latrines comprised simple wooden seating above tubs or a cess-pit, which would have required periodic emptying, and most people, especially those with accommodation above ground floor, were reliant upon public latrines and chamber pots.[76] As in more recent times, a virtue was made of necessity and sewage was put to a number of uses. Composted with other kitchen and household refuse it was spread on fields, while both tanners and fullers used human as well as animal excrement in their processes. Tanneries, at least, were generally kept away from centres of population, but at Pompeii, as presumably at other towns, fulling establishments shared street blocks with shops, cafés and houses.[77] Not just the fulleries themselves, but other parts of the town too must have been rank with the stench of stale urine, for the urine that fullers required for stiffening cloth was obtained in part from pots placed at street corners for the use of passers-by. The scale of the enterprise is apparent from the tax which the emperor Vespasian introduced on this most lowly of commodities. In just retribution for this pecuniary measure the collecting vessels became known thenceforth as 'Vespasiani'.[78]

Astonishingly, latrines were not infrequently situated within kitchens, as in the by no means impoverished houses of L. Ceius Secundus and C. Trebius Valens at Pompeii,[79] while sewage from chamber pots and latrines was sometimes buried in pits close to wells. Such arrangements provide the clearest possible evidence of the lack of perception amongst ordinary people of the importance of even the most basic hygienic measures. They contributed to the spread of disease, primarily bowel disorders; intestinal parasites, notably whipworm (*Trichuris* sp.) and roundworm (*Ascaris* sp.), as well as flies and their pupae, have been found in most analyses of sewage so far undertaken. Diarrhoea and dysentery, to judge from the frequency with which they were mentioned by medical writers,[80] must have been endemic in most places. Many people would have developed a resistance, but to those weakened by illness, to the aged and, above all, to young children and new-born infants these were dangerous, often fatal, diseases.

Although some among the wealthy had the time, the wish and the facilities to be fastidious over such things as hand-washing, bodily hygiene for most people would undoubtedly have meant no more than a regular or occasional visit to the baths. True soap was unknown, and additional efforts directed towards personal cleanliness were, on the whole, subordinated to those aimed at improving personal appearance. However, one concession to personal hygiene that was not restricted to the

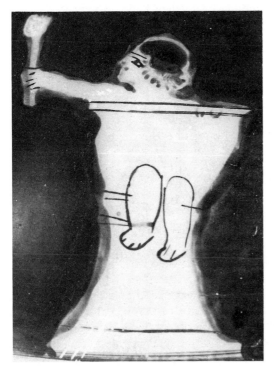

11 Baby on a potty. Scene from a red-figured vase made in Athens *c.* 440–430 BC. The potty chair comprises a tall base surmounted by a deep bowl with leg holes. The object in the child's hand is more probably a rattle than a cleansing sponge.

rich was the carrying of a 'pocket set', a common Roman accoutrement somewhat akin to a modern manicure set. It comprised several small bronze instruments, usually a tooth-pick, nail-cleaner, ear-scoop and tweezers, held on a ring for suspension on a belt or clothing. Following the dictates of fashion or attempting to mask the evidence of advancing age sometimes had an indirectly beneficial effect on bodily hygiene. In the case of hairdressing, men were no less slaves to fashion than women, and both took their lead from the styles affected by the imperial family. For shaving, barbers used thin-bladed iron razors with water, but no soap or oil, and a frequent complaint was that they worked extremely slowly. The normal alternative was a speedy but careless barber who might inflict injury, and many a customer had recourse to Pliny's recipe for a plaster to be applied to razor cuts.[81] Hair was cut with small spring shears, while heated curling irons were used to create the ever more elaborate female coiffures which were curled, ringleted, braided or piled up according to the current trend. Premature hair loss was a constant worry for the fashion-conscious, and men employed various deceptions: 'You fob us off with fictitious hair by means of ointment, Phoebus, and your dirty bald scalp is covered with locks represented in paint. You need not call in a barber for your head; to give you a better clearance, a sponge, Phoebus, is the thing.'[82] Rich women often resorted to the use of wigs and hair-pieces, the black hair imported from India and ginger hair from Germany being particularly popular. Additionally, both their own and false hair could be dyed. A favourite shade was blonde, achieved through the use of *sapo*, a mixture of beech ash and goat's fat, also brought from Germany.[83]

While both women and men went to considerable lengths to retain the hair on their head, some also followed the fashion of removing the other body hair, by plucking or by use of depilatories. The latter comprised several different recipes, including one compounded from resin and pitch. Such vanity was a natural target for the Roman satirists like Juvenal and Martial, but short hairstyles, baldness, clean-shaven faces and the removal of body hair from the armpits and pubic region would have had a positively hygienic side-effect in helping to prevent infestation by body lice and other ectoparasites.[84] The most immediate benefit, often no doubt the incentive, would have been in the eradication of rashes and itching, but more significant would have been the decreased chance of contracting parasite-borne diseases like typhus.

Most of the other stages of a lady's toilet involved the application of cosmetics: forehead and arms were whitened using chalk or white lead; the cheeks and lips were reddened with wine-lees or ochre; and charcoal or powdered antimony (stibnite) were used to blacken the eyelids and eyebrows. On aged or ageing women, who might also avail themselves of false hair and false teeth in an attempt to create the illusion of youth, the effect struck some as ridiculous: 'Your tresses, Galla, are manufactured far away, you lay aside your teeth at night just as you do your silk dresses, and you lie stored away in a hundred caskets. Your face does not sleep with you yet you wink with that eyebrow which has been brought out for you this morning.'[85] Appearance apart, the use of some mineral-based cosmetics, like stibnite and white lead, could be positively dangerous: Vitruvius warned of the toxicity of white lead and Celsus had a remedy for poisoning by it.[86] Yet through ignorance or an overriding vanity their use continued.

Not all cosmetics were harmful, however, and society women commonly employed bean-meal plasters as a skin conditioner: 'Bean meal. 'Twill be a welcome gift, and one not without use to a wrinkled belly, if in broad daylight you go to Stephanus' bath.'[87] Bean-meal also had medical uses of a similar nature, and Celsus recommended it as an emollient for dispersing the discoloration and bruising from a blow on the face and as a heating poultice 'for drawing out the material of disease'.[88]

Despite regular bathing, body smells would have been all too evident whether in a provincial town or the imperial court in Rome. The usual response of the rich was to smother themselves in unguents and perfumes,[89] and, to judge by the ubiquity of perfume containers, this was a habit that was widely adopted lower down the social scale too. Perfumes were not just applied to the body but were also taken internally. Halitosis was a common problem in a society which thrived on wine and spicy fish sauces, in which people had almost no concept of oral hygiene and did not envisage the extraction of carious teeth until the pain became unbearable. Some sucked pastilles or even drank perfume neat or in wine in an often vain attempt to cure or obscure bad breath: 'That you may not smell strong of yesterday's wine, Fescennia, you devour immoderately Cosmus's pastilles. That snack discolours your teeth, but is no preventive when an eructation returns from your abysmal depths.'[90]

A flourishing trade in costly and exotic substances grew up, part of an extensive drug market to which many Roman writers took exception. Blamed for all kinds of ills, in particular for contributing to the lowering of morals,[91] the excessive use of perfumes was often condemned. Seneca piously claimed: 'I have ... throughout my life avoided perfumes; because the best scent for the person is no scent at all'. The sentiment, similarly expressed by Martial and Plautus,[92] was admirable, but the reality must have been less so.

In summary, it is difficult to over-estimate how important it was for the individual to maintain good health. In an age when both drugs and doctors were of uncertain quality, few illnesses were easily cured, and their prevention was therefore paramount. Leaving aside the rich, however, the preservation of health was hardly within the control of the individual. Those who made a living in towns and cities might have access to public baths and running water as well as the dubious benefit of a choice of several self-professed physicians. However, there were many less enticing aspects of urban life, in particular the problems of waste disposal, over-crowding, and the increased susceptibility to contagious diseases. Those who laboured in small rural communities might be spared these urban blights. They had space and fresh air and were arguably less liable to the effects of food shortages, but sanitation was often basic or almost non-existent, and for medical advice or care most country-dwellers would have been dependent upon local lore, prayers to healing deities, a doctor in the nearest town or, perhaps, the occasional visit of a 'circuit doctor'.

While the rich might suffer from self-inflicted diseases they nonetheless had the best opportunity to maintain their own health. The advice to their peers of medical writers like Celsus and Galen shows what was possible. However, it should not be allowed to obscure the evidence from other quarters, that ill health was a real and ever-present hazard of ordinary people, and one which the poor, above all, were least able to resist.

Chapter 3

Physicians and their medicine

In 46 BC Julius Caesar granted citizenship to foreign doctors working in Rome, and at about the same time in Ephesus doctors were honoured with the conferment of tax-immunity.[1] Such legislation reflected an increased awareness of the physician's importance in the community. In Rome especially, but also in the Western Empire generally, the majority of physicians, then and for centuries to come, were Greek or of Greek descent.[2] In the first century BC most were slaves, freed slaves or their descendants, who brought the knowledge and practice of medicine to Roman households. We occasionally glimpse their faces on tombstones cut in the severe sculptural style of the period. Some were simply practitioners of medicine ministering to the needs of the family, from the master down to fellow slaves. Others were men of wide learning, whose worth was measured as much in their ability to converse knowledgeably on subjects such as philosophy as in their ability to treat illness. They were chosen by the wealthy as learned companions, friends whose influence and knowledge belied their low official status.[3]

An exceptional case was Antonius Musa, a former slave and freedman of Mark Antony, who was a follower of Asclepiades of Bithynia and his principles of medicine. Musa and his brother Euphorbus, who was physician to King Juba II of Mauretania, developed a new system of cold water treatment, and Musa was rocketed to fame in 23 BC when he employed this system to good effect in curing the emperor Augustus of a serious illness.[4] Despite subsequent less satisfactory applications of his hydrotherapy Musa remained in high esteem with Augustus and he was handsomely rewarded. His success also earned him, and all those of his profession, immunity from taxation.

Not all Greek doctors were slaves or freedmen. Many were Roman citizens, like Galen, the most famous of all Greek and Roman doctors, who was Marcus Aurelius' personal physician. Another was Caius Stertinius Xenophon, who became immensely wealthy as court physician to the emperor Claudius. Born into an Asclepiad family on the island of Cos, Xenophon acquired Roman citizenship and came to Rome to practise medicine. His wealth came not just from imperial patronage in Rome, but also from a highly successful medical practice at the most fashionable of all Roman spa resorts, Baiae, on the north side of the Bay of Naples. His influence also extended to politics, and he took every opportunity to plead Greek causes, above all those of his native Cos. Through Xenophon Claudius released the island from taxation, and the sanctuary of Asklepios attained a peak of prosperity. Although Tacitus was later to implicate Xenophon in the death of Claudius, his reputation at the time seems to have been unharmed.[5] His benefactions to the Coan sanctuary included the construction of new buildings, the restoration of existing ones and the establishment of a library. For their part the Coans honoured him with titles, offices, statues, inscriptions, even a coin issue bearing his portrait.

In addition to the independent practitioners, and those attached to families or to the emperor's retinue, there was another group of physicians, those who were employed by civic authorities. A further legacy of Greek medicine, these public physicians were paid a retainer by the town council to provide medical treatment for all who required it. Privileges usually included immunity from taxes and, like other physicians, exemption from compulsory service, although some doctors found that in practice they had to struggle to obtain the latter.[6] Premises might also be provided,[7] while a successful doctor, though expressly forbidden from requesting a fee, might often receive money from a grateful patient, and there was scope for the public doctors in particular to achieve a comfortable living standard. However, within a society in which land-ownership was the measure of real wealth, a medical practice was seldom the means to a fortune, despite popular opinion at the time.[8] Some doctors certainly found fame or attained high office, like Criton, the emperor Trajan's physician, who wrote the official history of the Dacian Wars. Others occasionally received astronomical fees, like the four hundred gold pieces Galen was paid for a single operation, but these were the exceptions rather than the rule.[9]

Nevertheless, because of the considerable attraction of tax-immunity, there would have been no shortage of candidates for the civic posts. Indeed, around the year AD 160, probably because of the increasing financial burden they put on the local tax-payers, the emperor Antoninus Pius introduced a statute restricting the number of these privileged physicians: no more than ten for capital cities, seven for large towns, and five for small towns. Furthermore, by the fourth century AD state doctors in Rome had to be chosen by at least seven other doctors.[10] If this proliferation can be interpreted as an indication of success rather than abuse, then doctors as a group certainly failed in another respect – their public image. For doctors were denigrated by many authors:

> There is no doubt that all these [physicians], in their hunt for popularity by means of some novelty, did not hesitate to buy it with our lives. Hence those wretched, quarrelsome consultations at the bedside of the patient, no consultant agreeing with another lest he should appear to acknowledge a superior. Hence too that gloomy inscription on monuments: 'It was the crowd of physicians that killed me.' (Pliny, *Natural History* XXIX, v, 11; trans. Rackham *et al.*)

> Socles, promising to set Diodorus' crooked back straight, piled three solid stones, each four feet square, on the hunch-back's spine. He was crushed and died, but he became straighter than a ruler. (*Greek Anthology* IV, 129; trans. W. R. Paton)

> Lately was Diaulus a doctor, now he is an undertaker. What the undertaker now does the doctor, too, did before. (Martial, *Epigrams* I, xlvii; trans. W. C. A. Ker)

It was Martial's robust candour that won him his reputation. Pliny the Younger thought his writings 'remarkable for their combination of sincerity with pungency and wit',[11] and there is no doubt that this traditional and long-standing caricature of the unscrupulous or incompetent doctor served Martial's purpose admirably. Few were spared in his satirical picture of Roman society, and those who visited doctors were mocked, too, for the cure or help they sought. However, the epigrams would have had no force if there was not some truth in the portraits.

One of the fundamental criticisms made by Martial and other lay writers, and also by some medical authors, was the ease with which a man could establish himself as a doctor, like the quack in one of Phaedrus' verse fables who had previously been a cobbler. The 'schools' of medicine, loose associations of those who held similar medical doctrines, operated quite differently from today's medical schools, and they provided no formal system of teaching.[12] Intelligent and dedicated aspiring physicians from a wealthy background might travel widely to gain experience at medical centres like Alexandria, Smyrna and Ephesus, or at the home of famous physicians. However there was no legal requirement to do so, and you could become a doctor, man or woman, merely by proclaiming yourself to be one. More scrupulous would-be doctors joined an established physician, observing and helping him in his work. This system is revealed in another of Martial's wry epigrams: 'I was sickening; but you at once attended me Symmachus, with a train of a hundred apprentices. A hundred hands frosted by the North wind have pawed me; I had no fever before, Symmachus; now I have.'[13]

The apprenticeship system was deeply rooted in Roman society and applied to all of the arts and crafts, whether carpentry, sculpture or medicine. Apprenticeship was a two-way process, the apprentice learning his craft or art while providing the master with another pair of hands, and, as medical literature records, physicians and surgeons required at least one assistant in their work. Often the apprentice was a son or other young relative, as had been the case from earliest times in the 'families of Asklepios'. If not a relative, the trainee or his father would have been required to pay the physician an apprenticeship fee, and it would appear that Martial's Symmachus, doubtless like many another doctor, profited by taking on a large number of apprentices.

The need for this form of training, where knowledge was imparted by demonstration and by word of mouth, arose particularly from the restricted access to written works. In a world where books had to be laboriously and expensively copied, only the wealthy could afford to acquire medical texts of any length, and even they would often have had difficulty in locating certain works to copy for their private libraries, especially if they did not live in or near one of the larger cities. This scarcity of texts enhanced the importance of the great public libraries, most notably those of Alexandria and Pergamum, Athens, Rome and Ephesus, but again, travel to these centres was a luxury mainly restricted to the rich.

Like other craftsmen, doctors had the right to form their own craft association or guild (*collegium*), and *collegia* of doctors are known at Turin and Beneventum in Italy. At Aventicum (Avenches, Switzerland) it comes as no surprise to find doctors united with teachers in one guild, for healing and teaching were activities traditionally undertaken by people of Greek extraction and their interests must often have overlapped. Despite the criticism that some received, doctors, like teachers, were regarded corporately as learned men, and one of the emblems of the medical profession was the scroll often to be seen on doctors' tombstones and in other medical depictions (17).[14]

The guild aims were mainly social, notably in the provision of club dinners and proper burial for members, and they had none of the political power of modern trades unions, although their support was often sought by candidates for political office. However, they also held meetings to discuss work-related matters and to give advice and instruction where necessary. At Ephesus the doctors organised medical contests.[15] In these ways the interests of members were protected and their activities regulated. Such guidance was particularly important in view of the 'bad press' doctors frequently received. A code of practice already existed in several parts of the Hippocratic Corpus, where it was recommended that a physician should:

> look healthy, and as plump as nature intended him to be; for the common crowd consider those who are not of this excellent bodily condition to be unable to take care of others. Then he must be clean in person, well dressed, and anointed with sweet-smelling unguents ... In appearance let him be of a serious but not harsh countenance; for harshness is taken to mean arrogance and unkindness, while a man of uncontrolled laughter and excessive gaiety is considered vulgar, and vulgarity must be avoided.
> (*The Physician*; trans. Jones and Withington)

Particular stress was laid upon the physician's conduct in his relations with a patient: 'The intimacy also between physician and patient is close. Patients in fact put themselves into the hands of their physician, and at every moment he meets women, maidens and possessions very precious indeed. So towards all these self-control must be used.' The point is reiterated in *The Oath*: 'Into whatsoever houses I enter, I will enter to help the sick, and I will abstain from all intentional wrong-doing and harm, especially from abusing the bodies of man or woman, slave or free' (trans. Jones and Withington).

Several centuries later Celsus also had firm views on the manner in which a doctor went about this work: 'in all theorizing over a subject it is possible to argue on either side, and so cleverness and fluency may get the best of it; it is not, however, by eloquence but by remedies that diseases are treated. A man of few words who learns by practice to discern well, would make an altogether better practitioner than he who, unpractised, over-cultivates his tongue.'[16]

According to Galen, a physician should also be skilled in the three branches of philosophy: logic, the science of how to think; physics, the science of 'nature'; and ethics, the science of what to do.[17] He should also have considerable energy and stamina in order to digest the work of his predecessors and undertake his own research into disease, while self-control, a disregard for money and abstention from immoderate living were almost taken as read.

The wish, at least, to aspire to these high professional and moral standards may be discerned in most surviving depictions, where doctors are portrayed as serene, attentive, sober or scholarly bearded men of middle or advanced age (15, 17). The reality may often have been less admirable, and in Martial's and Pliny's day the stock literary figure of a doctor was still that of an adulterous swindler and charlatan who might well poison those who stood in his way.[18] Even the Roman historian Tacitus relates a story which shows a doctor in the worst possible light. It concerns the death of Claudius some fifty years earlier and the role of his personal physician C. Stertinius Xenophon: 'Agrippina ... had already secured the complicity of the emperor's doctor Xenophon; and now she called him in. The story is that, while pretending to help Claudius to vomit, he put a feather dipped in a quick poison down his throat. Xenophon knew that major crimes, though hazardous to undertake, are profitable to achieve.'[19] Similarly, the doctor Posidippus was said to have helped contrive the murder of Lucius Verus, Marcus Aurelius' co-emperor, by bleeding him at an inopportune moment.[20]

Such scurrilous gossip and anecdotes, of course, made lively reading, while tales of virtue and success doubtless held less literary appeal. Against the views of the detractors, however, may be set the testimony of Seneca, who valued the skill, care, concern and, above all, the friendship of his physician:

> He spent more than the average doctor on me; it was for my sake that he took precautions, not to preserve the reputation of his art; he sat beside those in distress; he was always present in times of crisis; no duty burdened him, none sickened him; he heard my groans with sympathy; amid a crowd of patients, my health was his first concern; he attended others only when my health permitted it; I was bound to him, not as to a doctor, but by ties of friendship. (Seneca, *On Benefits* VI 15, 4; trans. in Nutton 1986, 32)

Seneca took the trouble to write in praise of his physician, but there must have been many others who received from their physician treatment of a similarly professional standard without immortalising it in print. The Younger Pliny, though not as effusive as Seneca, nonetheless had faith in the ability of his doctors. He praised and rewarded their care and attentiveness, and when ill he trusted them to the extent that he would do or take nothing without their permission. However, he also understood their human frailties and the limitations of their medicine: 'Illness is the same in a slave as in a free man', he remarked to a friend, 'but you will have observed how a doctor will treat the free man with more kindness and consideration.' Discussing the illness of another friend, he asserted: 'The doctors are in fact reassuring in their promises; it only remains for the gods to confirm these.'[21]

Nevertheless, even some medical writers took doctors to task, though more normally for incompetence than deliberate malpractice. Perhaps the most outspoken critic was Galen, who found that few medical authorities measured up to his high standards and who considered that most practising physicians were quite inadequately prepared for their profession. There is no doubt that few would have had his determination and means, quite apart from the natural aptitude, to pursue their medical studies in the way that he did. Although he lived in the Roman Empire, his native tongue was Greek, and it was through his prolific writings that Graeco-Roman medicine was to steer the course of European medicine for the next fifteen hundred years.

Galen was born in AD 129 at Pergamum, a great cultural centre in Asia, the richest province of the Roman Empire. His father Nikon, an architect, belonged to the upper tier of Pergamene society, and Galen took full advantage of the privileges his wealthy background bestowed upon him. His early studies included Greek language, rhetoric and philosophy, through which he became an authority on the works of Aristotle. When he was sixteen he embarked on the study of medicine, first at Pergamum with the eminent physician Satyros, then at Smyrna, where he studied anatomy. Later he went to Corinth, and finally to Alexandria, still one of the foremost medical centres and home of the school that he later singled out for especial praise. He was clearly an avid student and he did not feel over-awed by the medical men with whom he was in contact. At Alexandria, for instance, he wrote scorching criticisms of the doctors Lycus and Julian.[22] This long period of medical study, some twelve years, was exceptional, and sets him apart from any other Greek or Roman physician.

At the age of twenty-eight Galen returned to Pergamum, where he was appointed surgeon to a school of gladiators by the High Priest of Asia. Although the post may have been an honorary one acquired by nepotism, Galen would nonetheless have had the opportunity, which he is unlikely to have missed, to observe and operate upon a wide range of wounds, to extend his knowledge of anatomy and to experiment in diet and exercise. Certainly by AD 162, when he travelled to Rome, he was already famed as a philosopher-physician, and while in the capital he consolidated and increased his renown, both as an effective practitioner and a brilliant anatomist. He correctly predicted the recovery of the philosopher Eudemus from a fever that other doctors had regarded with despair, and he cured the wife of Flavius Boethus when other physicians had failed to do so.[23] Boethus, who was of consular rank and had influence with the emperor, became Galen's friend and sponsor, and the dedicatee of some of his books. Thus by his skill and his connections Galen was introduced to the highest level of Rome society. However, he soon became unpopular in medical circles, for he did not shrink from denouncing fellow physicians whose standards were less stringent than his own. Some of these were doctors of high repute and influence, and although he received imperial patronage Galen created such considerable hostility that his precipitate departure for Pergamum in AD 166, perhaps to avoid an outbreak of plague in Rome, probably saved his life in more ways than one. Nevertheless, he returned to Rome only three years later at the specific request of the co-emperors Marcus Aurelius and Lucius Verus, who appointed him a court physician.

It is to this period that his most significant medical works belong. His output was prodigious, both in medicine and philosophy, and the twenty-one volumes now in existence, which may represent only about a third of what he wrote, are together twice the length of the complete Hippocratic Corpus. They have a strong philosophical component, indeed they are pervaded by Aristotelian and Platonic ideas, and if it can be said that Hippocrates separated medicine from philosophy then Galen once more united them. In fact, classical medicine always had a philosophical background more or less prominent in different authorities and at different times and levels.

The very scale of Galen's work, and the survival of a significant proportion of it, makes it difficult to compare meaningfully with the fragmented texts of other medical authors, such as Rufus of Ephesus, an older contemporary of Galen. Only parts of Rufus' work survive, but he was clearly an excellent physician and a noted authority on anatomy. His terminology for many parts of the eye is still used today. Galen's claim was to have perfected the principles of 'ancient medicine' in a way that had never before been achieved,[24] and it is true that the interpretation of earlier works, most notably the commentaries on Hippocratic treatises, constituted a large part of his written endeavours. His most fundamental achievement, however, and one which gave his work an enduring importance, was his ability to set medicine in context. He had the capacity to embrace the whole of medicine, to synthesise all that was best, developing a system that countered the prevalent move towards specialisation and rose above the dissension of rival sects, an affliction that was, he believed, 'harder to heal than any itch!'[25]

While he advocated the necessity for a reasoned system of medicine, Galen nonetheless appreciated the need to treat patients as individuals. Nor in his respect of early medical authorities did he follow them slavishly, and he was constantly reassessing, revising and correcting their conclusions according to his own research. Some of his greatest contributions were in anatomy and physiology, fields of medicine upon which he had concentrated during his long and comprehensive training. His key to success was a keen mind and acute observation applied to dissection, and although he has left no unequivocal statement on whether or not he practised human dissection, there are clues to suggest he did have access to human cadavers on occasion. Normally, however, he describes experiments on animals, especially those species which he regarded as 'near to man', notably Barbary apes, dogs, and pigs. Referring, for example, to the stomach and the womb Galen asks:

> What prevents us, then, from taking up these first and considering their activities, conducting the enquiry on our own persons in regard to those activities which are obvious without dissection, and, in the case of those which are more obscure, dissecting animals which are near to man; not that even animals unlike him will not show, in a general way, the faculty in question, but because in this manner we may find out at once what is common to all and what is peculiar to ourselves, and so may become more resourceful in the diagnosis and treatment of disease. (*On the Natural Faculties* III, ii, 146–7; trans. A. J. Brock)

He had a sound understanding of the role of blood in tissue-nutrition, and although he failed to comprehend the circulatory system he was able to demonstrate that the arteries, as well as the veins, were vessels for blood, not air (*pneuma*).[26] Of particular importance in neurology was his discovery of the recurrent laryngeal nerve, for although the research of Herophilus and Erasistratus, over four centuries earlier, had demonstrated the central role of the brain in controlling the body, those who chose to follow Aristotle in endowing the heart with that function could still support their case by pointing out that the voice issued from the chest. By tracing the course of the recurrent laryngeal nerves from the spinal cord to the chest and thence to the larynx, where they control the movement of cartilaginous plates, Galen was able to close the argument by proving conclusively that the brain was also the controlling organism of speech.[27] He also clarified the perception of respiration by building on the research of one of his teachers, Pelops. Pelops had defined the action of the diaphragm, to which Galen added a description of the function of the intercostal muscles.

Both of these discoveries lent themselves well to demonstration by public display, a form of teaching in which Galen excelled. By severing the recurrent laryngeal nerves on live animals, especially those with loud or raucous voices, Galen could prove unequivocally and dramatically that the brain controlled the voice.[28] Amongst other animal vivisections was his demonstration of digestion:

Now, I have personally, on countless occasions, divided the peritoneum of a still living animal and have always found all the intestines contracting peristaltically upon their contents. The condition of the stomach, however, is found less simple; as regards the substances freshly swallowed, it had grasped these accurately both above and below, in fact at every point, and was as devoid of movement as though it had grown round and become united with the food. At the same time I found the pylorus persistently closed and accurately shut, like the os uteri on the foetus. In the cases, however, where digestion had been completed the pylorus had opened, and the stomach was undergoing peristaltic movements, similar to those of the intestines. (*On the Natural Faculties* III, iv, 157; trans. A. J. Brock)

Such displays were attended not only by medical authorities, practitioners and students, but also by philosophers, gymnastic trainers and those simply attracted by the spectacle, and Galen could be accused of the kind of sensationalism that he deprecated in others. In fact, by his own account, he had given up public dissections by AD 163. Certainly, while his dissections were brilliantly performed they were nonetheless often intended to discredit a rival. Galen must have been an awesome opponent in terms of both his wide learning and his overbearing character. Few were spared his polemic, even the small number of his predecessors whose work he generally approved, and those who dared to contradict him or simply differed from his views were submitted to a severe verbal bludgeoning:

Asclepiades is absurd when he states that the quality of the digested food never shows itself either in eructations or in the vomited matter or on dissection . . . Erasistratus, however, is still more foolish and absurd, either through not perceiving in what sense the Ancients said that digestion is similar to the process of boiling, or because he purposely confused himself with sophistries. It is, he says, inconceivable that digestion, involving as it does such trifling warmth, should be related to the boiling process. This is as if we were to suppose that it was necessary to put the fires of Etna under the stomach before it could manage to alter the food. (*On the Natural Faculties* III, vii, 166; trans. A. J. Brock)

Since the early days of Greek science the principle of analogy as a means of clarifying or fortifying abstract arguments had been widely adopted. Galen had a special fondness for its use, and because of his broad outlook he was able to employ the technique with considerable success. He was also an accurate logician, and these qualities, together with a persuasive rhetoric, made him a fine teacher of medicine. In addition to those books presenting his own theories and research, there were others in which he collected and assessed existing knowledge on a particular subject, as, for example, *On Anatomical Procedures* and *On the Method of Healing*. These were intended as 'textbooks' for practising physicians, while others, like *On Pulses for Beginners*, were specifically written as introductions for students of medicine.

While he dealt with phlebotomy – blood-letting – in several books, Galen, despite his expertise as a surgeon and anatomist, wrote no separate work on surgery, although he had intended to do so. Nevertheless, there are sufficient references throughout his other works to demonstrate the wide variety of surgical operations he performed, many during his term as physician to the gladiators at Pergamum.[29] However, elective (non-essential) surgery was never undertaken lightly, especially in Galen's medical system in which the four humours reigned supreme:

> Now in reference to the genesis of the humours, I do not know that any-one could add anything wiser than what has been said by Hippocrates, Aristotle, Praxagoras, Philotimus and many others among the Ancients. These men demonstrated that when the nutriment becomes altered in the veins by the innate heat, blood is produced when it is in moderation, and the other humours when it is not in proper proportion. And all the observed facts agree with this argument. Thus, those articles of food, which are by nature warmer are more productive of bile, while those which are colder produce more phlegm. Similarly of the periods of life, those which are naturally warmer tend more to bile, and the colder more to phlegm. Of occupations also, localities and seasons, and, above all, of natures themselves, the colder are more phlegmatic, and the warmer more bilious. Also cold diseases result from phlegm, and warmer ones from yellow bile. There is not a single thing to be found which does not bear witness to the truth of this account. How could it be otherwise? For, seeing that every part functions in its own special way because of the manner in which the four qualities are compounded, it is absolutely neces-sary that the function [activity] should be either completely destroyed, or, at least hampered, by any damage to the qualities, and that thus the animal should fall ill, either as a whole, or in certain of its parts. (*On the Natural Faculties* II, viii, 117–18; trans. A. J. Brock)

Health was to be restored by correcting the balance through diet, regimen, drugs and blood-letting, and serious operations should be considered only as a last resort. This return to Hippocratic humoral theory, which had been rejected by Erasistratus centuries before, fitted somewhat uneasily with Galen's own research and discoveries, especially in physiology. However he never abandoned it, and it remained as one of the cornerstones of his medical system. Treated with the same extreme reverence that Galen himself had accorded Hippocrates, Galenic medicine largely determined the direction and make-up of European medicine from the eleventh to the seventeenth centuries.

Galen probably died around the year AD 210, a rich and successful physician, yet, surprisingly, he is not commemorated by a single surviving statue.[30] Nor are any inscriptions known, from Pergamum or elsewhere, recording public benefactions of the kind normally made by wealthy individuals. Many explanations for this absence are possible, and it may be that in time something of the kind will be discovered. However, by his own account Galen spent most of his inherited wealth on books and scribes. The latter were required as amanuenses, for Galen's vast literary output was due in large part to his method of composition. He did not write but dictated his work, quoting other medical authors at some length as a basis from which to develop the results of his own research and expound his own theories. He also set the scribes to copy borrowed medical books for his extensive personal library.[31]

Living at the court of Marcus Aurelius, Galen had both the time and the facilities to continue his research and writing as well as attending to the medical needs of the emperor and his immediate family. Other doctors led a rather less secure existence. Those who attended the rich were at their beck and call and dependent upon their whim for payment, for there was no scale of charges. This worked both ways, for it allowed no legal redress if treatment was unsuccessful or even damaging. Normally, however, a doctor's reputation determined his prosperity. In a small town conspicuous success would soon become widely known, while news of a failure would spread equally fast.[32] In the latter case popular opinion might put a doctor out of business. Galen relates the story of a young Pergamene doctor of high repute who attempted to treat the wife of a wealthy townsman for childlessness.[33] The stakes were high – a huge fee had been promised if treatment succeeded – but this was the sort of gamble that most medical writers discouraged.[34] Better to decline an uncertain case than risk opprobrium and ruin. In the event the woman suffered a severe stomach disorder, the doctor's fee was forfeited, and he was forced to leave Pergamum in disgrace. Even then his reputation preceded him and wherever he went he was pilloried and shunned, despite his expertise in other fields of medicine. Thus in the absence of formal checks and control a levelling mechanism did nonetheless exist for the regulation of medical treatment, even if it was not always a completely fair system. How far down the social scale this extended is difficult to say, for as literacy decreases so our evidence is reduced, but it is probable that expectations, and therefore quality of treatment, were lower amongst the poor.

The place of treatment also varied according to social rank. The rich were normally attended in their own home by resident or visiting physicians. Many doctors, however, including the 'public' physicians, provided their services in premises within the town. Sometimes these might take the form of a room or suite of rooms in their own house. On other occasions surgeries were rented or were provided by the civic authority. Some, the *tabernae medicae*, were small street-side shops of the kind occupied by an assortment of traders and craftsmen. Serving soldiers were treated in military hospitals in forts and fortresses, but no civilian hospital has yet been certainly identified. Nevertheless, though they were probably never common, their existence can be inferred from occasional written references.[35] Just as military hospitals evolved to safeguard the health of a large, concentrated and, most critically, valuable body of men, so similar, though undoubtedly less satisfactory arrangements would have been made for the maintenance of the large slave work-force, the assets of private landowners on the huge estates (*latifundia*) of late Republican Italy. To avoid any expense on medical care particularly ruthless masters left sick slaves at temples of healing, notably at the temple of Aesculapius on the Tiber Island outside Rome. Clinics and nursing homes might also have been run in their own houses by private doctors, especially those who had had experience of supervising the military hospitals. However, in the pre-antisepsis era hospitals would have been a mixed blessing, and practice must have shown them to be inappropriate to the needs of most free civilian patients.[36]

Few surgeries or consulting rooms, either, have been positively identified, for the ground-plan of an excavated building seldom betrays its precise original use. A doctor's surgery depended far more on its furnishings and contents than its architectural design, and the sort of evidence that aids identification, medical texts or equipment, is very rarely found. Ancient written works, on papyrus and other perishable

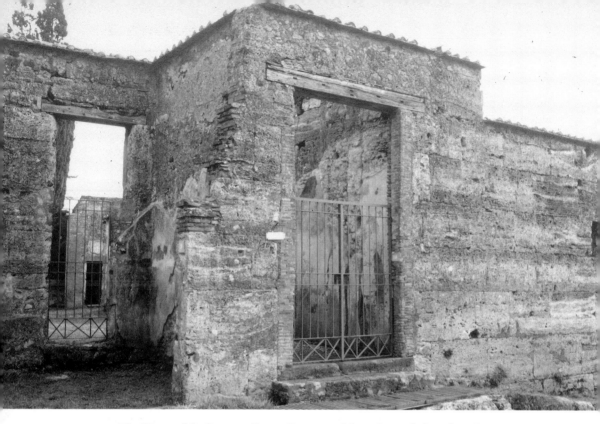

12 The House of the Surgeon, Pompeii, so named from the profusion of medical instruments discovered there in the early 19th century.

materials, have normally survived only through continued use, care and copying, while medical instruments, though found in some numbers throughout the ancient world, are infrequently discovered in direct association with buildings. This, of course, is hardly surprising. Both books and instruments were of considerable value and would only be abandoned under such exceptional circumstances as the Vesuvian disaster of AD 79.

The most famous medical discovery at Pompeii is that of the so-called House of the Surgeon on one of the main streets, the Via Consolare. The identification rests on the discovery there of a very considerable number of surgical and medical instruments, dropped on the dining-room floor in the terror and chaos of the eruption. This is probably an example of a doctor practising from his private residence, though no clue was found as to which room or rooms comprised the surgery. Unfortunately, the house was uncovered during the early excavations when archaeological techniques were still very primitive. The exact position of the instruments was not recorded, and the method of injecting plaster of Paris into cavities in the lava and ash had not been developed, so that the evidence from casts of objects made of wood or other organic materials, was missed and destroyed.

Amongst other evidence of medical practice at Pompeii is a *taberna medica* on the busy Via dell'Abbondanza. Medical instruments and bottles and jars, some of which still contained the residue of medicaments, were found strewn across the floor. Above the door was painted the name of the doctor, A. Pumponius Magonianus. The Surgery of Polydeukes has also been identified at Perge in Pamphylia.[37]

These few discoveries can be supplemented by evidence from other archaeological and written sources. The key requirement of a doctor's surgery was that it was well lit, as detailed in the Hippocratic Corpus:

> The operator whether seated or standing should be placed conveniently to himself, to the part being operated upon and to the light. Now, there are two kinds of light, the ordinary and the artificial, and while the ordinary is not in our power the artificial is in our power. Each may be used in two ways, as direct light and as oblique light. Oblique light is rarely used, and the suitable amount is obvious. With direct light, so far as available and beneficial, turn the part operated upon towards the brightest light – except such parts as should be unexposed and are indecent to look at – thus while the part operated upon faces the light, the surgeon faces the part, but not so as to overshadow it. (*In the Surgery* III, 1–16; trans. Jones and Withington)

Both physician and specialist surgeon alike required assistants who were to receive and prepare the patient, hand instruments to the physician and 'present the part for operation as you want it, and hold fast the rest of the body so as to be all steady, keeping silence and obeying their superior.'[38]

Thus a room of sufficient size to accommodate at least three people was required, and often the numbers would have been greater. A well-known scene on a Greek pot, the 'Clinic-painter' vase, shows a physician at work in his surgery (13). To judge from the number of people present his must have been a flourishing practice in premises of some size. His assistant, a dwarf, ushers in prospective clients, while the young doctor operates on a patient's arm. Another patient with a bandaged upper arm is seated nearby.

13 A doctor's surgery. The seated Greek physician operates on a male patient. He seems poised to incise a vein on the arm prior to the application of a cupping vessel, three of which are shown hanging on the wall behind him. A man with a bandaged arm is seated opposite, while to the left further patients await their turn. Vase-painting, *c.* 470 BC.

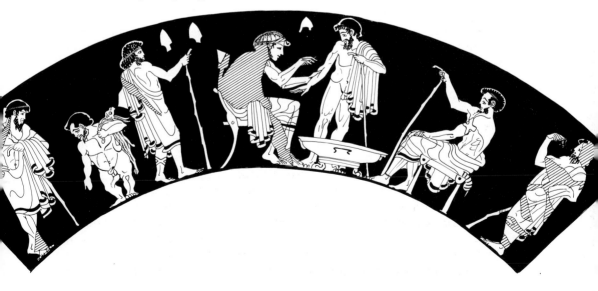

The treatment of wounds and injuries, especially to arms and legs, must have accounted for a large part of the physician's time. The mildly antiseptic property of wine and vinegar, and the stronger action of pitch and turpentine, were known by Greek and Roman medical writers, and they also understood and described in detail the importance of correct bandaging. However, if a wound was not treated in time or if it received the attention of a less knowledgeable doctor, as must have occurred on countless occasions, septic infection and ulceration might result. Some wounds would have become gangrenous, necessitating amputation, and the sight of women and children, as well as men, with missing limbs would have been a common one. Most would have managed with a stick, crutch or simple wooden 'peg', but for those that could afford it artificial limbs were available, though it is unlikely that any comprised moving joints or working parts. A skeleton with an artificial leg was discovered in a tomb of about 300 BC at Capua. Realistically modelled in sheet bronze over a wooden core, it stretched from knee to ankle and incorporated a support for the stump of the thigh. Pliny records another prosthesis, that of Marcus Sergius Silus, a battle-scarred veteran of the second Punic War (218–201 BC), who lost his right hand in action and had an 'iron hand' made to replace it.[39]

The doctor in the 'Clinic-painter' vase scene, painted at about the time of Hippocrates, operates in the seated position recommended in one of the treatises of the Hippocratic Corpus: 'when seated his feet should be in a vertical line straight up

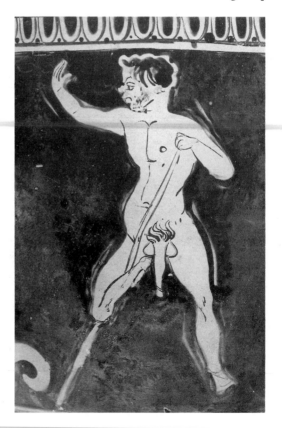

14 A grotesque male, probably a satyr or a comic actor playing the part of a man with an amputated leg. The right thigh is supported by a simple peg fastened below the knee, while the lower leg is bent back tightly against the thigh. Vase-painting, 2nd century BC.

as regards the knees, and be brought together with a slight interval. Knees a little higher than the groins and the interval between them such as may support and leave room for the elbows.'[40] Such detailed attention to posture was not mere whim but sound advice intended to give the doctor the stability required in delicate and precise treatment, and it is a position adopted in other depictions of Greek and Roman doctors at work. When a preliminary examination was being carried out the position was less critical, and on a marble relief showing the doctor Jason examining his patient, the attitude is rather more relaxed (15). His bearing appears kindly, if scholarly, as though to gain the confidence of the patient, whose fear of visiting or being visited by a doctor must have been considerable in an age when death was 'the occupational hazard of being a patient'.[41]

Celsus gave sound advice on how a physician should seek to reassure his patient: 'a practitioner of experience does not seize the patient's forearm with his hand, as soon as he comes, but first sits down and with a cheerful countenance asks how the patient finds himself; and if the patient has any fear, he calms him with entertaining talk, and only after that moves his hand to touch the patient.'[42] Next, by predicting the course of the illness – *prognosis* – the doctor could increase the trust of his patient before attempting a cure. When severe pain was involved he could further assist and impress by administering a pain-killer or sleeping-draught. Pliny and Dioscorides describe the use of a powerful anodyne made by boiling the root of white mandrake,

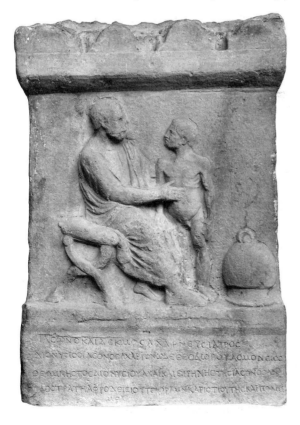

15 A physician at work. Jason, an Athenian physician, examines a young man with a swollen abdomen. The outsized cupping vessel on the right would have been instantly recognisable as a symbol of the medical craft. Tombstone, 2nd century AD.

and a decoction from henbane, a mild narcotic of the belladonna family, was also used. However, Celsus' preference was for those preparations whose main ingredient was 'poppy tears', the opium-bearing juice derived from the head of the wild poppy. A draught of one, he claimed, would alleviate the pain of 'headache or ulceration or ophthalmia or toothache or difficulty in breathing or intestinal gripings or inflammation of the womb or pain in the hips or liver or spleen or ribs'.[43] Celsus did not mention the cultivated poppy (*Papaver somniferum*), which yielded opium in a stronger form, but it was certainly known to Dioscorides and to Galen, who prescribed it for Marcus Aurelius though he was aware of the problems of addiction.

Diagnosing and curing an illness presented the physician with his greatest challenge, for knowledge of bacteria and viruses was denied to early doctors, and disease was difficult enough to characterise, let alone to comprehend. Still today, despite the prodigious resources of the medical profession, the cause of many a disease eludes discovery. It is no surprise that in the past disease was a real and ever-present source of fear. Seemingly trivial symptoms might quickly develop into serious or mortal conditions. The normal response of Greek and Roman doctors was to observe and record the symptoms and the stages of the illness, and to draw on experience of apparently similar cases in order both to predict the course and to assist in a recovery. However, the pre-eminence of the humoral theory of disease largely dictated the form of treatment. A return to health involved a restoration of the critical balance of the bodily fluids, for which doctors normally had recourse to the time-honoured methods of purging, blood-letting or drug therapy, and the doctor who purged and bled his patient to distraction, whatever the illness, was one of the Roman satirist's stock characters.

Celsus mentions several purgatives, including aloes and hellebore, but he was averse to their unrestricted use, especially by those 'who by ejecting every day achieve a capacity for gormandizing'. Though he accepted purging as a method for 'thinning' patients, he was aware of the side-effects and favoured instead the administration of enemas:

> purgatives ... whilst necessary at times, when frequently used entail danger; for the body becomes subject to malnutrition, since a weakened state leaves it exposed to maladies of all sorts.

> For the most part the bowel preferably is to be clystered; the practice was limited by Asclepiades though still kept, but I see that in our time it is usually neglected. But the limitation which he seems to have adopted is most fitting; that this remedy should not be tried often, and yet we should not omit to use it once, or at most twice. (*De Medicina* I, 3, 26; I, 12; trans. W. G. Spencer)

Even more entrenched in Graeco-Roman medicine was blood-letting (phlebotomy, venesection, wet-cupping), which was believed to cure or alleviate almost every known ill, especially those which resulted from a 'constriction', 'superabundance' or 'corruption' of bodily materials. Celsus summarised the technique and its application as it had evolved by the first century AD:

To let blood by incising a vein is no novelty; what is novel is that there should be scarcely any malady in which blood may not be let ... For it matters not what is the age, nor whether there is pregnancy, but what may be the patient's strength ... Therefore severe fever, when the bodily surface is reddened, and the blood-vessels full and swollen, requires withdrawal of blood; so too diseases of the viscera, also paralysis and rigor and spasm of sinews, in fact whatever strangulates the throat by causing difficulty of breathing, whatever suppresses the voice suddenly, whenever there is intolerable pain, and whenever there is from any cause rupture and contusion of internal organs; so also a bad habit of body and all acute diseases, provided ... they are doing harm, not by weakness, but by overloading ... If the cause affects the body as a whole, blood should be let from the arm; if some part, then actually from that part, or at any rate from a spot as near as may be, for it is not possible to let blood from everywhere, but only from the temples, arms and near the ankles

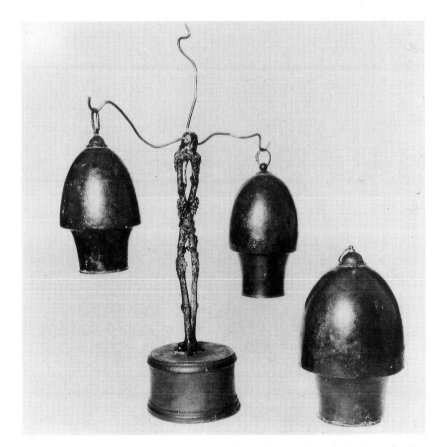

16 Three bronze cupping vessels and their stand, part of the extensive set of medical instruments found in a grave of the late 1st or early 2nd century AD at Bingen. The extraction of 'vicious humours' by dry and wet cupping was one of the mainstays of Greek and Roman medical practice.

... Practice itself, however, seems to have taught that for a broken head blood should be let preferably from the arm; when the pain is situated in one upper limb, then from the arm opposite; I believe because, if anything goes wrong, those parts are more liable to take harm which are already in a bad state ... Now blood-letting, whilst it may be very speedily done by one practised in it, yet for one without experience is very difficult, for to the vein is joined an artery, and to both sinews. Hence should the scalpel strike a sinew, spasm follows, and this makes a cruel end to the patient. Again, when an artery is cut into, it neither coalesces nor heals; it even sometimes happens that a violent outburst of blood results. Thus many things make difficult to one who is unskilled what to one experienced is very easy. The vein ought to be cut half through. As the blood streams out its colour and character should be noted. For when the blood is thick and black, it is vitiated, and therefore shed with advantage, if red and translucent it is sound, and that blood-letting, so far from being beneficial, is even harmful; and the blood should be stopped at once. (*De Medicina* II, 10, 1–17; trans. W. G. Spencer)

Diversionary bleeding was also commonly employed as one of the many measures to staunch the flow of blood in a wound: 'For bleeding from a place where it is not desired ceases after something is applied to stop it there, when the blood is given another exit.'[44] As Celsus noted, blood was normally drawn from the arms, and the patient being attended in the 'Clinic-painter' vase scene appears to be having a vein cut prior to the application of a bleeding cup, several of which are to be seen hanging on the wall behind the physician (13). Celsus describes two varieties, of horn and bronze, but suggests that a drinking cup or narrow-mouthed bowl might be pressed into service, while at the other extreme some doctors used cups made of silver. Antyllos, a doctor of the third century AD, recommended glass cupping vessels which allowed the flow of blood to be more closely monitored. Few glass cups have been recognised, nor, as yet, any of horn, but those of bronze are known in some numbers. They are among the few Greek medical instruments to have survived, and examples are known from contexts dating as far back as the fifth century BC.[45] Their distinctive form was already fully developed and altered very little over the next thousand years – a bell-shaped body with narrow neck. The mouth often had a carefully rolled rim to ensure a comfortable and even contact with the skin, while at the other end there was usually a ring attachment to allow the cup to be suspended on a hook or stand when not in use (16). From its resemblance to a gourd (*cucurbita*) the Romans called the bleeding cup *cucurbitula*, 'little gourd'.[46]

The cupping technique was a simple one which remained popular in European medicine up to the beginning of the nineteenth century. Suction was achieved through the creation of a vacuum:

Now there are two kinds of cups, one made of bronze, the other of horn. The bronze cup is open at one end, closed at the other; the horn one, likewise at one end open, has at the other a small hole. Into the bronze cup is put burning lint, and in this state its mouth is applied and pressed to the body until it adheres. The horn cup is applied as it is to the body, and when the air is withdrawn by the mouth through the small hole at the end, and after the hole has been closed by applying wax over it, the horn cup likewise adheres. (Celsus, *De Medicina* II, 11, 1–2; trans. W. G. Spencer)

Sometimes the 'vicious humour' could be extracted by dry-cupping, which depended on suction alone without the need to let blood. On other occasions leeches were used to draw blood in place of cups,[47] a technique that became increasingly popular in medieval medicine and has continued sporadically down to the present day. However, blood-letting with cups was by far the most frequently practised method and already in Greek times the bleeding cup had become the symbol *par excellence* of the medical profession. It was often depicted on doctors' tombstones and other reliefs, sometimes alongside a box of surgical instruments (15, 28).[48]

Bowls of various sizes were also required by physicians for a range of tasks. Some have been discovered with sets of instruments, while others are depicted in several medical scenes. That shown at the feet of doctor and patient in the 'Clinic-painter' vase scene may have been used to catch the blood in phlebotomy. Another one shown on a fragmentary terracotta relief from the tomb of a doctor, M. Ulpius Amerimnus, appears to be being used in the bathing of a wound.[49] The patient has his right foot in the bowl while the doctor applies a sponge to his lower leg.

Most Roman houses were sparsely furnished by modern standards, and this would also have applied to doctors' consulting rooms and surgeries. Nonetheless, doctors would have required chairs, tables and couches for the examination of patients,

17 A physician reads from a scroll, probably a medical work, in front of a cabinet. The opened double doors reveal two shelves on which are further scrolls and a bowl. A small hinged box on top of the cabinet is conveniently opened to display a set of surgical instruments. Marble sarcophagus, 4th century AD.

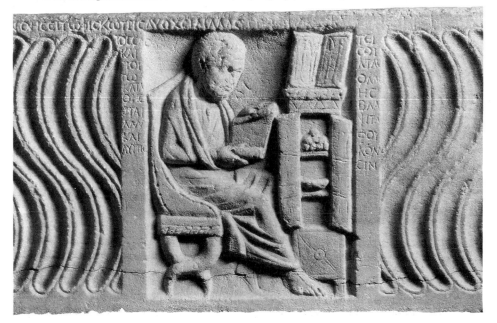

as well as wall-hooks, shelves and cupboards to accommodate their medical instruments and apparatus, and a fine example of a doctor's cabinet is depicted on the side of a marble sarcophagus from Ostia (17).[50]

Cupboards and shelves would also have been filled with a variety of herbs and drugs in jars, pots and boxes, for patients also went to *tabernae* for draughts of medicine. A patient might gaze in awe at the bewildering array of medical substances, an impression of which can be gained from a description by the Roman physician Dioscorides:

> Flowers and such parts that have a sweet-smelling fragrance should be laid down in small dry boxes of limewood, but occasionally they can be serviceably wrapped in papyrus or leaves to preserve their seeds. As for moist drugs, any container made from silver, glass, or horn will be suitable. An earthenware vessel is well adapted provided that it is not too thin, and, among wooden containers, those of boxwood. Copper vessels will be suitable for moist eye-drugs and for drugs prepared with vinegar, raw pitch or juniper-oil. But stow animal fats and marrows in tin containers.
> (*De Materia Medica* Preface, 9; trans. in Scarborough and Nutton 1982)

In addition, there would have been the paraphernalia of drug preparation – pestle and mortar, fine balances, scales and weights, marble palettes for rolling pills, bottles, scoops, spoons, and spatulae. Glass and ceramic pots filled with animal fats and beeswax, the base for most ointments, would jostle for space with flasks of olive oil, used as a lubricant, and jars of wine, water, milk and honey, with which medicines were often mixed.

Most medicines were specifics and panaceas, preparations derived in the main from herbs and vegetables, but also from a wide range of inorganic and animal organic substances, sometimes mixed with spices. Although some had active ingredients, many would probably have had little or no direct effect, other than psychosomatic, upon the patient. Furthermore, because neither disease nor human physiology were properly understood, the majority of medications were for external application, where their effect could be closely observed and monitored. Even so, the active ingredient of a drug could not necessarily be pinpointed, for many medicines were 'cocktails' composed of numerous ingredients: polypharmacy was the price of uncertainty. The few internal remedies were, apart from purgatives, mainly foods and drinks.

Although the medicines themselves have normally perished or deteriorated, their containers have occasionally been found. A characteristic type of rectangular box had a sliding outer lid and several internal compartments, each with its own hinged lid. This allowed the storage together of a small range of different medical substances without risk of contamination. Those examples that survive are normally made of bronze or sometimes ivory, but they must originally have been most common in wood. Another type of bronze box was long, narrow and cylindrical, rather like a modern cigar tube. Often several of them are found together, for they would normally have held only a single medicament, a powder, a semi-solid ointment, dried sticks or pills. A specialised type of drug storage comprised a stacking system of cylindrical bronze pots, the stepped base of each forming the lid of that beneath (27).[51] Many draughts and decoctions would have been individually prepared from dried substances, but for those potions and ointments that were stored in a liquid or semi-liquid form

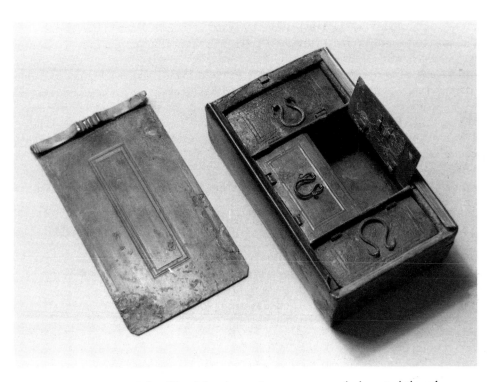

18 Bronze box with sliding lid and four internal compartments. A characteristic and long-lived Roman type which was often used for the storage of medical substances. Length 12.6 cm.

there was a range of glass vessels. Most common are slender glass phials and small, squat jars, but small 'dropper' juglets are also known.

Unfortunately, it has seldom proved possible to identify the residues which in rare instances have survived in the bottom of medicine containers, for even detailed scientific analysis often leaves many questions unanswered. Those substances that are least subject to deterioration and are most easily detected are metals, and they have been discovered on most occasions when pills or powders have been analysed. However, it is seldom clear how many other ingredients might originally have formed part of the medicine, nor the original proportions. Nevertheless, where results are available they demonstrate the use of copper, lead, zinc and iron in their various forms singly or in combination, and these are precisely the metals most frequently referred to in the ancient pharmacopoeias.[52] They were recommended particularly in the treatment of wounds and ulcerations – to stop haemorrhage, as astringents, caustics, cleansers, desiccants, erodents and emollients – and as ingredients in ointments for eye diseases.

The knowledge that certain plants and mineral and animal substances had healing properties is probably almost as old as the human race itself. In most cultures drug lore developed as a key part of folk medicine, and the rural basis of most societies up to recent times meant that the vast majority of the population knew the medical properties of at least those plants and other natural resources native to their own region. Knowledge was handed down by word of mouth from one generation to the next, a system geared to the needs of small scattered communities. However, with the territorial expansionism of Alexander the Great and the meteoric rise of the Roman Empire diverse cultures were brought together and it became possible to compare and exchange medical ideas. A flourishing trade in *materia medica* developed with a ready market in the towns, to which growing numbers of people were being attracted. Those medical writers who sought to bring order to pharmacology faced a task of immense proportions, the scale of which can be seen in their surviving works. Theophrastus, a pupil of Aristotle, described some 550 plants, Dioscorides assembled almost 600 remedies, Galen a similar number, whilst Pliny, in Books XX–XXXII of his *Natural History* recorded a staggering 900 substances.[53] Pliny highlighted some of the technical problems that were faced in compiling herbals:

> Crateuas, Dionysius and Metrodorus adopted a most attractive method, though one which makes clear little else except the difficulty of employing it. For they painted likenesses of the plants and then wrote under them their properties. But not only is a picture misleading when the colours are so many, particularly as the aim is to copy Nature, but besides this, much imperfection arises from the manifold hazards in the accuracy of copyists. In addition, it is not enough for each plant to be painted at one period only of its life, since it alters its appearance with the fourfold changes of the year. (*Natural History* XXV, 4; trans. Rackham *et al.*)

There were two key requirements of a herbal: ready access to the medical and botanical information it contained, and the recognition of individual plants. Despite Pliny's reservations on the quality of drawings, illustrated pharmacopoeias gave the reader the best chance of identifying plants, and they were popular throughout antiquity. The method of presenting the written information posed a still greater problem, and there were many differing approaches, from Pliny's loose arrangement by plant type to Celsus' well-ordered classification according to property. Others listed the plants alphabetically, while Dioscorides employed a system of 'drugs-by-affinity'.[54]

Pedanius Dioscorides, from Anazarbus in Cilicia, was the most famous pharmacologist of antiquity. He lived during the first century AD, a well-travelled physician who is thought to have spent part of his career as a military doctor during the reigns of Claudius and Nero. Although contemporaries, Dioscorides and Pliny did not know each other, nor did either know the other's work, although they drew on the same sources. Dioscorides' herbal, *De Materia Medica*, comprised five books written in Greek around the year AD 64, the product of a lifetime's study. Its systematic layout and detailed observations, combined with a rejection of superstition and magic, ensured its success. It even met with Galen's approval, and superseded all existing herbals to become a standard work, whose influence was felt up to recent times. The finest surviving copy is the 'Vienna Dioscorides', which was made in Constantinople around the year AD 512. A gift for the princess Anikia Iouliana, daughter of a former Roman emperor, it was the work of a Byzantine artist who illustrated it with coloured drawings, of varying accuracy, of the plants described. Later, after the invention of printing, the *Materia Medica* went through some seventy editions in Europe.

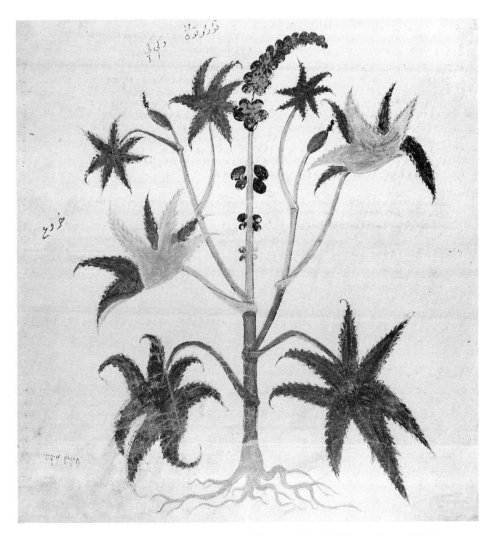

19 The castor-oil plant (*Ricinus communis*) as illustrated in the 'Vienna Dioscorides',
a copy of Dioscorides' herbal made in Constantinople *c.* AD 512.

Dioscorides, like Pliny, addressed the problem of plant recognition, but because of his pharmacological training his was a positive and practical solution:

> Anyone wanting experience in these matters must encounter the plants as shoots, newly emerged from the earth, plants in their prime, and plants in their decline. For someone who has come across the shoot alone cannot know the mature plant, nor if he has seen only the ripened plants can he recognise the young shoot as well. Great error is occasionally committed by those who have not made an appropriate inspection, as a result of the changes in the form of the leaves, the varying sizes of stems, flowers and fruits, and some other characteristics.

He also had strong views on the collecting of medical plants:

> Before anything else, it is appropriate to consider the storage and collecting of individual drugs in their proper seasons, for these matters in particular determine the weakness or efficacy of drugs. (*Materia Medica* Preface, 6–7; trans. in Scarborough and Nutton 1982)

While physicians would have been able to heed such advice with regard to those plants that grew in their neighbourhood, some difficulty was faced with the more exotic herbs. Those doctors rich enough to own land, if only the courtyard of their home, might cultivate a private herb garden, but climate would still have governed the range available. To acquire herbs from foreign lands those doctors who chose not to travel or were unable to do so (and they must surely have been the majority) had to turn to the drug markets. These were to be found in most large towns and echoed to the call of 'root cutters' (*rhizotomoi*), spice dealers (*aromatopoles*), ointment sellers (*unguentarii*) and dubious druggists (*pharmacopolae*), who had a myriad of rare and expensive commodities. Such centres were infamous, in particular the *seplasia* at Capua, which became a byword for luxury and vice. The patriotic Pliny deplored this development, as much for the suppression of traditional Italian self-sufficiency as for the exorbitant prices of imported herbs. However, there was clearly a ready market:

> the deceit of men and cunning profiteering led to the invention of the quack laboratories, in which each customer is promised a new lease of his own life at a price. At once compound prescriptions and mysterious mixtures are glibly repeated, Arabia and India are judged to be storehouses of remedies, and a small sore is charged with the cost of a medicine from the Red Sea, although the genuine remedies form the daily dinner of even the very poorest. But if remedies were to be sought in the kitchen-garden, or a plant or a shrub were to be procured thence, none of the arts would become cheaper than medicine ... But the reason why more herbs are not familiar is because experience of them is confined to illiterate country-folk, who form the only class living among them; moreover nobody cares to look for them when crowds of medical men are to be met everywhere. (*Natural History* XXIV, i, 4–5; XXV, vi, 16; trans. Rackham *et al.*)

Many other writers, including Martial and Phaedrus, joined Pliny in admonishing the public for its gullibility at the claims of doctors and druggists. Inevitably, however, the combination of greed, ignorance and credulity sustained the drug markets, while even some among the educated classes were prey to the extravagant claims of quack doctors, so hopeful were they of a cure.

One of the consequences of the profitable drug trade was the common occurrence of 'diluted' or bogus wares. Adulteration was rife and a doctor had very little control over the quality of his raw materials.[55] This would not only have deprived him of the full effect of those few substances that had active ingredients but, if contaminated or completely substituted, they might sometimes have a positively harmful, even lethal, result. It is hardly surprising, therefore, that to maintain their standing as eminent physicians men like Galen capitalised on every opportunity to cut out the middle-man and acquire raw materials at or near their source. Galen had both the wealth and the contacts in high places to enable this. In Rome he acquired herbs direct from the emperor's own suppliers; while on a visit to Syria he bought genuine 'balsam of Mecca' and, from a passing caravan on the Indian trade route, some of the highly prized Indian *lycium*. These were two of the most celebrated and expensive substances in early pharmacy, and the Roman emperors, to ensure their own top-quality supply of the former, owned balsam groves in Syria.

Opobalsamum was the name given to the secretion of a number of different balsam trees, the most famous being 'Mecca balsam' or 'balm of Gilead' from Arabia. Collected as exuded resin or obtained as an essence from boiling the leaves, seeds and branches, it had many applications. Celsus alone recommended its use externally for cleaning wounds, as an erodent, suppurative and emollient, as an ingredient in poultices, in an anodyne salve for the relief of neuralgia, in an eye ointment and, taken internally, as a diuretic.[56] It was also one of the thirty-seven constitutents of his version of the most famous ancient antidote, *mithridatium*. This was named after its inventor, the brilliant and learned king of Pontus, Mithridates VI (120–63 BC), who 'thought out the plan of drinking poison daily after first taking remedies in order that sheer custom might render it harmless.'[57] As Celsus soberly put it: 'Antidotes are ... chiefly necessary against poisons introduced into our bodies through bites or food or drink.'[58] Snake bites apart, the premature end of many a Roman emperor at the hands of those close to him makes Mithridates' fascination with antidotes understandable. Ironically, so successful were his experiments in immunity that when forced to take his own life poisons were ineffective and he had to die by the sword.

Lycium, like balsam, was obtained from several sources, from one of which, Lycia, in southern Asia Minor, it took its name. A tannin-rich shrub of the Boxthorn family, it was especially effective as an astringent, and its medical uses included the relief of ulcerations, the staunching of haemorrhage, and the checking of discharge in eyes, ears and nose.[59] Indian *lycium*, extracted from shrubs of the Berberis family, was regarded especially highly in the treatment of eye diseases. Scribonius Largus, a widely travelled physician who flourished about AD 14–54, rated the uncompounded use of Indian *lycium* above all other eye salves.[60] Its use continued up to recent times in India, whence, in the early nineteenth century, it was brought to Britain and found to be effective in the treatment of conjunctival ophthalmia.[61] Not all Roman doctors could obtain the genuine product, and there were substitutes with similar properties, like that mentioned by Pliny which was made from gentian.[62] Additionally, like most ancient drugs, *lycium* was subject to variation in its mode of preparation. Thus a few of the minute lead jars which contained this precious commodity have been found to bear proprietary Greek inscriptions. One was marked 'Jason's *lycium*', another, from Athens, '*lycium* according to the recipe of Musa', while 'Nymphodorus' *lycium*' was being used in Priene, on the south-west coast of Asia Minor, as early as the third or second century BC.[63]

Very few other labelled medicine containers have survived, presumably because most were dispensed in glassware or wooden boxes with attached papyrus labels or painted inscriptions. One interesting exception, however, was found at a Roman fortress of late Augustan date at Haltern, near Essen in northern Germany. It is the lid of a lead pot inscribed with the words EX RADICE BRITANICA (*sic*), 'extract of the root of Britan(n)ica'.[64] A passage in Pliny's *Natural History* not only confirms that what the box contained was a medicine but also describes the antiscorbutic use to which medicine of exactly that kind was put in a region close to Haltern a few years later in AD 16:

> When Germanicus Caesar had moved forward his camp across the Rhine, in a maritime district of Germany there was only one source of fresh water. To drink it caused within two years the teeth to fall out and the use of the knee-joints to fail. Physicians used to call these maladies stomacace and scelotyrbe. A remedy was found in the plant called britannica, which is good not only for the sinews and for diseases of the mouth, but also for the relief of quinsy and snake-bite. It has dark, rather long leaves, and a dark root. Its juice is extracted even from the root. It was pointed out to our men by the Frisians, at that time a loyal tribe, in whose territory our camp lay. Why the plant was so called I greatly wonder, unless perhaps, living on the shore of the British ocean, they have so named the britannica because it is, as it were, a near neighbour of Britain. It is certain that the plant was not so named because it grew abundantly in that island: Britain was at that time an independent state. (*Natural History* xxv, vi, 20–1; trans. Rackham *et al.*)

Stomacace and *scelotyrbe* are Greek words meaning, respectively, scurvy of the gums and disorder or paralysis of the legs, and the disease that afflicted Germanicus' army must have been scurvy. Its cause was not the water source but a vitamin C deficiency due to a lack of fresh fruit and vegetables, for the regular military supply system had probably been interrupted during the difficult campaigns in the forests and marshland of northern Germany. From Pliny's description the plant 'Britannica' has been identified as dock.[65] The episode underlines the value of Pliny's anecdotal method of composition and is illuminating in a number of respects, not least in showing the empirical medical knowledge that the Romans encountered and absorbed when entering new lands.

One of the striking things about the best Greek and Roman pharmacopoeias, those of Dioscorides, Celsus and Galen, is the common occurrence of preparations or ingredients that are chemically similar to some still in use today. *Auripigmentum*, for instance, which Celsus recommended for the cleaning of wounds, was variously orpiment or sandarac, in modern terms the sulphides of arsenic, which do have a mildly antiseptic property; and his *thymum* yielded the antiseptic *thymol*, akin to, though rather weaker than, the phenol (carbolic acid) used by Joseph Lister eighteen centuries later. In his prescriptions Celsus gives the amount as well as the name of the ingredients, thus permitting some assessment of their effectiveness. However, as there is no means of establishing the strength of the drugs accurate quantification and controlled experiment are impossible. One optimistic estimate is that perhaps as many as 40 per cent of the drugs prescribed by Dioscorides for a particular disease would have had a positively beneficial effect.[66] When one takes into consideration such things as the unreliability of supply of top-quality drugs and the physicians' variable success in diagnosis, the real figure is likely to have been rather lower, perhaps in the region of 20 per cent, though many of the remaining 80 per cent of remedies must have had a beneficial placebo effect on patients.

Even though the calculations are based upon use of the best pharmacopoeias and the best drugs by the best physicians, treatment that would only have been available to a small percentage of wealthy patients in certain parts of the Roman Empire, they imply a significant degree of success which was seldom bettered before recent times. Furthermore, they must represent a sizeable satisfied public whose silence compared to the vociferous comments of the critics, preserved especially in Martial's writings, may have helped to create a false impression of the Roman public's regard for its doctors. It is a common enough phenomenon that success may pass unnoticed while a single failure can bring forth a flood of indignant and angry criticism. So it is ironic that Pliny's drug remedies would probably have had a rather lower success rate than those of Dioscorides, Galen and Scribonius Largus, all members of the medical profession that he was so quick to deride.

The high cost of medical books would always have severely restricted the number in circulation, but it must also have preserved them for long periods and made the same books available to generations of doctors. If individual doctors were unable to acquire their own copy of pharmacopoeias, they may yet have had access to them at libraries or through their guild.[67] Pharmacopoeias would undoubtedly, too, have been amongst the medical books and manuals available to the military doctors who served in forts and fortresses throughout the provinces, and by these means pharmaceutical knowledge reached every corner of the Empire. Archaeology provides confirmation not only in the occasional discovery of pharmaceutical equipment and medicine containers with or without the residue of their contents, but also in the identification of plant remains and mineral substances used in medicine. The minerals include several lumps of realgar found at the Roman town of Silchester which, as *auripigmentum*, Celsus especially recommended as an antiseptic for the cleansing of wounds and ulcerations.[68]

Plant remains are a little more common, and seeds of dock, *Rumex obtusifolius*, already mentioned for its relief of scurvy, have been found at several Roman towns in Britain (Caerwent, Carmarthen, Southwark), while the wild celery from a latrine in the fort at Bearsden, Scotland, may have been used as a diuretic, as recommended by Celsus.[69] A most important discovery was made in the legionary hospital of the fortress at Neuss (Roman Novaesium), near Düsseldorf, Germany.[70] The many hundreds of plant seeds identified include species mentioned in the Greek and Roman pharmacopoeias: centaury, which was used to heal wounds, to cure eye diseases and as an antidote for snake bites; fenugreek, a decoction of which was heated as a poultice or was used as a soothing enema and was also an ingredient in a remedy for pleurisy and pneumonia; henbane, also found at the Roman towns of Silchester and Carmarthen, universally recommended as a pain-killer and sleeping-draught; plantain, which was administered for phthisis (pulmonary tuberculosis), haemorrhage, dysentery and elephantiasis; and St John's wort, used as a pastille to expel bladder stones and as an ingredient in the famous antidote, *mithridatium*. Foodstuffs often had medicinal uses; indeed, medicines were frequently taken as foods, and the figs whose remains have been found at many Roman sites, including Neuss and Bearsden, may often have been taken as a medicine. Cooked over charcoal, the fruit was recommended for coughs, while the sugar content of its juice helped to promote a thin discharge in wounds and ulcers.

Another means of administering medicines, and one which even in Dioscorides' time already had a long history, was in wine. In a fortress at the very limit of the empire, Carpow in Scotland, was found a fragment of a wine amphora on which was scratched the letters πPAC, part of the Greek word *prasion*.[71] This was horehound, with which the wine in the amphora had been infused, and it would have been very appropriate to the needs of soldiers in Scotland, for it was recommended by Dioscorides, Celsus and Pliny for chest complaints, especially as a cure for coughs. Equally appreciated by its recipients would have been the wine amphora marked AMINE sent to the fortress of Caerleon, South Wales,[72] for Aminean was one of the best-quality Italian wines. It was also recommended medicinally as a cure for diarrhoea and for the common cold, *gravedo*, so succinctly described by Celsus: 'This closes up the nostrils, renders the voice hoarse, excites a dry cough; in it the saliva is salt, there is a ringing in the ears, the blood-vessels in the head throb, the urine is turbid . . . These affections are commonly of short duration, but if neglected may last a long while.'[73]

Recipes for eye ointments comprise a distinct and substantial part of ancient pharmacopoeias,[74] and there is no doubt that eye diseases were among the most common afflictions of the time. In consequence the medical examination, undergone by all recruits to the Roman army, included an eye-test. Writers like Pliny the Younger were especially prone to eye troubles, and occasionally, too, serious eye disorders were realistically depicted in sculpted portraits.[75]

Many people of every class would have suffered from eye weaknesses such as myopia, for although the effect of artificial lenses was understood there is no evidence that they were adopted as an aid to vision, and it was not until the thirteenth century that spectacles began to gain general usage. Perhaps more class-specific were those complaints caused by irritants and infections which must have been especially easily spawned and spread in the unhygienic living conditions of the poor. As will be seen (chapter 5), certain complaints could be corrected or alleviated by surgery, but for the most part treatment was by medicament, normally applied as a salve. These were often known by the name of the inventor – 'the salve of Philo', 'the salve of Dionysius', 'the salve of Nileus' – or by the name of the principal ingredient – *dialibanum* (containing frankincense). Sometimes they were named after a special property – *authemerum* (curing within one day), or *achariston* ('ungrateful', because the salve caused such rapid relief that the patient felt no gratitude for his easy cure).[76]

Though many of these concoctions would have had little useful effect and a few could have been positively harmful, a number contained active ingredients still in use today or up to recent times.[77] Such is the salve of Axius, an oculist of the British Fleet, singled out for mention by Galen.[78] For use on 'ulcered corners of the eye, bad inflammation of the eye, intense irritation, and chronic condition', its ingredients included copper and zinc hydroxide, zinc carbonate, opium and mercuric sulphide. Galen described Axius as an *ophthalmikos*, that is to say he was a specialist eye doctor. He probably practised at one of the bases of the British Fleet, perhaps the main base at Dover, where he would have been part of a medical team ministering to the needs of a squadron of several hundred sailors and marines. From inscriptions on their tombstones, eye specialists (*medici ocularii*) are also known to have practised in Rome and several other cities of the Empire, and some acquired considerable riches.

However, the army and the cities were exceptional, the one comprising Rome's most valuable and most expensive asset, the other providing concentrated centres of wealth and population sufficient to support numbers of medical specialists. In most towns and regions the conditions did not exist for other than 'general practitioners'. Thus in Assisi P. Decimius Eros Merula amassed a small fortune by combining several specialisms, to judge by the inscription on his tombstone, where he is described as *medicus clinicus chirurgus ocularius*.[79] Many other doctors who treated eye diseases must have been known simply as *medicus*. In any case, there was no certainty that a specialist would give superior treatment for, like the medical profession in general, no qualification was required of those who sought to establish a practice, and reputation was the sole criterion by which the ability of a doctor or specialist might be gauged. It is hard to believe, for instance, that two *medici ocularii* in Rome had either an extensive knowledge or a wide experience of eye medicine: their tombstones record their age at death as seventeen years and nineteen years.[80] Eye doctors also suffered badly at the hands of satirical poets like Nicarchus, who is thought to have lived in Alexandria at the time of Nero: 'Before he anoints your eyes, Demostratus, say "Adieu dear light," so successful is Dion. Not only did he blind Olympicus, but through his treatment of him put out the eyes of the portrait of himself he had.'[81]

Archaeologically it is difficult to discern medical specialists, or the exact form their specialism took, but an exciting discovery made at Rheims, France, appears to have been the trousse of an oculist.[82] An extensive range of medical equipment was found with the remains of a large wooden box in a grave dated to the late second or early third century AD. In addition to the normal instruments of Roman surgery (scalpels, forceps, hooks and probes) and the usual apparatus of pharmacy (scales, bowls and flasks), there were nine handled needles and a stamp for impressing semi-solid 'sticks' of eye ointment, as well as many fragments of the desiccated ointment sticks (*collyria*) themselves. Here, then, was a doctor who was equipped to treat eye diseases with salves or by surgery. His *collyria* would have been prepared according to one of the many recipes in the pharmacopoeias.[83] The ingredients were mixed and then rolled like pastry into short lengths at which stage they were marked with a stamp and left to dry. The stamps were rectangular slabs of stone, rather smaller than a matchbox, bearing an engraved text on the flat face of each edge. The inscription was cut in reverse so that its impression could be read by the user of the *collyrium*, who may not have been the man who made it. The Rheims *collyrium* fragments, for instance, are marked with recipes which include one of Marcellinus, but none of G. Firmius Severus, whose name appears on the stamp, and the physician who used both stamp and *collyria* may have been neither of these men.

Unlike other medical apparatus, these *collyrium* stamps were not easily broken, and stone is seldom subject to destructive processes in the ground. Consequently many have survived, and to date some three hundred are known.[84] Although variable in content, the format of the inscriptions is very standard and normally consists of three parts: the name of an affliction, usually an eye disease; the name of a salve to be used for its treatment; and the name of a person associated with the salve, who may or may not have been the originator of the prescription or the user of the stamp. Thus one of the four inscribed faces of a stamp found in London reads: C SILVI TETRICI EVODES AD ASPRITUDINES, 'the fragrant lotion of Gaius Silvius Tetricus for trachoma'.[85] Study of the inscriptions on these stamps reveals some one hundred

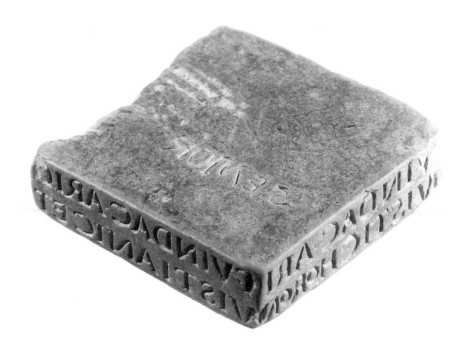

20 Collyrium stamp marked with the name of Titus Vindacius Ariovistus and his various preparations for the treatment of eye diseases. The inscriptions are cut in reverse so that they could be read when impressed into blocks of the prepared medicaments. The roughly incised word *Senior* may have been the name of a doctor who used the stamp. Length 3.9 cm. From Kenchester, England.

salves intended for the treatment of more than thirty ailments and diseases. However, many of these occur once only, while a few are encountered time and time again. The most frequently mentioned ailments are *aspritudines*, trachoma, chronic conjunctivitis; *lippitudines*, eye inflammation, ophthalmia; and *cicatrices*, corneal scars; while the commonest salves include *crocodes*, made from saffron dregs; *dialepidos*, made from copper oxide; *diamisus*, made from antimony sulphide; and *diasmyrnes*, made from myrrh.

Almost all of these stamps come from the Roman provinces of Gaul, Germany and Britain, and yet eye diseases were prevalent throughout the Roman Empire; indeed, one of the most serious, trachoma, was endemic in the eastern Mediterranean. One explanation of this is that it reflects a different method of packaging geared to the needs and conditions of two distinct regions. In the Mediterranean provinces, where the herbs and spices could be more readily obtained, freshly prepared eye salves were probably carried in bottles and tubes. However, in the north-western provinces, perhaps due to the greater difficulty of ensuring a regular supply of the eastern herbs which figured so prominently in eye remedies, large batches were prepared and stored in ready-made dried form. It is further possible that the stamping of salves was a fiscal requirement connected with customs duties, an early instance of protectionism perhaps. Certainly, it has been shown that the distribution of *collyrium* stamps coincides with the Roman tax region known as the Four Gauls.[86]

Whatever the exact reason, such a system would have permitted a doctor to carry a range of prepared and clearly marked *collyria* from which he could select the most appropriate for his patient and simply let it down in water, milk or egg-albumen to apply it as a salve. This would have worked particularly well if there were a number of doctors based at a single centre requiring the same range of eye medicines, and a convincing case has been made for the existence of circuit doctors, the *circuitores* known from literary sources.[87] There was a long tradition of travelling physicians extending back to the beginnings of Greek medicine, and the needs of the predominantly rural communities of the north-western provinces may have been met by a similar arrangement.

The concentration of *collyrium* stamps at particular towns may represent regional medical centres, from which panels of these *circuitores*, eye specialists or not, embarked on regular and set routes through the surrounding countryside, stopping at towns, villages, markets, healing shrines and other meeting places to treat the sick. Such a centre probably existed at Aventicum (Avenches, Switzerland), where a *collegium* of doctors and teachers is referred to on a stone inscription set up by two of its members, both *medici*, Q. Postumius Hyginus and his freedman Postumius Hermes.[88] For Postumius Hermes' name has been found again, on a *collyrium* stamp from Vidy, some fifty kilometres away.

The eye was not the only part of the human body that was subject to specialist treatment, and in subsequent chapters we shall look at the work of midwives, gynaecologists and surgeons. Galen mentions doctors who specialised in almost every part of the anatomy, in eye diseases, ear disorders or tooth troubles, and in operations for hernia, for bladder stone and for cataract. Others write of dieticians and hydrotherapists, doctors for fevers, for fistulae and for anal complaints. However, as with eye doctors, such specialists were rare in most places, and Galen himself asserts that only Rome and Alexandria could support such a range. Elsewhere a doctor, like Eros Merula of Assisi, might combine several specialisms, or he might attempt to treat the broad spectrum of illness and injury.

It is impossible fairly to estimate the effectiveness of Greek and Roman physicians. There were clearly cases of conspicuous success, and equally certainly many occasions when the doctor's client was more truly his victim than his patient. However, those doctors who followed the dictum of the best medical authorities, that treatment should be sparing, and that extreme measures should be avoided if at all possible, are likely to have met with the greatest success. For, despite the skill, ingenuity, dedication and high principles of some physicians, they were still faced with considerable difficulties in diagnosis and treatment. Furthermore, the ability of the body to cure itself of many diseases should not be underestimated. Even today, with the wealth of medical expertise, drugs and equipment at our disposal, spontaneous cures are an important element in healing. In antiquity, when a physician's limited resources made unpredictable all but the most straightforward of medical interventions, there was much to be said for restraint on his part.

Chapter 4

Women's diseases, birth and contraception

When Pliny compiled the medicinal plants section of his *Natural History* he noted that 'among a great number of the common people' women still retained the pre-eminent position that they had long occupied in folk medicine and sorcery.[1] However, in Pliny's day there were also women who practised a more scientific medicine, like Antiochis, daughter of Diodotos, who was given permission to erect a statue of herself at her home town of Tlos in Lycia.[2] This considerable honour was bestowed on her by 'the council and the people of Tlos in recognition of her skill as a medical practitioner', and she is almost certainly the same Antiochis whom Galen credited with the discovery of a medicine for rheumatism and sciatica.[3]

The practice of medicine was one of the few male activities open also to Roman women, and there are sufficient references to *medicae*, medical women, to show that many took up the challenge.[4] Furthermore, these female practitioners were not restricted to any one class but were drawn from several social tiers. Tacitus admired the actions of Agrippina, the wife of Germanicus, who, during her husband's German campaigns, raised morale at the base camp by dispensing clothes to needy soldiers and medical aid to the wounded. The satirists Juvenal and Martial also made mention of lady doctors who practised in Roman high society,[5] while lower down the social scale *medicae*, like their male counterparts, were often commemorated in funerary inscriptions. Many were of Greek origin or had Graeco-Latin names;[6] some were slaves or freed women;[7] others came from medical families, like Antiochis, whose father Diodotos was probably the doctor of that name mentioned by Dioscorides.[8] Some were sufficiently rich to fund the construction of large monuments or buildings, while a few, at least, became specialists or wrote medical treatises.[9] Many were held in high regard and affection – even Martial spared *medicae* his normal sarcasm – as in the case of Iulia Saturnina of Merida, whose epitaph, written by her husband, was to 'an incomparable wife, the best physician, a most virtuous woman', and of a certain Victoria, to whom, in the later fourth century AD, the imperial physician Theodorus Priscianus dedicated his book on gynaecology with the words 'artis meae dulce ministerium' (the sweet teacher of my art).[10]

Although there were doubtless exceptions, most female physicians, whether or not they were specialists, probably treated exclusively or predominantly women's diseases,[11] and the title *medica* may have been synonymous, or nearly so, with that branch of medicine. That is not to say that gynaecology was their sole preserve. Far from it, for most male medical authorities wrote on the subject, including Soranus of Ephesus, the most famous gynaecological and obstetrical writer of antiquity. Nevertheless, already in Hippocratic times women's diseases were regarded as very different to men's, and while a male physician, by careful questioning, might elicit sufficient information to allow successful diagnosis and treatment, it was recognised that gynaecology and obstetrics were a province in which specialists were required and in which women had a natural advantage over men. However, *medicae* were always less numerous than *medici* and, as Soranus records, midwives, *obstetrices*, often served in their stead: 'the public is wont to call in midwives in cases of sickness when the women suffer something peculiar which they do not have in common with men.'[12]

While we might assume that experienced midwives could have dealt effectively with most female conditions and disorders, they were often guided by consultant physicians. Boethus' wife, for example, whom Galen cured of a mysterious and trouble-some 'female flux',[13] was in the care of midwives who received direction from a number of male physicians. That some midwives were more than simply intermediaries who administered the treatment prescribed by doctors is evident however. Galen, like Theodorus Priscianus, dedicated an early work, *On the Anatomy of the Uterus*, to a midwife,[14] and it is clear that they were expected to read medical treatises. Indeed, Soranus' first requirement of those who intended to become midwives was that they

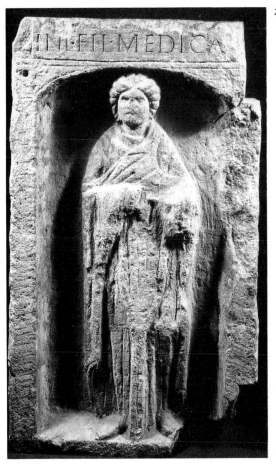

21 Tombstone of a woman doctor (*medica*) from Metz. Probably 1st century AD.

should be literate, and they were doubtless part of the intended readership of his textbook on gynaecology.[15]

Soranus was not only an eminent authority on gynaecology, but one of the greatest physicians of his day. Born in Ephesus, he studied at Alexandria, practised in Rome during the reigns of Trajan and Hadrian, and died around the time that Galen was born. Although he wrote almost twenty works on many aspects of biological and medical science, few have been preserved in their original Greek. A *Life of Hippocrates* is ascribed to him and there are short treatises *On Bandages* and *On Fractures*, the latter perhaps part of the lost *Surgery*, but for an assessment of Soranus as a medical writer and physician we are largely dependent on the *Gynaecology* and on another substantial treatise, *On Acute and Chronic Diseases*, which has been preserved in an excellent Latin paraphrase by Caelius Aurelianus, who lived in the fifth or sixth century AD.

Soranus was one of the best-known adherents of the Methodist school of medicine, whose principles are most apparent in his division of diseases into those that are chronic and those that are acute, and in his use of the cyclic form of treatment for chronic illnesses, as in his method for curing or easing dysmenorrhoea (painful periods).[16] He also followed Asclepiades in adopting a mechanistic approach to certain diseases, in particular in his use of passive exercises like rocking in a chair or carriage. However, he was an able and original thinker, and, like all of the greatest physicians, he was not constrained by any one set of doctrines, but was prepared to adapt to each situation as he observed it. In consequence the *Gynaecology*, though in contemporary terms a little uneven in quality, is one of the most impressive and significant medical works of antiquity. It is arranged in four books, the first two comprising a discussion of the qualities required of a midwife and an account of 'things normal', the second devoted to 'things abnormal'. 'Things normal' include a description of the female genitals, the hygiene of female sexual functions and pregnancy, normal labour and puerperium, and infant care and children's diseases. 'Things abnormal' are divided into those women's diseases to be treated by dietetics and those that require treatment by surgery or drugs. Throughout, the four books are particularly striking for their rationality, generally sound therapy and practical advice, a clear and succinct style, and, above all else, for a firm denunciation of superstition. Unlike Pliny, who criticised magic yet often endorsed magical beliefs and practices, Soranus' denunciation was consistent and unequivocal. He was at pains to eradicate superstition in medicine both because it was generally useless and because it often involved methods that were unpleasant, painful or even dangerous; on a few occasions his text is ambivalent, but the folk remedy in question was of a harmless nature.[17]

Soranus was not prepared to accept unreservedly the ideas and methods of earlier authorities, and he had no qualms over differing with even the most hallowed or eminent, such as Hippocrates, Diocles and Asclepiades, but, in contrast to Galen, he expressed these differences concisely and objectively, avoiding emotive terms, abrasive language or personal acrimony. He was capable of compromise: 'Some people say that some things are effective by antipathy, such as the magnet and the Assian stone and hare's rennet and certain other amulets to which we on our own part pay no attention. Yet one should not forbid their use; for even if the amulet has no direct effect, still through hope it will possibly make the patient more cheerful.'[18]

His own scepticism was unshaken but he was sufficiently realistic and sensitive to the needs of his patients to realise the psychological benefit that they might derive from such aids.

A measure of Soranus' medical standing is that even Galen acknowledged the importance of his work, despite the underlying Methodist concepts to which Galen was vehemently opposed. As Galen himself was to do later, Soranus synthesised the best existing works and added to them the results of his own experience and research. His *Gynaecology*, because of its essentially practical nature, was, above all, of profound and continuing importance, and in Greek and in Latin translation it influenced medical thought both in the east and the west of the Roman Empire. Via the gynaecological section of the work of Paul of Aegina, a Greek medical authority of the seventh century AD, an attenuated version of the *Gynaecology* passed into Arabic medicine. A little earlier it had been paraphrased by a Latin writer named Muscio, whose book retained its popularity throughout the Middle Ages and was itself transmitted to post-Rennaissance medical literature through German, French, English, Dutch and Spanish adaptations. Like some of the contemporary pharmacopoeias and herbals, it appears that Soranus' *Gynaecology* was illustrated, and it is believed that the drawings of the womb and the foetus *in utero* that accompany some copies of Muscio's text were derived from Soranus.

It is not difficult to see the appeal of Soranus' *Gynaecology*, especially to the patient, for, wherever possible, harsh or unpleasant methods were consistently avoided. More important, the obstetrical technique was excellent, and experience must have proved the value of his work to midwife and physician alike. Moreover, his account of the female anatomy, though occasionally inaccurate (he denied the existence of the hymen, for example),[19] was better than anything else at the time and includes a good description of the uterus. We do not know how often, if at all, Soranus dissected human cadavers, for although he had studied at Alexandria, where dissection was still practised, the Methodist sect rejected dissection as part of the 'useless' scientific research of the Dogmatists. It is probable, therefore, that he drew heavily on earlier treatises on human anatomy, notably that of Herophilus which retained its importance at least down to the time of Galen. Nevertheless, Soranus appears to have been the earliest author to note the cartilaginous joint of the female pubic bones, which allows extra movement in childbirth.[20]

Both Soranus and Galen broke with a very curious tradition in which the womb was regarded as a mobile entity that could traverse the abdomen or travel still further afield (this despite a knowledge of the diaphragm), causing pain through displacement or distortion. Some, like Plato, even believed the womb had its own animal-like existence,[21] and still in Galen's day a contemporary medical writer, Aretaeus of Cappadocia, maintained the Hippocratic doctrine of a 'wandering womb': 'In the middle of the flanks of women lies the womb, a female viscus, closely resembling an animal; for it is moved of itself hither and thither in the flanks, also upwards in a direct line to below the cartilage of the thorax, and also obliquely to the right or to the left, either to the liver or spleen; and it likewise is subject to prolapsus downwards, and, in a word, it is altogether erratic.'[22] The painful and unpleasant sensations, in particular the feeling of suffocation, that were attributed to such movements of the womb were regarded as hysteria in its original meaning as 'affections of the womb'.

Thus hysteria, which was believed to be a specifically female condition, had a very different meaning then to the modern term. However, Galen, at least, applying a keen mind and careful observation to two similar cases, one a lovesick young woman, the other an elderly male slave with a guilty conscience, recognised the primarily psychological nature of their conditions which might today be diagnosed as hysteria.[23]

Soranus defined hysteria as: 'obstructed respiration together with aphonia [loss of voice] and a seizure of the senses caused by some condition of the uterus. In most cases the disease is preceded by recurrent miscarriages, premature birth, long widowhood, retention of menses and the end of ordinary childbearing or inflation of the uterus.'[24] He recommended gentle measures, which included laying the patient down in a warm and moderately bright room, applying warm compresses, and sponging the face with warm water. If the voice was still not restored the groin and surrounding regions were to be dry-cupped and fomented with sweet olive oil, and the patient was to be rocked in a hammock. Later mouth-washes, poultices, relaxing baths, fomentations, suppositories and vaginal injections of olive oil might be necessary. Such mild treatment stood in contrast to that of many of his predecessors and contemporaries:

> the majority of the ancients and almost all followers of the other sects have made use of ill-smelling odours (such as burnt hair, extinguished lamp wicks, charred deer's horn, burnt wool, burnt flock, skins and rags, castoreum with which they anoint the nose and ears, pitch, cedar resin, bitumen, squashed bedbugs, and all substances which are supposed to have an oppressive smell) in the opinion that the uterus flees from evil smells ... Hippocrates ... believing that the uterus is twisted like the intestines are in intestinal obstruction, inserted a small pipe and blew air into the vagina by means of a blacksmith's bellow, thus causing dilation ... Xenophon proposes torchlight and prescribes the making of greater noise by whetting and beating metal plates. ... We, however, censure all these men who start by hurting the inflamed parts and cause torpor by the effluvia of ill-smelling substances. For the uterus does not issue forth like a wild animal from the lair, delighted by fragrant odours and fleeing bad odours; rather it is drawn together because of the stricture caused by the inflammation. Also upsetting the stomach, which suffers from sympathetic inflammation, with toxic and pungent potions makes trouble. Forcing air by means of the smith's bellows into the vagina – this inflation makes the uterus even more tense, which is already rendered sufficiently tense by reason of the inflammation ... Sounds and the noise of metal plates have an overpowering effect and irritate those who are made sensitive by inflammation. At any rate, even many healthy persons have been given headaches by such sounds. (*Gynaecology* III, 29; trans. O. Temkin)

Many other women's diseases and disorders were described by medical writers. They include inflammation of the uterus and vagina, uterine haemorrhage or, less specifically, 'uterine pain'; morbid uterine and vaginal discharges; ulceration of various parts of the reproductive tract; closure of the womb due to hardening of the cervix; prolapse of the uterus; and 'affections of the breast'. The accounts of breast complaints relate mainly to disorders in menstruation, pregnancy and lactation. Care was taken to avoid abscess of the nipples in pregnant women by loosening the breast band, while the treatment for inflammation and intumescence of the breasts included linseed and wheat or bread and honey-water poultices.[25] That there were specialists in breast disorders is confirmed by an inscription which refers to a lady doctor described as *medica a mammis*,[26] and Celsus included the female breast in his list of body parts most prone to 'carcinoma'.[27] Nevertheless, despite the difficulty of translating ancient medical terms, breast cancer appears to have been far less prevalent than it is today.

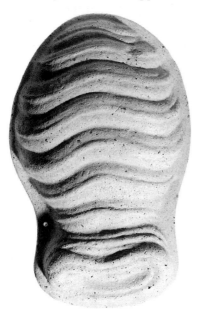

22 Terracotta votive model of a uterus. Length 17.5 cm. Roman, 3rd–1st century BC.

Treatment for women's diseases was often by dietetics, and Pliny lists many remedies to be taken in wine or water. External medication, in particular wax salves and plasters, was also commonly prescribed,[28] but many drugs were administered internally by means of fumigation, clysters or pessaries. The process of fumigation involved the heating of substances such as bitumen, human hair, medicinal plants and aromatic herbs in a metal or ceramic pot with a close-fitting lid. The lid was pierced by a hole in which was a reed or lead tube, the other end of which was inserted into the woman's vagina and through which the heated and supposedly healing vapours passed. Fumigation was especially favoured by those physicians like Aretaeus, who sought to manoeuvre the uterus back to its proper position by use of repellent and pleasant-smelling vapours applied variously to the nose or vagina. It is, of course, difficult to gauge the potential effectiveness of techniques that are alien to the practices of modern medicine, but Soranus' warning of the severe burning that might occur if fumigation was unskilfully undertaken serves as a reminder of the pain and danger to which patients were often subject.[29]

The basic principle of clystering was little different to that of fumigation, namely the introduction of 'healing' substances, in this case liquids, into a bodily orifice. Clysters were used to instil medicaments into the ear and the nose, but the commonest varieties were those used to treat the bladder, rectum, vagina and uterus. The rectal clyster, like its modern counterpart, was used especially to inject enemas, for example during labour,[30] while the bladder clyster was often recommended for irrigation of the urethra or an ulcerated bladder. A vaginal or uterine clyster was described in a passage of Hippocrates.[31] It comprised a pouch, made from the bladder or skin of an animal, fastened to the top of a smooth metal tube whose lower end terminated in one or more perforations above a solid, rounded tip. The patient guided the clyster into position herself at which point the physician expelled the medicament by squeezing the pouch in which it was held. The clyster was also used as an irrigator, and vaginal douching was a common ancient expedient for many ills.

The uterine clyster evidently changed little over the next half-millennium, for an instrument buried by the Vesuvian eruption of AD 79 exactly fits the Hippocratic description.[32] Occasionally true syringes were stipulated for uterine or vaginal treatment, and an ear-syringe was recommended in the treatment of infants suffering from 'a flux of the bowels'.[33] Although Roman medical instruments were usually of extremely fine workmanship, and those intended for internal work were very carefully smoothed, as instructed by the medical authors, one cannot but feel that the common insertion of such instruments into the body in an attempt to heal must sometimes have had the opposite effect, and they may have been responsible for some of the 'ulcers' so frequently referred to. Despite this, injections into the vagina and the uterus using clysters and syringes remained a common practice down to the early nineteenth century.

Pessaries, a form of vaginal suppository, are commonly referred to in the medical literature. Celsus wrote: 'there are other useful compositions, such as those which are introduced into women from below, the Greeks call them pessoi. Their characteristic is that the component medicaments are taken up in soft wool, and this wool is inserted into the genitals.'[34] He described the composition of several pessaries which were to induce menstruation, to soften the womb, to treat inflammation of the womb, to render the expulsion of a dead foetus and to relieve hysterical fits, and Pliny listed many more for a similar range of disorders.[35] As in other forms of medication, the ingredients include some that could have helped as well as many that would not. Some were exotic, and it is hard to imagine that many women who had difficulty conceiving would have had access to the treatment recommended by Celsus, a pessary made from rose oil and lion's fat.[36] It is still harder to imagine that those who did would have found their unfortunate condition improved.

Pessaries were occasionally used as a mechanical support, worn in the vagina to remedy uterine displacements, as in Soranus' and Diocles' treatments for a prolapsed uterus.[37] Tents (lint plugs) were also employed, as, for example, to promote healing in a suppurating womb or to stop uterine haemorrhage,[38] while a metal tube was usually inserted after operations on the vagina to prevent contraction or adhesion, and to introduce medication, as Celsus stipulated in the treatment following his operation for occlusion of the vagina: 'as soon as it begins to heal, a lead tube smeared with a cicatrizing ointment is passed in, and over this the same application applied until the cut surface has cicatrized.'[39]

Another common gynaecological technique was dilation of the cervix, recommended amongst other things for treating hysteria, and graduated sets of tapered wooden or metal rods must have been a basic component of the *instrumentarium* of women's doctors. However, the diagnosis of, and application of remedies to, many vaginal and uterine disorders was facilitated by a much more sophisticated dilator, one of the most spectacular Graeco-Roman medical instruments, the *dioptra* or vaginal speculum. Although Soranus is one of the first authors to mention it, noting that in haemorrhage of the uterus, 'one can determine the affected part more safely by using a speculum',[40] the discovery of three examples at Pompeii demonstrates that it was, in fact, known well before Soranus' time. The Pompeii specula are expertly made precision instruments. They comprise a projecting *priapiscus* composed of three (or in one case four) prongs operated by a screw-threaded handle and crossbar mechanism. When closed, the prismatic internal faces of the blades dovetail together to present a solid phallic shape with rounded tip and immaculately smooth surface, and in that respect they are superior to the European Renaissance specula which had a more pointed *priapiscus*.[41]

Archigenes of Apamea, a contemporary of Soranus who also practised in Rome, has left an instructive account of the use of the speculum which has been preserved in the medical compilation of the late Greek writer, Paul of Aegina:

> The operator is to make the examination with a speculum proportioned to the age of the patient. The person using the speculum should measure with a probe the depth of the woman's vagina, lest the priapiscus of the speculum being too long it should happen that the uterus be pressed on. If it be ascertained that the tube is longer than the woman's vagina, folded compresses are to be laid on the labia in order that the speculum may be laid on them. The priapiscus is to be introduced while the screw is uppermost. The speculum is to be held by the operator. The screw is to be turned by the assistant, so that the blades of the tube being separated, the vagina may be expanded. (Paulus Aegineta VI, lxxiii; trans. F. Adams)

23 Bronze quadrivalve speculum, used to dilate the vagina and facilitate treatment of the uterus. A modern copy of the instrument found at Pompeii. Length 28.5 cm.

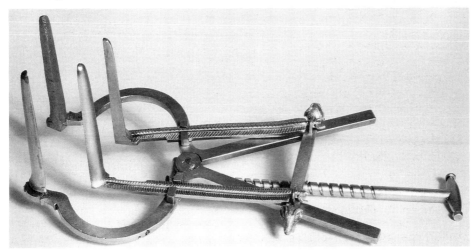

Archigenes' operation was for abscess of the womb, and for this and many other conditions effective treatment, such as curetting the uterus, would have been rendered far more difficult and haphazard without a speculum. It would have been a costly and correspondingly rare medical instrument, though,[42] and, despite its specific recommendation by authorities like Soranus and Galen, its use must have been restricted largely to wealthy patients.

Of all women's diseases menstrual disorders are probably those most frequently referred to, and there were many remedies in the pharmacopoeias, especially that of Pliny, to cure or to ease them. Soranus wrote at some length on the function of menstruation and generally his account is both perceptive and sound:

> Menstruation, in most cases, first appears around the fourteenth year, at the time of puberty and swelling of the breasts. Beginning from little, the amount of secretion increases and after remaining the same for some time, it diminishes again and so it finally comes to an end, usually not earlier than forty, nor later than fifty years . . .
> One has to infer approaching menstruation from the fact that at the expected time of the period it becomes trying to move and there develops heaviness of the loins, sometimes pain as well, sluggishness, continual yawning, and tension of the limbs, sometimes also a flush of the cheeks which either remains or, having been dispersed, reappears after an interval; and in some cases approaching menstruation must be inferred from the fact that the stomach is prone to nausea and it lacks appetite. (*Gynaecology* I, 20, 24; trans. O. Temkin)

Differing from the commonly held view that menstruation was a purging process which helped to preserve the health of the whole female body, Soranus concluded that it 'does not contribute to their health, but is useful for childbearing only; for conception does not take place without menstruation'.[43] He regarded virginity, rather than menstruation, as a positive aid to female health: 'For pregnancy and parturition exhaust the female body and make it waste greatly away, whereas virginity, safeguarding women from such injuries, may suitably be called healthful.'[44] Nevertheless, he conceded the natural desire for sexual intercourse and procreation, and maintained that 'the function of the uterus is menstruation, conception, pregnancy and, after its completion, parturition', and that 'women usually are married for the sake of children and succession, and not for mere enjoyment'![45] In view of the threat to health, or even life, that pregnancy might pose, Soranus devoted a chapter of his *Gynaecology* to advice on the appropriate time for first intercourse:

> Since the male merely discharges seed he does not run any risk from the first intercourse. Since the female on the other hand also receives seed and conceives it into the substance of the living being . . . in this respect one finds her endangered if led to defloration earlier or later than necessary . . . It is good to preserve the state of virginity until menstruation begins by itself. For this will be a definite sign that the uterus is already able to fulfil its proper functions . . . As a matter of fact in most instances the first appearance of menstruation takes place around the 14th year. This age then is really the natural one indicating the time for defloration. (*Gynaecology* I, 33; trans. O. Temkin)

Although Herophilus had identified the ovaries and the Fallopian tubes, neither he nor Soranus was aware of their function or the process of ovulation. Consequently, while Soranus distinguished between conception and pregnancy, recognition of the former was problematic. Various symptoms or techniques were believed to show whether a woman had conceived,[46] and Soranus advocated an assessment of 'many signs lumped together', but it was not until the early stages of pregnancy that he could point to 'facts', such as the interruption of the menstrual cycle. Such imprecision probably accounts for the occasional reference to excessively brief or excessively long pregnancies. It may also explain Soranus' curious advice, also adopted by many subsequent medical writers, on the time at which women were most likely to conceive: 'The best time for fruitful intercourse is when menstruation is ending and abating . . . for the time before menstruation is not suitable, the uterus already being overburdened and in an unresponsive state . . . consequently the only suitable time is at the waning of the menses'.[47]

Soranus identified three stages in the care of pregnant women, 'preservation of the injected seed', alleviation of the subsequent symptoms of pregnancy, especially pica, the unpredictable appetite which can include a strong desire for extraordinary items of food, and 'perfection of the embryo and a ready endurance of parturition'. For the first he recommended an avoidance of any excess or sudden change. The seed, he believed, might be evacuated through physical stress, caused by vigorous exercise, by lifting heavy objects, by falling over, even by coughing or sneezing. It might also be lost through dietary stresses such as drunkenness, indigestion, diarrhoea and malnutrition, or through blood-letting or the use of drugs. All these things were to be avoided, but Soranus also understood the adverse effects of mental stress and he cautioned that 'if there is any bodily agitation, one must completely remove it; one must appease the soul, if the worries of life have troubled it'.[48]

Pica, he believed, began around the fortieth day and persisted generally for some four months. He noted the nausea, sickness and stomach disorders that were often suffered as well as the 'appetite for things not customary like earth, charcoal, tendrils of the vine, unripe and acid fruit'. In addition to gentle exercise and poultices, he advocated a carefully chosen diet which was easily digestible and good for the stomach. Like his modern counterpart, Soranus stipulated that 'one must not pay attention to the popular saying that it is necessary to provide food as for two organisms'. His commonsense approach, too, to those who deviated from their prescribed diet is hardly less appropriate today than it was then: 'One must oppose the desires of pregnant women for harmful things first by arguing that the damage from the things that satisfy the desires in an unreasonable way harms the foetus just as it harms the stomach; because the foetus obtains food which is neither clean nor suitable, but only such foods as a body in bad condition can supply.'[49] In the final months of pregnancy care was to be taken through diet and exercise to build up the strength of the woman, so that she might more readily endure the rigours of childbirth. Frequent relaxing baths were also prescribed, and the need to 'generally divert her mind' was recognised. To relieve discomfort a support made from broad linen bandages was to be employed 'if the bulk of the abdomen is hanging down under its weight'.

Even among the well-to-do, best able to follow Soranus' advice, miscarriage was not uncommon,[50] as may be seen in a letter from the Younger Pliny:

> I know how anxious you are for us to give you a great-grandchild, so
> you will be all the more sorry to hear that your granddaughter has had
> a miscarriage. Being young and inexperienced she did not realize she was
> pregnant, failed to take proper precautions, and did several things which
> were better left undone. She has had a severe lesson, and paid for her
> mistake by seriously endangering her life; so that although you must inevi-
> tably feel it hard for your old age to be robbed of a descendant already
> on the way, you should thank the gods for sparing your granddaughter's
> life even though they denied you the child for the present. They will
> surely grant us children later on, and we may take hope from this evidence
> of her fertility though the proof has been unfortunate. (*Letters* 8, 10; trans.
> B. Radice)

Pliny does not specify the precise cause of his wife's miscarriage, but it sounds as
though he believed it to have been from some form of physical exertion. Such hazards,
as also the especial vulnerability of the foetus and pregnant woman to disease, meant
that those who could afford to do so employed a midwife throughout pregnancy.
She might well be summoned at the outset to offer an opinion as to whether conception
had taken place. A physical examination to check for pregnancy was certainly among
the duties that midwives were sometimes called upon to perform: 'Where a woman
denies that she is pregnant by her husband, the latter is permitted to make an examination of her, and appoint persons to watch her. The physical examination of the
woman is made by five midwives, and the decision of the majority shall be held
to be true.'[51]

There is no doubt that there was as much variation in the status and ability
of midwives as there was in physicians. Some would have been the village 'sage-femme',
while a few were eminent authorities in their own right.[52] Many began as slave-
midwives who continued their profession even after gaining their freedom.[53] Some
were clearly quite elderly, like Claudia Trophima, a Rome midwife, who may still
have been practising at her death at the age of seventy-five, and many started young
like Poblicia Aphe, also of Rome, who had gained her freedom and was a practising
midwife when she died at the age of twenty-one.[54] As already seen, the realm of
the midwife went beyond obstetrics alone to include gynaecology, and although Soranus believed there was no necessity for a midwife to have given birth herself, he
did expect her to be literate:

> A suitable person will be literate, with her wits about her, possessed of
> a good memory, loving work, respectable and generally not unduly handi-
> capped as regards her senses, sound of limb, robust, and, according to
> some people, endowed with long slim fingers and short nails at her finger-
> tips . . . she will be unperturbed, unafraid in danger, able to state clearly
> the reasons for her measures, she will bring reassurance to her patients,
> and be sympathetic . . . She must be robust on account of her duties but
> not necessarily young as some people maintain, for sometimes young per-
> sons are weak whereas on the contrary older persons may be robust. She
> will be well disciplined and always sober, since it is uncertain when she
> may be summoned to those in danger. She will have a quiet disposition,
> for she will have to share many secrets of life. She must not be greedy
> for money, lest she give an abortive wickedly for payment; she will be

free from superstition so as not to overlook salutary measures on account of a dream or omen or some customary rite or vulgar superstition. She must also keep her hands soft, abstaining from such woolworking as may make them hard, and she must acquire softness by means of ointments if it is not present naturally . . .

Now generally speaking we call a midwife faultless if she merely carries out her medical task; whereas we call her the best midwife if she goes further and in addition to her management of cases is well versed in theory. And more particularly, we call a person the best midwife if she is trained in all branches of therapy (for some cases must be treated by diet, others by surgery, while still others must be cured by drugs). (*Gynaecology* I, 3–4; trans. O. Temkin)

A woman who possessed such a combination of physique, virtue, skill and learning must have been difficult to find, and it is interesting to note the three grades of 'best midwife' that Soranus specifies. The first was technically proficient; the second had read up on the theory of gynaecology and obstetrics; but the third might more reasonably be called a medical specialist, having received training 'in all branches of therapy', before concentrating on midwifery. To this latter category probably belonged Salpe of Lemnos, who wrote on women's diseases and was mentioned several times by Pliny.[55] Pliny himself valued nobility and a quiet and inconspicuous disposition in a midwife, and these qualities are, in fact, stressed in the epitaph of several midwives. The simple inscription on the tombstone of Julia Pieris from Trier, for example, reads: 'Iulia Pieris *obstetrix*. Here she lies. She was in life no burden to anyone'.

Delivery was almost invariably in the home of the pregnant woman, and the midwife had to ensure that the requisite items and equipment were available at the start of labour. According to Soranus they included: 'Oil for injection and lubrication; warm water in order that the parts may be cleansed; warm fomentations for alleviation of the pains; sea sponges for sponging off; pieces of wool in order that the woman's parts be covered, bandages that the newborn may be swaddled; a pillow that the infant may be placed upon it below the parturient woman, till the afterbirth has also been taken care of; and things to smell (such as pennyroyal . . . and apple . . . a quince)'.[56]

Although a physician might be present to oversee the proceedings, the birth was usually controlled by the midwife. She reported progress to the physician and presumably received more or less guidance according to her standing and experience. In difficult labour Soranus advised that the foetus should be extracted with the woman lying down, but in normal labour a birthing chair was recommended:

The midwife, however, does not make the parturient woman get up at once and sit down on the [obstetric] chair, but she begins by palpating the os as it gradually dilates, and the first thing she says is that it has dilated 'enough to admit the little finger', then that 'it is bigger now', and as we make inquiries from time to time, she answers that the size of the dilatation is increasing. And when it is sufficient to allow of the transit of the foetus, she then makes the patient get up from her bed and sit on the chair, and bids her make every effort to expel the child. (Galen, *On the Natural Faculties*, III, iii; trans. A. J. Brock)

Soranus gave a detailed description of the 'midwife's stool'.[57] As a part of her midwifery equipment it was necessary that it might be adapted to women of different sizes. Thus the seat had a crescent-shaped cavity of medium size, 'neither too big so that the woman sinks down to the hips, nor, on the contrary, narrow so that the vagina is compressed'. Below the seat the sides comprised solid boards for support, while above they incorporated a handle grip, 'on which to press the hands in straining'. For the same reason the seat was provided with a back. Of the three assistants that Soranus recommended to help restrain the woman during labour (one at each side, one at the back of the chair), two would probably have been servants or friends of the mother-to-be. The third, of whom at least some knowledge of midwifery was required, might be another midwife, the midwife's daughter, or a trainee. Soranus stipulated of the birthing chair that beneath the seat it was to be open at front and back to allow access for the midwife and her assistant:

> the midwife, after having covered herself properly with an apron above and below, should sit down opposite and below the laboring woman; for the extraction of the fetus must take place from a higher towards a lower plane ... the rear is occupied by the assistant for necessary service; for by placing a pledget underneath she must restrain the anus of the gravida because of the prolapses and ruptures which occur in straining. Further- more it is proper that the face of the gravida should be visible to the midwife who shall allay her anxiety, assuring her that there is nothing to fear and that delivery will be easy.
>
> Next, one must advise her to drive her breath into the flanks without screaming, rather with groaning and detention of the breath ... Whence, for the unhindered passage of the breath, it is necessary to loosen their girdles as well as to free the chest of any binder ...
>
> Thus one must advise the women to compress their breath and not to give in to the pains, but to strain themselves most when they are present ...
>
> And with a circular movement of her finger the midwife should dilate the orifice of the uterus [and] the labia ...
>
> ... she must insert the fingers gently at the time of dilatation and pull the fetus forward, giving way when the uterus draws itself together, but pulling lightly when it dilates. For to do this at the time of contraction produces inflammation, or hemorrhage of the uterus, or drags it down- wards. And the servants standing at the sides should softly press the mass down towards the lower parts with their hands. Finally the midwife herself should receive the infant, having first covered her hands with pieces of cloth or, as those in Egypt do, with scraps of thin papyrus, so that it may neither slip off nor be squeezed, but rest softly. (*Gynaecology* II, 5–6; trans. O. Temkin)

Almost contemporary with this description and matching it closely in detail is a childbirth scene from Ostia.[58] It is on a terracotta relief from a tomb commemorat- ing Scribonia Attice, whose husband, M. Ulpius Amerimnus, was a physician-surgeon. Scribonia herself was a midwife and she is shown in the midst of delivery. The labouring woman grips the handles of the birthing chair on which she is seated, while the midwife's assistant stands behind to help restrain her. Scribonia, wearing a simple tunic with bare arms, sits, as advised, on a low stool in front of the labouring woman. Her face is turned away, probably in deference to the modesty of the latter, a concession made also by Soranus: 'The midwife should beware of fixing her gaze steadfastly on the genitals of the labouring woman, lest being ashamed, her body become contracted.'[59]

Soranus' account continues with instruction for the delivery of the afterbirth and much sound advice on the post-natal care of mother and infant. Censuring the many superstitious beliefs that surrounded the cutting of the umbilical cord, he recommended a simple and hygienic procedure. Equally he condemned the barbaric custom of 'the Germans and Scythians and even some of the Hellenes' of plunging new-born infants into cold water to toughen them or 'to let die, as not worth rearing one that cannot bear the chilling but becomes livid or convulsed'.[60] There is a detailed description of swaddling techniques, with advice on how to prevent ulceration, while the infant's crib and bedding are also discussed. Treatment is described for teething

24 Childbirth scene. The midwife Scribonia Attice and her assistant deliver a woman on a birthing chair. Terracotta relief from Ostia. 2nd century AD.

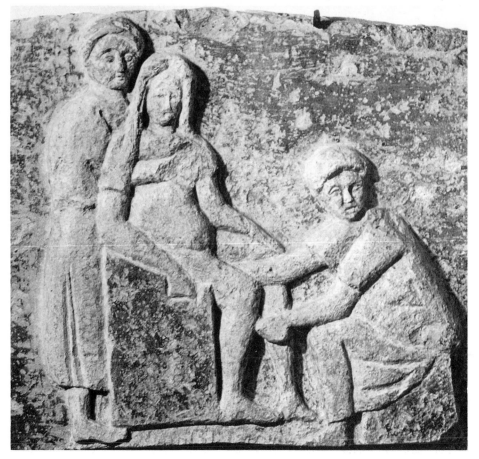

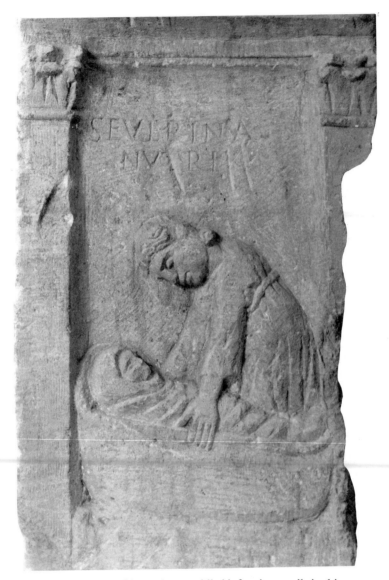

25a Severina, a wet-nurse (*nutrix*), tends a swaddled infant in a cradle in this scene from her tombstone. From Cologne, 3rd century AD.

pains and for several of the most common children's ailments, and there is even a reference to a 'chair on wheels' to assist a child learning to walk.[61]

Not unnaturally, much space is devoted to the critical matter of the infant's diet, when and how often to feed, and Soranus chided those women who indulged in certain timeless ploys to quieten a crying baby:

> one must give it milk several times, but not incessantly, not before the bath, and far less during the bath itself, as women obstinately do who wish to silence an infant that cries easily.

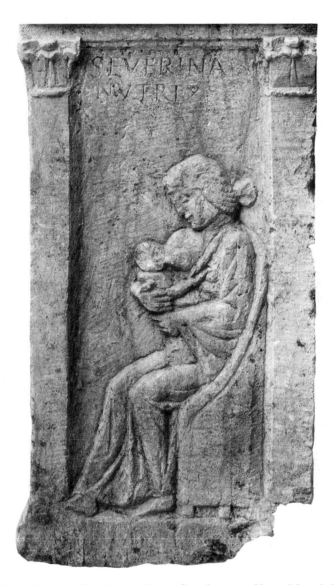

25b In another scene from her tombstone Severina, seated in a wicker chair,
    suckles her tiny charge.

...One must, indeed, pay rather strict attention to the bath so that
the newborn be neither bathed continually nor be much softened by dous-
ing. This is what most women do. For they give it three baths day and
night and pour water over it to the point of exhaustion, delighting in
the fact that when it has grown weary after the bath it keeps quiet and
falls asleep. But this is harmful, for the body becomes weak, susceptible
to disease, easily cooled and easily affected by any harm...

If, however, the newborn cries constantly after nursing, the wet nurse should hold it in her arms, and soothe its wailing by patting, babbling, and making gentle sounds, without, however, in addition frightening or disquieting it by loud noises or other threats. (*Gynaecology* II, 38, 30, 40; trans. O. Temkin)

Although Soranus favoured maternal breast-feeding, he believed that this should not begin until some three weeks after birth in order to allow time for the mother's body to regain health. Only then would she produce wholesome milk. In the interim a wet-nurse (*nutrix*) was to be employed, and in some cases Soranus allowed that a wet-nurse might be needed for the whole period of breast-feeding: 'To be sure, other things being equal, it is better to feed the child with maternal milk; for this is more suited to it, and the mothers become more sympathetic towards the offspring, and it is more natural to be fed from the mother after parturition just as before parturition. But if anything prevents it one must choose the best wet-nurse, lest the mother grow prematurely old, having spent herself through the daily suckling.'[62] As in more recent times, wet-nurses were sometimes employed by the wealthy, who took care to make arrangements well in advance so that they might avoid the dangers involved in using such substitutes as honey diluted with water or goat's milk. However, there is also evidence that slave wet-nurses were given the infants of their fellow slaves to rear, a practice involving coercion rather than volition, hard-nosed economics in place of sensitivities.[63] Among the many *nutrices* known from their tombstones are Prima, a freedwoman of the emperor Tiberius and wet-nurse to his grand-daughter Julia Livilla, and Severina, a wet-nurse from Cologne, who is shown with her charge in two scenes on the sides of her tombstone (25a & b). In one she stoops attentively over the swaddled infant in its cradle, rocking it to sleep perhaps; in the other the infant feeds at her breast.[64]

Great importance was attached to the selection of a suitable woman who should be 'not younger than twenty nor older than forty years, who has already given birth twice or thrice, who is healthy, of good habitus, of large frame, and of a good color. Her breasts should be of medium size, lax, soft and unwrinkled, the nipples neither big nor too small and neither too compact nor too porous and discharging milk over-abundantly.' In addition to these physical requirements there were aspects of personal behaviour and character that weighed just as heavily: 'She should be self-controlled, sympathetic and not ill-tempered, a Greek, and tidy ... "self-controlled" so as to abstain from coitus, drinking, lewdness, and any other such pleasure and incontinence. For coitus cools the affection toward [the] nursling by the diversion of sexual pleasure and moreover spoils and diminishes the milk or suppresses it entirely.'[65]

Excepting slave wet-nurses, who usually must have had no say in the matter, it might be thought that comparatively few women would satisfy such stringent regulations nor indeed submit to them, but for those that did there were many compensating factors. Over and above their pay they would either have been comfortably accommodated at the infant's home or would have been provided with sufficient means to ensure a healthy regimen in nursing the infant in their own home. Furthermore, because their health directly affected that of their charge considerable care was taken to provide wet-nurses with a plentiful and healthful diet, doubtless better than most could normally have afforded.

A number of papyrus documents relating to wet-nurses have survived. One from Oxyrhyncus, Egypt, dated AD 187, demonstrates the commercial use of a slave *nutrix*. It is addressed to 'Tanenteris daughter of Thonis' from 'Chosion son of Sarapion'. Chosion acknowledges receipt of '400 silver drachmae of Imperial coin for nurse's wages, oil, clothing, and all other expenses of the two years for which my slave Sarapias nursed your daughter Helena ... whom you have received back after having been weaned and treated with every attention.'[66] Another, written exactly two centuries earlier, is a hiring contract for a free nurse:

> Didyma agrees to nurse and suckle, outside at her own home in the city, with her own milk pure and untainted, for a period of sixteen months ... the foundling infant slave child ... which Isidora has given out to her, receiving from her, Isidora, as wages for milk and nursing ten silver drachmae and two cotylae of oil every month. So long as she is duly paid she shall take proper care both of herself and of the child, not injuring her milk nor sleeping with a man nor becoming pregnant nor suckling another child...
>
> Didyma shall visit Isidora every month regularly on four separate days bringing the child to be inspected by her. (Berlin Papyrus 1107; trans. in Hunt and Edgar 1932, 46–51, no. 16)

The periods of nursing involved, two years and sixteen months respectively, correspond with that recommended by Soranus, who suggested that: 'As soon as the infant takes cereal food readily and when the growth of the teeth assures the division and trituration of more solid things (which in the majority of cases takes place around the third or fourth half-year), one must stealthily and gradually take it off the breast and wean it by adding constantly to the amount of other food but diminishing the quantity of milk.'[67] The reason for a lengthy period of breast-feeding is not difficult to understand. It was the safest diet that could be provided in a world devoid of sterile conditions, and Soranus underlined the need to return a weaned infant to breast milk if it fell ill. Pliny, in his 'remedies from women', included many bodily ills and ailments that could be cured by drinking or applying 'woman's milk', the best being that from a mother who had just weaned twin boys.[68]

Despite every care many babies must have fallen victim to diseases, above all to gastric disorders, diarrhoea and dysentery.[69] Of dysentery Celsus recorded that 'this disease carries off mostly children up to the age of ten; other ages bear it more easily. Also a pregnant woman can be swept away by such an event, and even if she herself recovers, yet she loses the child.'[70] The organisms of these diseases are found in cow's or goat's milk, and a baby fed with these substitutes, because its mother died in childbirth or was otherwise unable to breast-feed or to afford a wet-nurse, must have had a poor chance of survival. Aristotle paints a grim picture of the situation in his day, when children were not named until a week after birth, because most perished before that time.[71] Many factors influence life expectancy, and we have insufficient data for the Roman period to attempt even regional analyses, let alone an assessment of general chronological trends. Infant mortality was evidently high, but it should be remembered that there was little improvement until the recent past. In the period 1762–71, for example, the London Bills of Mortality reveal that around 50 per cent of children died before reaching the age of two years.[72]

It was not only newborn babies and infants that were at risk. Even if the mother survived the hazards of pregnancy, she still faced considerable danger if complications developed at birth. Dystocia, difficult labour, is treated at some length by Soranus and is among the most revered parts of his *Gynaecology*. He divided the causes into those of a psychological nature, those that arose from the foetus, and those that concerned the birth canal. The main indicators of impending danger were abnormal respiration and pulse, and in these cases the physician was advised to question the midwife before deciding on a course of action. He was neither to 'have immediate recourse to surgery nor allow the midwife long to dilate the uterus forcibly', but might use 'greasy substances' to soften and relax the neck of the uterus. Some doctors resorted to crude and brutal methods: 'some have raised the legs of the bed at the head and, fastening the patient to the bedstead by means of a bandage around the chest, have ordered an assistant to lift the foot end of the bed with his hands and let it fall down to the floor ... others have advised that somebody standing behind the parturient should put his hands under her armpits and lift and shake her vigorously.'[73] Such 'vigorous shaking' was rejected by Soranus, not least because of the potential danger of rupture or prolapse.

If difficulties persisted after the cervix had been dilated surgery might be required:

> One should push aside a tumor with ointment if it lies close by. If not, one should cut it out surgically whether it be a warty excrescence, or a calloused swelling, or a dividing membrane, or a growth of flesh, or any other such obstacle. If the excreta have been kept back, one should get rid of the faeces by introducing an enema of water mixed with oil or hydromel, while the urine should be removed by means of the catheter if the bladder is full of urine. If a wedged-in stone is the cause, one must push the stone with the catheter out of the neck of the bladder and drive it back into the cavity. One should carefully cut through with the lancet a chorion that does not open, having first made a depression at some place with the finger. If, however, the fluid has already drained forth, one should instill some greasy fluid into the vagina by means of a small syringe. (Soranus, *Gynaecology* IV, 7; trans. O. Temkin)

Head presentation with arms along the legs was considered the only normal position of the foetus, and every attempt was made by manipulation to correct malpositions. Difficulties also arose in the case of multiple births or an abnormally large or dead foetus. There is no evidence for the use of obstetrical forceps, an instrument first known to have been used by Arab physicians around AD 1000, but whose introduction to Europe, shrouded in secrecy, did not occur until the late seventeenth century. Soranus counselled: 'One should do everything gently and without bruising, and should continually anoint the parts with oil, so that the parturient remains free from sympathetic trouble and the infant healthy; for we see many alive who have thus been born with difficulty.'[74] If the foetus did not respond to manual traction the physician resorted to one of a range of fearsome instruments for mechanical extraction.

These would have inflicted grievous wounds to the foetus, which by this stage was given up for dead, but they might save the mother. Various forms of hooked knife were used to dismember a dead foetus in the womb and thus ease delivery. In deep transverse arrest, for example, the head was to be delivered first after severing it with a decapitator.[75] The internal use of any instrument, however, in particular blades, involved severe risks and Soranus preferred to amputate parts of the foetus as they presented.[76] This was not possible in the case of an excessively large foetal head, which had to be split with an embryotome or crushed by hand or with a cranioclast, taking great care to ensure that no fragments of bone were left in the womb. The cranioclast was mentioned as early as Hippocrates, and a broken example was found amongst a group of instruments from Ephesus.[77] Like its modern equivalent, it was a metal forceps with jagged teeth along the inner edge of its bowed jaws.

More commonly used was the traction hook, several examples of which were found at Pompeii,[78] and it is described by the authors of the three most important extant early works on obstetrics, Hippocrates, Celsus and Soranus. As a preliminary, Celsus urged the surgeon to make every attempt to turn the foetus to a head or foot presentation:

> Then if the head is nearest, a hook must be inserted which is completely smooth, with a short point, and this it is right to fix into any eye or ear or the mouth, even at times into the forehead, then this is pulled upon and extracts the foetus. But not every moment is proper for the extraction; for should this be attempted when the mouth of the womb is contracted, as there is no way out, the foetus is torn away from the hook, and its point then slips into the mouth of the womb itself; and there follows spasm of the sinews and great risk of death. Therefore whilst the mouth is contracted we should wait, and draw gently on the hook when it dilates, and so at these opportunities gradually extract the foetus. (*De Medicina* VII, 29, 4–5; trans W. G. Spencer)

Soranus' account is similar, though he adds that two hooks should be used in opposition to allow more balanced traction. According to the early Christian writer Tertullian (*c.* 160–*c.* 225), a vaginal speculum might be used in conjunction with the foregoing instruments:

> an infant is sometimes by an act of necessary cruelty destroyed when yet in the womb, when owing to an oblique presentation at birth delivery is made impossible and the child would cause the death of the mother unless it were doomed itself to die. And accordingly there is among the appliances of medical men an instrument by which the private parts are dilated with a priapiscus worked by a screw, and also a ring-knife whereby the limbs are cut off in the womb with judicious care, and a blunt hook by which the whole mass is extracted and a violent form of delivery in this way effected. (*De Anima*, trans. Milne 1907, 158)

The destruction of the foetus to save the mother nevertheless subjected her to severe physical stress, and Soranus underlined the importance of those measures concerned with her safety. He stressed the need for lubrication of instruments and the hands of physician and midwife and even recommended warming the traction hooks. He also specified experienced assistants in difficult cases, a demand all too easily understood when we read of the complications that might otherwise occur: 'Often, however, because of the traction exerted upon the feet by inexperienced persons, the head is torn off and is hard to grasp because of its rounded shape and because it slips away into the uterine cavity.'[79]

Despite the attention of the very best obstetricians, uterine haemorrhage and inflammation were a constant danger in childbirth and must have killed many women.[80] No figures are available, but the order of magnitude may be inferred from the rate of maternal mortality in a region of rural England between the sixteenth and eighteenth centuries. There, it has been calculated, haemorrhage and puerperal sepsis may have accounted for some 25 maternal deaths per 1,000 baptisms.[81] Assuming the situation was not markedly better in Roman times, it is understandable that many women sought divine protection either by direct prayer to the goddesses of childbirth or by the use of charms or amulets. Soranus, as already seen, had no faith in amulets but did not reject their use, believing they could at least be of psychological benefit, while lists of amulets and charms with their supposed effects were included in the works of many ancient authors, including some medical writers.[82] A fascinating example of a fertility or childbirth amulet was found in a Roman building at Dicket Mead near Welwyn, England.[83] Dating probably to the fourth century, it is a tiny oval stone made of haematite and engraved on both sides. The complicated design and text include a serpent devouring its own tail (an Egyptian symbol of Eternity), the goddess Isis, a scarabaeus (sacred beetle), an invocation in Greek to Typhon (a monster that typified elemental force), and the names of Ororiouth (a protector spirit of women's diseases) and Iao, Jewish *Jahweh*. Most interesting is the depiction of a human womb, which appears to include the Fallopian tubes, described by Galen[84] and rediscovered in the sixteenth century. Below is a key which symbolised the locking and unlocking of the womb in pregnancy and delivery. The combination of motifs and words drawn from Greek, Egyptian and Semitic beliefs concentrated magical power in the amulet, which was probably sewn into clothing or hung from the neck in a pouch.

Roman girls married young, often by the age of fifteen, and, taking into consideration the Roman and Christian ideal of marriage as an institution for the procreation of children, it might be expected that large families were the norm. However, there were many limiting factors which would have made a family of even five children a comparatively unusual event. The reproductive life of women in early populations was probably rather shorter than it is now, sometimes perhaps as short as fifteen years, while prolonged lactation would have reduced the chance of another pregnancy within two or three years of a live birth. When allowance is made, too, for still births and for a spontaneous miscarriage rate of about 20 per cent of all pregnancies, it could be that a woman would not easily attain even five or six live births. Occasionally, in recent years, estimations of parity (the number of children a woman has borne) have been made using skeletal remains, as at the fourth-century Roman cemetery at Bath Gate, Cirencester, where thirteen women had probably produced about sixty children.[85] Although three of these women may only have given birth to a single child, the majority appear to have undergone between five and seven full-term pregnancies, while one may have achieved ten live births. It is of course impossible to tell how long their babies survived, but, as already seen, as many as half of them may have died before the age of two. In western Asia Minor in the early fourth century AD nine families recorded in the census lists had just seventeen children between them, including orphans and young relatives in their care, and the largest single family was a husband and wife with three boys and one girl.[86]

Whatever the birth-rate was in a fourth-century provincial town, large families were exceptional amongst the upper classes of Rome at the time of Augustus. Marriage had become increasingly infrequent, childlessness was common, and even those couples with children seldom had more than three.[87] Augustus sought to increase the fertility and to raise the moral standards of the aristocracy in Rome and native Italians in Italy by passing a series of 'social' laws in 18 BC and AD 9. There were harsh penalties for adultery, which was rife, while incentives for marriage and parenthood included the reduction of the minimum age qualifications for patricians to senior posts by one year for each child born before the age of thirty. Not surprisingly, the laws were unpopular and change was slow, for, in addition to those virtually irremediable limiting factors already mentioned, there were several widespread and longstanding means of deliberately minimising family size, contraception, abortion, infanticide and exposure.

The barbarity of infanticide and exposure stimulated legislation from earliest times, as in a section of the laws attributed to Romulus in eighth-century BC Rome. Written down later but thought to retain much of the original, they state that all male children and the first-born female child were to be reared, and no other child could be killed unless it was crippled or deformed at birth. Even those children that the law permitted to be exposed had first to be shown to five neighbours whose sanction was required. Despite the repugnance of the law-makers, however, infanticide and exposure were always the most effective means of disposing of unwanted children, especially amongst the poor, and the practice continued throughout the period of the Roman Republic and Empire. Juvenal, one of many writers who refers to exposure of children, demonstrates that the laws were flouted even in Rome itself.[88] There was, in fact, a tacit acceptance of the low value put on a baby's life in the exclusion of infants from the law that required all burials to be made outside the limits of a town. In excavations infant skeletons have frequently been found under the floors of houses, even in rubbish pits, while the custom of placing a new-born infant in the foundation deposit of a new building was also prevalent.[89]

If exposure and infanticide, albeit outside the law, allowed the poor to dispose of children they could not afford to rear, the mother had still to endure pregnancy and the perils of childbirth, so a different form of birth-control, as Juvenal records, was preferred by many, especially amongst the wealthy:

> poor women ... endure the perils of child-birth, and all the troubles of nursing to which their lot condemns them; but how often does a gilded bed contain a woman that is lying in? So great is the skill, so powerful the drugs, of the abortionist, paid to murder mankind within the womb. Rejoice, poor wretch; give her the stuff to drink whatever it be, with your own hand: for were she willing to get big and trouble her womb with bouncing babes, you might perhaps find yourself the father of an Ethiopian; and some day a coloured heir, whom you would rather not

meet by daylight, would fill all the places in your will. (*Satires* VI, 592–601; trans. G. G. Ramsay)

Indeed, of all references to birth-control abortion is by far the most frequent, for adultery, fornication and prostitution continued despite the Augustan laws. While a 'back-street' abortionist could often be found, the medical profession claimed for itself at least some sort of ethic on abortion. Indeed, the Hippocratic *Oath* forbade a physician to give a woman 'an abortive suppository'. However, as on a number of other issues, the Hippocratic writings incorporated apparently contradictory views on abortion, for in the work *On the Nature of the Child* a girl thought to be in the sixth day of pregnancy is advised that in order to expel the 'seed' she should leap strenuously enough that on descent her heels touch her buttocks. Soranus noted that some physicians had reconciled these two seemingly opposing views by labelling as an 'expulsive' the leaping technique, which Hippocrates tolerated, and an 'abortive' those means reliant on drugs, which he did not. In Soranus' day some physicians discerned two stages to conception, namely reception of the 'seed' and conception of the embryo, and even if they had qualms over sanctioning abortion they probably had little compunction over prescribing a means to expel the 'seed'. Moreover, although there were physicians who did refuse to give abortives, there were others who advocated their responsible and selective use, not 'when a person wishes to destroy the embryo because of adultery or out of consideration for youthful beauty; but only to prevent subsequent danger in parturition if the uterus is small and not capable of accommodating the complete development, or if the uterus at its orifice has knobby swellings and fissures, or if some similar difficulty is involved.'[90] In reality many physicians, whatever their personal view, may have found it difficult to refuse to prescribe an abortive, for their patient was generally also effectively their employer, whom they would have been unwilling to alienate.

One of the ways in which physicians tried to induce an abortion was to reverse the advice they normally gave to pregnant women who wished to avoid a miscarriage. Thus Soranus recommended that a woman who wanted an abortion should take violent exercise, should be jolted and shaken in a carriage, and should 'carry things which are heavy beyond her strength'. Other measures include vigorous massage, the consumption of spicy foods, the use of diuretics and of 'pungent clysters' to empty and purge the abdomen, and a wide range of poultices and vaginal injections. If these were without effect protracted baths were prescribed, prior to the removal, by venesection, of 'a relatively great quantity of blood', in accordance with the Hippocratic dictum that 'a pregnant woman, if bled, miscarries'. Soranus' last resort was to drugs, administered in the form of vaginal suppositories. There are many different prescriptions for this form of abortive in the medical literature, but Soranus recommends just three 'which are not too pungent, that they may not cause too great a sympathetic reaction and heat' and which would bring about abortion 'with relatively little danger'.

The inclusion of these abortives must mean that Soranus was one of those physicians who did not rule out their use but believed that they might be prescribed with discretion. It is possible too that, since he was evidently a realist, he knew that there would occasionally be irresistible pressure put on physicians and midwives to give an abortive, and that in his own work, intended for these practitioners, he could at least recommend the less dangerous ones. In any case, a discerning reader would not have had difficulty in distinguishing his advice on abortion from his exhortation that a midwife 'must not be greedy for money, lest she give an abortive wickedly for payment'. Soranus not only discouraged the prescribing of dangerous abortive suppositories but also warned against the use of instruments which destroyed the foetus *in utero*: 'many different things have been mentioned by others; one must, however, beware of . . . separating the embryo by means of something sharp-edged, for danger arises that some of the adjacent parts be wounded'.[91] That he did not entirely exclude their use is implied by Tertullian. Arguing that the foetus is already a living being in the uterus, he noted that even some of the most eminent physicians believed there to be legitimate reasons, occasionally, for producing the death of the foetus, as, in particular, before a forced delivery: 'There is also a bronze sound with which a secret death is inflicted. They call it the foeticide from its use in procuring abortions, as being fatal to a live child. Hippocrates, Asclepiades and Erasistratus had it, as also among the ancients did Herophilus the anatomist. Soranus too, a man of more tender nature who, when sure that a living creature had been conceived, mercifully judged that an ill-omened infant of this kind should be destroyed before birth to save it from being mangled alive.'[92] Although the 'foeticide' is named as the instrument used to pierce the amniotic membrane around the foetus, this operation might have been performed to equal effect with a uterine sound (probe), an example of which was found at Hockwold, England.[93] A rare survivor of what must have been a common class of Roman surgical instrument, the Hockwold sound is made of bronze with a decorated handle and slender cylindrical shaft. In length, curve, calibre and flexibility it differs little from its modern counterpart.

The Roman methods of birth-control described so far have all involved destruction of the newborn infant or the foetus. Infanticide and exposure were responses to the birth of unwanted children, while abortion was sometimes an expedient of those who neither wanted a child nor wished to suffer a pregnancy. However, there was also a knowledge of contraception. Soranus believed it to be the best form of birth-control, 'since it is safer to prevent conception from taking place than to destroy the foetus' and consequently his account of it immediately preceded his discussion of abortion. Intercourse was to be avoided at those periods which he had said were suitable for conception, while:

> during the sexual act, at the critical moment of coitus when the man is about to discharge the seed, the woman must hold her breath and draw herself away a little, so that the seed may not be hurled too deep into the cavity of the uterus. And getting up immediately and squatting down, she should induce sneezing and carefully wipe the vagina all around; she might even drink something cold. It also aids in preventing conception to smear the orifice of the uterus all over before with old olive oil or honey or cedar resin or juice of the balsam tree, alone or together with white lead; or with a moist cerate containing myrtle oil and white lead; or before the act with moist alum, or with galbanum together with wine; or to put a lock of fine wool into the orifice of the uterus; or, before sexual relations to use vaginal suppositories which have the power to contract and to condense. For such of these things as are styptic, clogging,

and cooling cause the orifice of the uterus to shut before the time of coitus and do not let the seed pass into the fundus. (*Gynaecology* I, 61; trans. O. Temkin)

Predictably, all put the onus of prevention on the woman. It has been suggested that many of these methods could have worked, and some were still being used in Western countries well into the present century.[94] Mobility of the sperm would have been reduced by the application of olive oil and the various sticky substances recommended, while alum, at least, is spermicidal. However, even Soranus, who was the most sound of all early medical writers on contraception, included measures that would have been ineffective. Few, if any, of Dioscorides' prescriptions to cause 'childlessness' would have been found to work, while in Pliny, any good advice would have been virtually impossible to disentangle from such superstitious nonsense as the 'hairy spider' amulet: 'There is also a third kind of phalangium, a hairy spider with an enormous head. When this is cut open, there are said to be found inside two little worms, which, tied in deer skin as an amulet on women before sunrise, act as a contraceptive, as Caecilius has told us in his *Commentarii*. They retain this property for a year. Of all such preventives this only would it be right for me to mention, to help those women who are so prolific that they stand in need of such a respite.'[95]

Although contraception was mentioned by several other medical writers, including Hippocrates, Aristotle and Paul of Aegina, those who did not derive their methods from Soranus often resorted to amulets and charms. Thus advice on contraception would have reached the literate rich, amongst whom medical literature circulated comparatively freely, but much of that advice would have been found sadly lacking in practice. A plethora of 'recipes' for vaginal plugs and occlusive pessaries was probably aimed at the rich, but for the great majority of the population contraception, if it impinged at all upon their lives, would probably have been in the form of amulets or charms hawked by quacks and charlatans. One such, written in Greek and preserved on a fourth-century papyrus, is advertised proudly as: 'Contraceptive, the only one in the wide world'.[96]

Two 'natural' contraceptive techniques, requiring no costly medication, might also have been practised by the poor, continency and *coitus interruptus*. However, their effectiveness is still more difficult to gauge than the other methods, for there is little evidence from which to judge how widely known and used they were. Continency was among the methods recommended by Soranus, although unfortunately he selected the least appropriate time, but he wrote nothing of *coitus interruptus*. Even though it was a non-medical method, it seems unlikely that he would have omitted a reference if he knew of it and believed it to be effective, especially as continency received a mention. Almost the only evidence for its practice are a few early Greek references, not without ambiguity,[97] and the brief references in the fifth-century *Confessions* of Augustine and in the writings of Epiphanius, a bishop in Cyprus in the fourth century, who included it, significantly, amongst the sexual aberrations of the Eastern heretics, the Gnostics.[98] Although it is tempting to believe that such an obvious technique would have been in common use, and as such would warrant little comment in the medical literature, research carried out on other pre-industrial societies demonstrates that this would be an unjustifiable assumption.

Disillusionment, as well as increasing Christian influence, may explain why Soranus' section on contraceptives was omitted by those who later adapted or translated his *Gynaecology*. For, with the imprecision over the time of conception, even those contraceptives that were sometimes found to be effective would simply not have been predictable. Some people may have reacted by using several different contraceptive methods together – amulet, vaginal plug, douching and sneezing, for example – in an attempt to counteract the weaknesses of any single method. Others, however, may have felt little incentive to use any form of contraception, regardless of the degree of motivation to avoid pregnancy, especially as most methods were inconvenient, or were unpleasant to apply. When so little was certain and chance played such an important role, it must have been difficult for a physician to disprove magic. Thus a charm might have appeared successful while a rational medical method might have been seen to fail. Furthermore, even some medical writers, including Dioscorides, were confused about the difference between an abortive and a contraceptive, and Soranus found it necessary to spell out the difference to his readership. It is therefore hardly surprising that contraception appears to have had a comparatively restricted impact on Roman society, even though the best theories and techniques available surpassed anything that followed until the nineteenth century. Despite the pain and danger of abortion and the revulsion that many writers expressed at infanticide and exposure, their results were fairly predictable and effective and they therefore continued to take precedence over contraceptive methods.

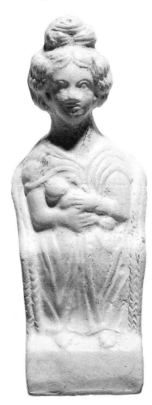

26 A mother feeds her child. Pipeclay figurine of a mother goddess suckling an infant. Height 14.5 cm. From Welwyn, England, 2nd century AD.

Chapter 5

The surgeon and the army

A few decades after the birth of Christ the Roman author Celsus, in the medical section of his encyclopaedia, described what he saw as the ideal surgeon:

> Now a surgeon should be youthful or at any rate nearer youth than age; with a strong and steady hand which never trembles, and ready to use the left hand as well as the right; with vision sharp and clear, and spirit undaunted; filled with pity so that he wishes to cure his patient yet is not moved by his cries, to go too fast, or cut less than is necessary; but he does everything just as if the cries of pain cause him no emotion. (Celsus, *De Medicina* VII Prooemium, 4; trans. W. G. Spencer)

Manual dexterity and a firm resolve are still important qualities in a surgeon, but in almost every other respect there is little similarity between today's surgeons and those of Imperial Rome. In comparison to his modern counterpart Celsus' surgeon was vastly disadvantaged, and he would have operated infrequently and usually with some trepidation. Excepting a few specific conditions, attempts to restore health would normally have been by means of exercise, diet or prescription. Surgery would be envisaged only if a cure could not be achieved by these other means. It is not difficult to understand the reasons for this. As Celsus pointed out, it was the branch of medicine in which the work of the doctor was most clearly seen. The hand of the surgeon, both metaphorically and literally, could be seen to be directly responsible for any change in the condition of the patient. Recovery might be attributed to the skill of the surgeon and would doubtless enhance his reputation. But success could certainly not be guaranteed, even in operations which would today be considered as minor. Knowledge of anatomy was incomplete and often faulty, due to the many constraints on human dissection. Except during the brief flowering of the Alexandrian school, it was rarely encouraged, and it was frequently the cause of vehement attacks on surgeons. By the first century AD human dissection seems to have ceased almost entirely. Consequently, a good deal of exploratory work took place before surgery, and in response an extensive range of probes and sounds was developed.

In addition to this imperfect knowledge of anatomy, the Roman surgeon was faced with a further major impediment: the lack of anaesthetics. Decoctions from the opium poppy and henbane were used as sedatives and pain-killers and, as Pliny records, a draught of white mandrake, the root of which yields hyoscine and atropine, was especially recommended before surgery: 'When the mandrake is used as a sleeping draught the quantity administered should be proportioned to the strength of the patient, a moderate dose being one cyathus. It is also taken in drink for snake bite, and before surgical operations and punctures to produce anaesthesia. For this purpose some find it enough to put themselves to sleep by the smell.'[1]

However, the absence of a true anaesthetic meant that speed was of the essence in all operations, and remained so until the introduction of anaesthesia in 1846. Robert Liston, the great nineteenth-century surgeon, is reputed to have cut for stone in just two minutes, while over a century earlier William Cheselden claimed to have performed the same operation in less than a minute. On another occasion a speedy leg amputation by a surgeon of the Liston era is said to have resulted in the removal not only of that limb, but of one of the patient's testicles and two of the assistant's fingers. Apart from such unfortunate consequences, the requirement of speed imposed severe limitations on the quality of the surgery, no less so in the Roman period than in Liston's day.[2]

Perhaps the most serious deficiency was the lack of powerful antiseptics, although some medical writers did know of the antiseptic qualities of pitch and turpentine.[3] Septicaemia was a major hazard and a disincentive to surgery, especially that of the abdomen, and it must frequently have been the cause of death and of amputation following gangrene. As late as the mid-nineteenth century the mortality rate for those operated upon in hospitals was often higher than one in two. (Only after 1867 and antisepsis could this horrific figure be reduced.) There was a partial understanding of the necessity to clean wounds and instruments, but no standard procedure existed, and even basic levels of hygiene will have varied tremendously from place to place, through time, and from one social stratum to another. In consequence, as early as Hippocrates, specific instructions were given to physicians not to attempt to treat those patients whose condition was seen to be terminal for fear that relations or observers would think the patient had been killed by his physician. The Hippocratic aim was not so much to protect the individual physician as to safeguard the art of medicine from its critics.

Where surgery was necessary it must often have been undertaken by a physician. Occasionally however, notably in Rome and the larger cities of the Empire, doctors who specialised as surgeons or even in a particular type of surgery, might be found. By the early Empire surgery had become highly esteemed and it was only later that it came to be regarded as a low-status craft, the poor relation of the medical profession. The environment in which a surgeon operated was essentially the same as that of the physician, differing in the contents, fixtures and fittings rather than in the architecture of the surgery. Thus the main requirements were space, light, assistant(s), apparatus and instruments. The operations that took place in such surgeries or in the patient's home may be gauged both from written accounts and from the instruments themselves.

Surgical instruments have been found widely but not evenly throughout the Roman Empire. Few date earlier than the first century AD, and the unique assemblage recovered from the Vesuvian towns of Pompeii and Herculaneum, destroyed in AD 79, is the largest and one of the earliest known. Other groups have been found in military hospitals, but apart from these and one or two more exceptional finds, like that of the so-called 'Paris Surgeon', most sets have been found in graves.[4]

Of the craftsmen who made medical instruments little is known. Nor is there a clear understanding of the organisation of their trade. However, it seems probable that some specialised in the manufacture of medical instruments, while others made them on a less regular basis. The single most striking feature of surviving instruments is their quality. Some are exquisitely decorated and some are plain, but almost without exception they are precision tools developed for a specific task or range of tasks.

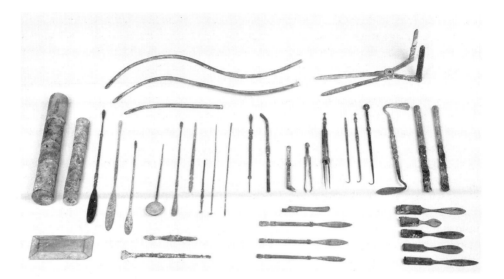

27 A doctor's instruments. One of the most extensive known sets of Roman medical and surgical instruments. It includes scalpel handles, hooks, forceps, probes, needles, catheters, bone chisels, drug boxes and a dilator. From Italy, 1st or 2nd century AD.

A few are made of iron, but most are of copper and its alloys, principally bronze and brass, which could be cast, forged or cold-worked. For bonding purposes tin-lead solder was used. Iron, chosen especially where strength was required, was always forged. Roman blacksmiths knew the technique of carburisation and produced steeled tools, but in certain regions the ore yielded a natural steel, and Galen amongst others was aware that the best quality of steel for surgical instruments, especially blades, came from the Alpine province of Noricum.[5]

The metalworker's mastery over his raw materials would certainly have helped the surgeon to overcome some of the difficulties he faced, and the quality of Roman medical instruments was not surpassed until recent times. Whether they gave any comfort to prospective patients we cannot be sure. But in spite of, or perhaps because of, the assertions of the second-century satirist Lucian[6] that he preferred a knowledgeable surgeon with a rusty knife to a charlatan with fancy equipment, we may assume that the fears of many a less discerning client were allayed by the use of fine instruments. In any case, although some decoration was purely ostentatious, much of it had a function, in particular the fine mouldings on slender-stemmed instruments which ensured a firm grip.

The core of a surgeon's *instrumentarium* comprised scalpels, forceps, hooks and probes, normally in some numbers. The scalpel soon acquired a standard form with an iron blade and a bronze handle. Like many Roman surgical instruments, it was double-ended, and the handle usually terminated in a spatula used above all for blunt dissection. In addition to the common 'bellied' type of blade, a variety of other shapes is known, including straight-edged, concave, convex and hooked types in a variety of sizes. When the blade broke or wore out it was possible to remove it from the handle and fit a new one. To have this done a surgeon could have gone to a blacksmith, a specialist instrument-maker or a cutler. A tombstone from Ostia of a smith who specialised in making or sharpening blades shows amongst his wares two scalpels in a box, which may have been sent to him for reconditioning.[7]

Other depictions on stone, together with archaeological remains, demonstrate that sets of scalpels were most commonly kept in hinged wooden cases.[8] Sometimes other instruments were contained in the same case, notably forceps and hooks. Forceps, essentially a mechanical extension of the fingers, were usually single-ended instruments made of bronze, although occasionally they were combined with a second forceps or another instrument. Several specialised types were used, but those most frequently found are pointed-jawed, plain fixation or toothed fixation forceps, with all three of which the surgeon could cover most eventualities. A ring-slide on the fixation forceps enabled the jaws to be locked for a firm and prolonged grip when fixing and raising skin or tissue, while the rifled faceting on the inner face of the tips of some pointed-jawed forceps, like that on modern anatomical forceps, also permitted a secure grip, but without causing tissue damage.[9]

Wound edges were held apart with retractors, small sharp hooks on slender handles, and a surgeon would have possessed several. They were also used to raise and excise small pieces of tissue, as in tonsillectomy. To ensure a firm grip the narrow handle was often decorated with elaborate mouldings or finely cut facets.

The other indispensable component of a surgeon's 'black bag' was his set of

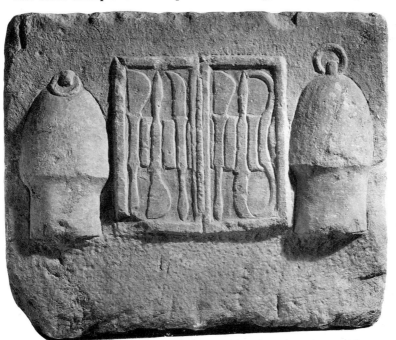

28 A marble votive relief showing a folding case of surgical instruments flanked by two cupping vessels. The instruments comprise five scalpels and what may be a bone lever. Roman, from the Asklepieion, Athens.

probes. As mentioned earlier, these were of especial importance in the preliminaries to any operation, particularly those on internal parts. The lack of detailed anatomical information meant that each operation involved a high degree of risk. This could be reduced by careful exploration using a range of probes and sounds. The tactile sense of some practitioners must have become very highly developed, to judge by such written accounts as Celsus' instructions for the sounding of fistulae arising from abscesses or ulceration:

> first of all, however, it is proper to pass a probe into the fistula that we may learn both its direction and depth, and at the same time whether it is moist or rather dry ... if what is touched by the end of the probe is soft, the disease is still limited to the flesh; if it meets with more resistance, the fistula has reached the bone. But when the probe slides smoothly, there is not yet decay; if it does not so slide, but meets with an even surface, there is some decay although still slight; if what underlies is uneven also and rough, the bone has become more seriously eaten away. (*De Medicina* V, 28, 12C–D; trans. W. G. Spencer)

Very fine flexible bronze probes were used for this sort of work, but in addition stouter probes, spatulae, scoops, spoons and needles were used both for preparing and applying medications and for a host of medical and surgical manipulations.

One of the few instruments that was normally made of iron was the cautery. Very few have survived, but that their use was extensive there is no doubt, for Greek and Roman medical authors frequently recommended them. In Celsus alone numerous different applications are described, from cauterisation of varicose veins to the destruction of diseased bone; from the checking of gangrene to the removal of a carbuncle or from the promotion of discharge in dropsy to the treatment of the bite of a mad dog. If use of the cautery was widespread it was not indiscriminate, and Celsus, at least, regarded cauterisation, excepting certain specialised treatments, as 'the ultimate measure'. Thus in the staunching of a flow of blood cauterisation is placed at the end of a long list of increasingly drastic measures. For those patients who feared the scalpel it was regarded as the lesser of two evils, and as a 'bloodless knife' the cautery remained popular with surgeons throughout the Roman and medieval periods and beyond. Its success must have been due in large part to the fact that through heat the incidence of infection was minimised.[10]

Most physicians and surgeons would have had several examples of each of the foregoing types of instrument, with which they could have operated on most of the commoner diseases and afflictions. The small set of instruments carried by a Pompeian doctor, one of the victims of the Vesuvian eruption, comprised four scalpels, two forceps, two hooks, six probes, and two needles. This was probably his portable set, which, as recommended in the Hippocratic Corpus, every doctor should possess for use away from the surgery.[11] A prosperous established surgeon would have had additional equipment for more specialised operations.

Fractures must have been commonplace, and their treatment was mastered from earliest times, though knowledge of a technique and its widespread application did not necessarily go hand-in-hand. Hippocrates wrote at length on fractures and displacements, and much of this was incorporated in Celsus' work on the same subject several centuries later. The manipulation, extension, reduction and splinting of fractures described in these books generally accords well with modern practice and when employed could have resulted in near perfect bone union. Bone surgery is one part of ancient medicine whose results can be comparatively readily discerned in the skeletons from contemporary cemeteries, and where detailed work has taken place the promise of this area of study has been confirmed. Nevertheless, there are many problems and pitfalls. For instance, whilst an untreated or poorly set fracture which has healed out of position is easily recognised, a properly united fracture once healed may be identified only with the greatest difficulty: the better the treatment the less easily it may be seen. Nor can the majority of the equipment used for healing fractures be illustrated by archaeology, comprising as it did largely wooden apparatus, although sets of surgical instruments sometimes include stout bronze and iron levers used for the manipulation of displaced and fractured bones, while fine sequestrum forceps have been found at Herculaneum and at Luzzi (near Cosenza, south Italy).[12]

In addition to the treatment of fractures and other injuries, elective surgery occasionally took place, normally for a restricted range of conditions. One of the most spectacular operations was trephination, a surgical procedure of the greatest antiquity even by the time of Celsus. He records its use in the removal of damaged cranial bone, but it is possible too that it was occasionally used as a therapeutic measure to relieve 'pains produced by diseases of the head', which Pliny included in his list of the three most painful diseases of mankind, '. . . these being about the only diseases that are responsible for suicides'.[13] Surprising as it may seem, the operation was a comparatively straightforward one which could be carried out with a minimum of equipment, simply a sharp blade. With little overlying flesh the risk of haemorrhage was not great, although infection was always a danger.[14]

Celsus therefore viewed trephination as a last resort to be used only after nonsurgical methods had been tried without success. He advocated extreme caution in the removal of the cranial bone whether by boring or cutting, and underlined the potentially lethal consequences of damage to the cerebral membrane which lay immediately below. For excising large areas of damaged bone he recommended that the area be surrounded by a circle of drilled holes using a bow- or strap-drill and the intervening bone be cut through with a small chisel (27). Even with a special metal guard designed to protect the cerebrum from a misplaced chisel stroke it is not difficult to understand Celsus' reservations, and many patients must have perished at the hands of less than excellent practitioners; skeletons found with an unhealed trephined hole in the skull are a gaunt reminder of those casualties.

For the excision of small areas of bone Celsus described a specialised instrument, a surgical modiolus or crown trephine:

> The modiolus is a hollow cylindrical iron instrument with its lower edges serrated; in the middle of which is fixed a pin . . . a small pit is made with the angle of a chisel for the reception of the pin, so that, the pin being fixed, the modiolus when rotated cannot slip; it is then rotated . . . by means of a strap. The pressure must be such that it both bores and rotates; for if pressed lightly it makes little advance, if heavily it does not rotate . . . When a way has been cut by the modiolus the central pin is taken out, and the modiolus worked by itself. (De Medicina VIII, 3; trans. W. G. Spencer)

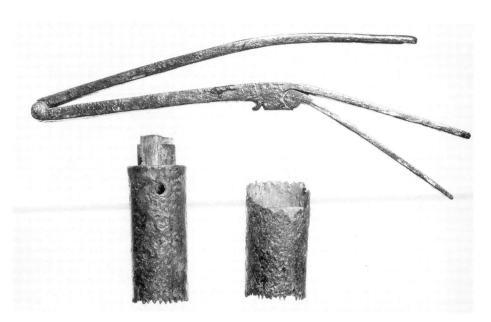

29 Two bronze crown trephines and the folding bronze handle used to rotate them. From the large set of instruments found in a grave at Bingen, Germany, late 1st or early 2nd century AD. Diameter of trephines 2.2 cm, 2.5 cm.

Similar crown trephines were used as recently as the late 1700s but they were by no means safe, and Celsus did not encourage their use except as a last resort. Two crown trephines of precisely the kind described above were found in a large and remarkable set of medical instruments in a tomb at Bingen, near Mainz, in Germany.[15] With them was the folding bronze handle or bow which, when threaded with a thin cord, provided the power which rotated them. The number and quality of the other instruments of the set suggest that it had belonged to a surgeon of some importance, quite probably the individual with whom it had been interred.

It is not possible to determine the success with which the Bingen surgeon employed his crown trephines, but the hand of another Roman bone surgeon has been detected on a skull from one of the Roman cemeteries in York.[16] Examination revealed a drilled circle with a tiny central 'pit', consistent with the use of a crown trephine with centre-pin. In this case the surgeon had stopped short of removing the disc of bone which appears undamaged, and the operation may have been carried out to combat chronic headache (Pliny's 'pains of the head') rather than to excise diseased bone. This is one of those rare instances in which evidence may be culled not only from classical written sources and finds of ancient instruments but also from the very skeletons of the people themselves, the mute testimony of otherwise unknown patients.

Many of those doctors who specialised in bone surgery doubtless were active, too, in the related field of dentistry. Martial lists with other medical specialists one

Cascellius, who 'draws or stops the decayed tooth',[17] and Celsus gives detailed instructions for tooth extraction:

> if a tooth gives pain and it is decided to extract it because medicaments afford no relief, the tooth should be scraped round in order that the gum may become separated from it; then the tooth is to be shaken. And this is to be done until it is quite moveable: for it is very dangerous to extract a tooth that is tight ... Then the tooth is to be extracted, by hand, if possible, failing that with forceps. But if the tooth is decayed, the cavity should be neatly filled first, whether with lint or with lead, so that the tooth does not break in pieces under the forceps. The forceps is pulled straight upwards, lest if the roots are bent, the thin bone to which the tooth is attached should break at some part. And this procedure is not altogether free from danger, especially in the case of the short teeth, which generally have shorter roots, for often when the forceps cannot grip the tooth, or does not do so properly, it grips and breaks the bone under the gum. But as soon as there is a large flow of blood it is clear that something has been broken off the bone. It is necessary therefore to search with a probe for the scale of bone which has been separated, and to extract it with a small forceps ... And whenever, after extraction, a root has been left behind, this too must be at once removed by the forceps made for the purpose which the Greeks call rhizagra. (*De Medicina* VII, 12; trans. W. G. Spencer)

Occasionally in sets of surgeons' instruments dental forceps have been found, both stout examples of iron for extracting the tooth, and fine bronze splinter forceps for removing broken fragments,[18] and many other surgical instruments would have had dental applications. Although a number of tombstones from Rome bear engraved pictures of dental forceps and teeth, presumably to signify that they commemorated dentists,[19] tooth extraction must usually have fallen within the realm of the surgeon-physician. Celsus, at least, regarded it as a part of that branch of medicine.

As Celsus indicates, every attempt was made to retain teeth: 'When a tooth

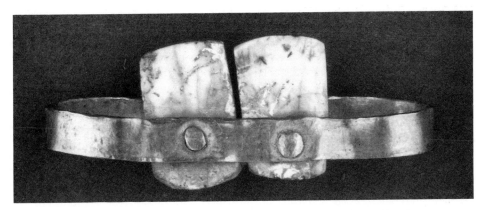

30 Etruscan dental bridgework. The skilful use of fine drills and thin gold bands, wire and rivets were techniques the Etruscans bequeathed to Rome.

decays, there is no hurry to extract it, unless it cannot be helped.'[20] Without teeth one's diet would have been restricted, and there is as yet no evidence for the existence of properly functioning sets of false teeth. Gold was the normal medium for dental repairs, and for those who could afford it loosened teeth could be satisfactorily treated: 'if teeth become loosened by a blow, or any other accident, they are to be tied by gold wire to firmly fixed teeth'.[21] There have been rare finds of skeletons with gold-capped teeth, a reminder of the ancient Roman law that forbade the burial of gold with a body except where it had been used to repair teeth.[22]

Bridgework, like that of the Etruscans, was also employed, the normal technique being to rivet the replacement tooth or teeth to a thin band of gold which was then attached by a loop at each end to the sound teeth adjacent to the gap (30).[23] The replacements might be actual teeth with the root sawn off or artificial teeth of ivory or bone, the latter being all too apparent under the cruel gaze of Martial: 'Thais has black, Laecania snowy teeth. What is the reason? One has those she purchased, the other her own.'[24]

If dental treatment left a lot to be desired by today's standards, then the Roman patient had at least one advantage over his modern counterpart. Examination of the skeletons in Roman cemeteries has shown that tooth decay was a much rarer phenomenon then than it is now. At Cirencester dental caries was detected in just 5.1 per cent of the skeletons as compared to a figure over five times that amount for the people of eighteenth-century England.[25] However, this had nothing to do with oral hygiene but was a passive dietary effect, the result of a low intake of honey and dried fruit, and a complete absence of sugar and fine-milled flour. The coarseness of the diet, especially that of the poor, had other less fortunate effects both in the build-up of tartar on the side of the teeth and in the attrition of the biting surfaces. The teeth of older people are frequently found to have been worn down to the pulp, occasionally causing periodontal disease, notably the development of abscesses, though these must also have occurred as a result of gum infection.[26]

For those who had the time and the inclination there were several means available for cleaning the teeth. The most common was undoubtedly the humble toothpick, which is frequently mentioned in Roman texts and was usually one of the components of the 'pocket-sets' of toilet instruments so beloved of the Romans. Martial believed that 'Mastic is better; but if pointed wood be not forthcoming, a quill can relieve your teeth.' Mastic, a gum or resin exuded from the bark of the tree *Pistacia lentiscus*, was recommended for aural ulceration, but it was also used as a chewing-gum to sweeten the breath. More rarely dentifrices were used, and they appear in several of the pharmacopoeias. Dioscorides, for example, listed the uses of emery (*Smuris lithos*) as a jeweller's stone polish, a caustic medicine, and a tooth cleanser! Slightly less abrasive would have been that made of the ashes of dogs' teeth mixed with honey, mentioned by Pliny, who also recorded the use of pumice.[27]

However, it is unlikely that there was any real concept of oral hygiene amongst the masses, and what few measures were taken appear to have been largely cosmetic in intent. Ovid's advice to those with bad teeth was simply not to laugh.[28] Despite Martial's reference to the stopping of teeth, no example of a true filling is known, and if a tooth deteriorated it was retained as long as was bearable and then extracted. Toothache must have been common and few would disagree with Celsus' assertion

that 'pain in the teeth ... can be counted among the greatest of torments'. In consequence many of the ancient anodynes, including the most powerful, were recommended for the relief of toothache. Celsus advised 'for more severe pain ... certain
medicaments held in the mouth and frequently changed ... hyoscyamus root either
in vinegar and water, or in wine, with the addition of a little salt, also poppy-head
skins not too dry and mandragora root in the same condition'. Not surprisingly,
he sounded the note of caution that 'the patient should carefully avoid swallowing
the fluid in the mouth'. Dioscorides and Pliny also recommended henbane (*Hyoscyamus*) as a toothache cure, while Scribonius Largus believed that by inhaling the vapour
from henbane seeds sprinkled on hot coals the 'tooth-worms' that caused decay would
be driven out.[29]

It has already been seen how common were eye complaints in the ancient world,
and Galen records well over one hundred. Many of these were treated with salves
and ointments, but surgery also played a large part. Like trachoma, granular ophthalmia seems to have been endemic, and, troublesome in itself, it often led to trichiasis,
abnormal ingrowing eyelashes which caused irritation of the eyeball. The minor operation to remove the eyelashes is mentioned by several ancient medical writers and
must have been one of the commonest pieces of surgery. The eyelid was everted
and the offending lashes plucked out with a special forceps, after which the root
was cauterised with a fine iron needle. Needles were widely used in eye surgery
as cauteries, as perforators, and in the removal of small tumours, and the oculist's
trousse from Rheims (see p. 83) included, in addition to scalpels, hooks, forceps and
probes, nine handled needles.[30]

From the written accounts of eye operations it is clear that while the patient
required great courage and fortitude, the eye surgeon had to be both accurate and
dextrous. He had to operate quickly and precisely and needed a light but steady
touch, never more so than in the delicate operation for cataract. Celsus' description
of this operation lays great stress on the careful procedures to be followed, not least
the preliminaries:

> the patient ... is to be seated opposite the surgeon in a light room facing
> the light, while the surgeon sits on a slightly higher seat; the assistant
> from behind holds the head so that the patient does not move; for vision
> can be destroyed permanently by a slight movement. In order also that
> the eye to be treated may be held more still, wool is put over the opposite
> eye and bandaged on: further the left eye should be operated upon with
> the right hand, and the right eye with the left hand.

The need for the surgeon to be ambidextrous, advantageous in many operations
but essential in this one, had long been recognised, and Hippocrates, Celsus and
others encouraged trainees to practise with either hand, while the necessity for a
well-lit surgery has already been noted. To be noted also is the role of the assistant.
In the absence of anaesthetics the task of holding the patient still was of vital importance
and must often have been both onerous and harrowing. Celsus' account continues:

> Thereupon a needle is to be taken pointed enough to penetrate, yet not
> too fine; and this is to be inserted straight through the two outer tunics

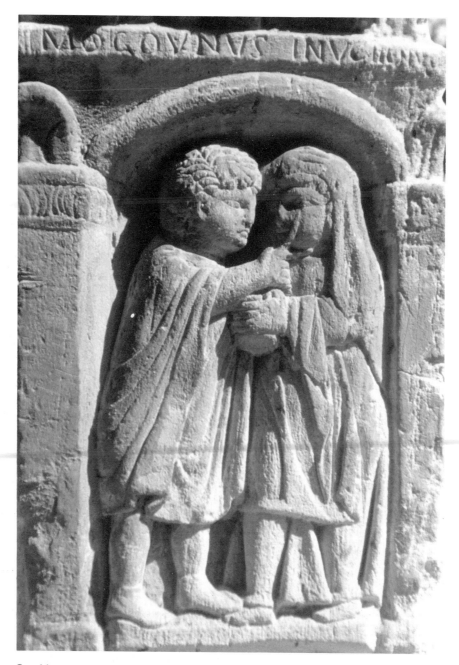

31 Couching cataract? A doctor treats or examines the eye of a female patient. He steadies her head with his left hand while operating with the right. The instrument is probably a needle or knife but may alternatively be a spatula. The woman's hands appear to be bound together, probably to prevent injury from a reflex movement. Detail of a stone relief found at Malmaison, France, thought to be from a shrine of the healing deity Apollo-Grannus, 3rd–4th century AD.

at a spot intermediate between the pupil of the eye and the angle adjacent to the temple, away from the middle of the cataract in such a way that no vein is wounded. The needle should not be, however, entered timidly ... When the spot is reached, the needle is to be sloped against the suffusion itself and should gently rotate there and little by little guide it below the region of the pupil; when the cataract has passed below the pupil it is pressed upon more firmly in order that it may settle below. If it sticks there the cure is accomplished; if it returns to some extent it is to be cut up with the same needle and separated into several pieces, which can be the more easily stowed away singly and form smaller obstacles to vision. After this the needle is drawn straight out; and soft wool soaked in white of egg is to be put on, and above this something to check inflammation; and then bandages. (*De Medicina* VII, 7, 14; trans. W. G. Spencer)

Although the operation was delicate and dangerous, it was nonetheless comparatively straightforward for an experienced surgeon and required little specialist equipment. More important than its simplicity was the low incidence of septic infection which follows this operation, allowing a good chance of success, and this method of moving – couching – cataract remained popular up to recent times.

Several of the bronze cataract needles themselves have been identified, including one in a set of instruments dropped by a fugitive from the Vesuvian eruption of AD 79.[31] Three more, discovered recently at Montbellet, France, were found together with two needles of an extraordinary design.[32] They comprise a long, thin needle within an extremely slender, close-fitting tube with a tiny eye at the tip. In effect they are needle syringes which were used to break up the cataract and then extract the pieces by suction, an operation alluded to by several Roman and Arabic medical writers.[33] Such advanced and audacious surgery cannot fail to impress, but the instruments would have been expensive and difficult to make, while the surgeon's technique would have been still more critical than in the operation to couch cataract. In consequence it seems probable that cataract extraction was always a much rarer and more hazardous operation than couching. Nevertheless, cataract was the one major impediment to vision that could be successfully corrected, and the surgeon who could restore sight in this way must have been held in high esteem. It is probable that some city surgeons specialised in this one operation, though most oculists doubtless operated on and dispensed for the broad spectrum of eye diseases.

Several dozen inscriptions, mostly from Rome and Italy, name eye doctors, *medici ocularii*, some of whom had become rich through specialising.[34] Martial had a less than respectful regard for some: 'You are now a gladiator: you were an eye specialist before. You did as doctor what you do now as gladiator.'[35] In another famous epigram he names a number of surgical specialists including Hyginus, whose forte was the operation for trichiasis: 'Cascellius draws or stops the decayed tooth; the hairs that wound the eyes you, Hyginus, sear; without cutting Fannius heals a suppurating uvula; the degrading brands on slaves Eros obliterates; of hernia Hermes is a very Podalirius'.[36]

The reference to the obliteration of slaves' brands highlights another area of treatment that would now be termed cosmetic surgery. Despite the many inequalities of the Roman world, there was nonetheless scope for betterment from almost every level and some slaves achieved a meteoric rise in fortune. For these people their former status doubtless proved an embarrassment and many will have turned to surgeons like Eros to solve their problem. It is easy to imagine very large sums of money changing hands in this peripheral branch of surgery: personal appearance was no less important then than it is today. Other remedial treatment included operations for healing diseased pierced ears, for circumcision and counter-circumcision, for raising slack eyelids, and for excising and patching mutilations to ears, lips and nose. The latter are the earliest instances of plastic surgery.[37]

Another of the surgeons listed by Martial, Fannius, is credited with the treatment of diseased uvulae. It might seem strange today that the uvula, the small fleshy appendage which hangs at the back of the throat, should require the attention of a specialist surgeon. In antiquity, however, with the very low levels of hygiene that prevailed almost universally, infections of the throat were commonplace and many different kinds are recorded. Fever often accompanied such infections and they were regarded with the greatest concern by the medical writers. One such that has been identified is erysipelas, an acute infectious disease accompanied by fever and constitutional disturbances. One of the consequences was an inflamed uvula, and care had to be taken that suffocation did not occur.

Through this and other causes the uvula often became elongated and diseased and required removal by either medical or surgical means. The latter was carried out using an instrument known by its Greek name, *staphylagra*. This was a specialised forceps whose long slender handles allowed easy access to the throat, but whose scissor-action provided the considerable leverage required to clamp the jaws closed immediately above the diseased part of the uvula. The jaws themselves were hollowed and

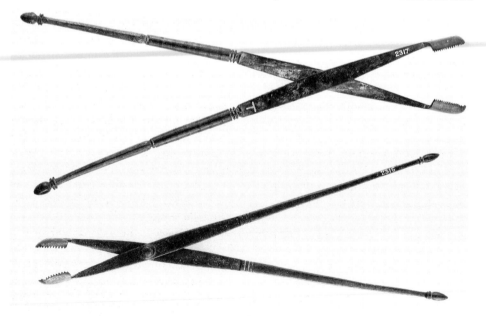

32 Two examples of the *staphylagra*, a bronze forceps used both for removing the uvula and crushing haemorrhoids.

large enough to enclose the uvula, while their upper rim was set with finely cut inter-locking teeth. These crushed the neck of the uvula destroying it within a short time and thus avoiding haemorrhage and its attendant problems that would have occurred if the tissue had simply been cut. Examples of the *staphylagra* have been found widely, suggesting this form of operation was not restricted to Rome or any particular part of the Roman world.[38]

However, their presence might be taken to indicate another comparatively common surgical operation, for the *staphylagra* was also used to strangle haemorrhoids. This disconcerting double use is not as odd as first appears. As a pilecrusher, the forceps carried out a near identical operation, the removal of a structure by means other than direct excision with a scalpel. As access to external haemorrhoids was not hindered, long handles were not as important, and other forms of sprung fixation forceps with a locking ring could also be used.

Haemorrhoids seem to have been as troublesome in the past as they are today and their causes are not far to seek. The uncertainty of diet and inadequacy of both public and personal hygiene combined with the frequency of horse-riding must have resulted in a range of complaints including, in addition to haemorrhoids, such things as anal ulceration and anal fistula. One of Martial's epigrams is dedicated to a padded saddle used to prevent piles, whilst a less orthodox measure was recommended by Cato: 'To prevent chafing: when you set out on a journey, keep a small branch of Pontic wormwood under the anus.'[39]

For examination and treatment of both fistula and internal haemorrhoids access to the rectum was necessary, and a rectal speculum is referred to as far back as Hippocrates. A few of the instruments themselves have survived, bivalve dilators of bronze, finely made but fearsome in appearance (27). Without anaesthesia their use must have occasioned the patient considerable discomfort and pain, yet a measure of their success as a surgical aid is the use of almost identical instruments as late as the eighteenth century.[40]

Dietary deficiencies and low levels of hygiene may also be regarded as major contributory factors to the urinary disorders and diseases mentioned with some frequency by Greek and Roman medical writers. Strangury, a symptom of various disorders, in which urine is passed only slowly, painfully and with difficulty was a common affliction which saw in response the development of a specialised instrument, the catheter, whose invention was attributed to Erasistratus in the third century BC.[41] Although few of the delicate bronze instruments themselves have survived, their appearance and use is frequently described in Greek and Roman medical treatises alike, and they can be seen to differ little from modern catheters (27). Celsus recommended a graded set with three for male, two for female patients.[42]

In addition to releasing urine in cases of strangury, the catheter could also be used to move a bladder stone lodged at the neck of the bladder, but the operation to excise bladder stone, lithotomy, was a much more complex and dangerous piece of surgery. One of the scourges of the past, urethral calculus remained common, especially in boys, until recent times. Pliny labelled it the most painful of diseases: 'the experience of time has concluded that the disease causing the sharpest agony is strangury from stone in the bladder',[43] and Celsus' description of the operation for lithotomy is one of the longest and most involved passages in his book on surgery.

Curiously, in the Hippocratic Corpus doctors were expressly forbidden to cut for stone. Indeed, along with poisons and abortifacients, it was singled out for censure in *The Oath*: 'I will not cut, even for the stone, but I will leave such procedures to the practitioners of that craft.'[44] The phraseology holds the clue, however, and it is probable that from earliest times the operation was the preserve of specialists. In Hippocratic times, even in the hands of experienced practitioners, lithotomy would have been extremely hazardous, as was any surgery of the abdomen until the introduction of antisepsis and anaesthesia. It was not so much the incision as the resulting hole which posed the threat, for it would have been especially hard to heal up given the presence of urine. By leaving this and other surgery to 'practitioners of that craft', strictly outside the medical profession, physicians and 'the Art' of medicine could avoid the disrepute into which they might be brought by the death, following surgery, of large numbers of lithotomy patients.

By the time of Celsus advances in medical knowledge, based in large part on the researches of the Alexandrian school of Hellenistic medicine, placed surgery alongside other specialities, such as ophthalmology and gynaecology, as a legitimate and respectable branch of medicine. Even more so than the operation for cataract, however, lithotomy must have remained a speciality within surgery and one which attracted few quacks. There can never have been many practitioners sufficiently bold, skilful and experienced to perform the operation successfully, but for those that did so the rewards would have been tangible enough. The release from Pliny's 'disease causing the sharpest agony' must have been so welcome as to cause rich patients to part with considerable wealth.[45]

While civilian doctors would have avoided abdominal surgery whenever possible, battle-wounds would often have presented the military surgeon with little alternative other than to attempt a cure through surgery. The generally poor chance of survival from serious internal wounds would have been common enough knowledge amongst the soldiery, and such mortal wounds resulted in a number of celebrated instances of conspicuous bravery. The Greek historian Dio Cassius immortalised the courage of a Roman auxiliary soldier who fought in the second Dacian War of the emperor Trajan in AD 105: 'It was here that a cavalryman, who had been badly wounded, was carried from the battle, in the hope that he could be healed. When he discovered that he was incurable, he dashed from the tent (the shock had not yet affected him) and took his place again in the line, and died, after displaying great feats.'[46]

However, many internal wounds were operable and a successful outcome to complex operations is recorded on more than one occasion. Plutarch[47] recorded the accomplishment of Cleanthes, a military doctor who, in treating a lower chest wound, replaced the entrails which had spilled out, stopped haemorrhage, stitched, and finally bandaged the wound confident that the patient would recover. The procedure for a similar operation is given in some detail by Celsus: 'Sometimes the abdomen is penetrated by a stab of some sort, and it follows that intestines roll out. When this happens we must first examine whether they are uninjured and then whether their proper colour persists.'[48] He warns that recovery is unlikely if the intestines themselves are wounded but that the larger intestine at least may be sutured, 'not with any certain assurance, but because a doubtful hope is preferable to certain despair'. He also advises lubrication, with water and a little oil, of intestines which have become

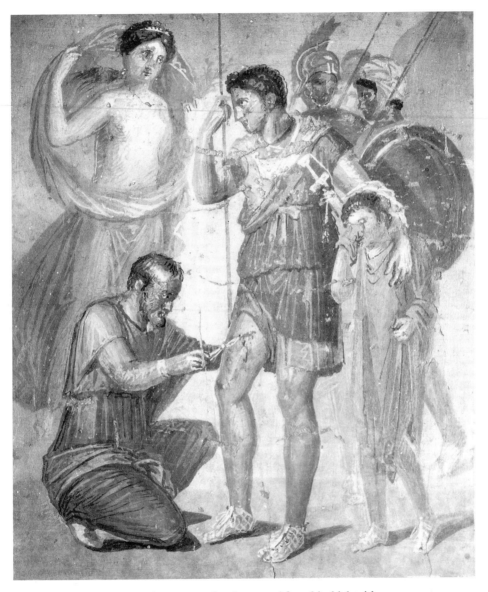

33 The wounded Aeneas has an arrowhead removed from his thigh with a cross-legged forceps. Wall-painting, Pompeii, 1st century AD.

too dry and underlines the importance of replacing them quickly and as nearly as possible in their original position. His account closes with a full description of the stitching of the wound, and elsewhere he details the method of bandaging, excellent by any standards:

The bandage too for binding up a wound is best made of linen, and it should be so wide as to cover in a single turn, not the wound alone but

127

somewhat of its edges on either side. If the flesh has receded more from one edge, the traction is better made from that side. If equally from both, the bandage, put crosswise, should press the margins together ... Moreover, the wound is to be bandaged so that it is held together, yet not constricted ... In winter there should be more turns of the bandage, in summer just those necessary; finally, the end of the bandage is to be stitched by means of a needle to the deeper turns; for a knot hurts the wound, unless, indeed, it is at a distance from it. (Celsus, *De Medicina* v, 26, 24; trans. W. G. Spencer)

There is little doubt that successful treatment of serious internal injuries was exceptional. More frequently battle injuries were flesh wounds caused by cutting weapons (swords, lances, daggers) and by projectiles (arrows, spears, sling bullets and artillery bolts), and from these the chance of recovery was far greater. Celsus devotes several chapters to the methods of treatment, laying great stress on the care to be taken to arrest haemorrhage, prevent inflammation and promote agglutination. He describes the use of specialised instruments, notably a type of 'glove-stretcher' forceps to facilitate the removal of arrow-heads, as well as a two-piece instrument for the extraction of larger projectile heads:

if it is a broad weapon which has been embedded, it is not expedient to extract it through a counter opening, lest we add a second large wound to one already large. It is therefore to be pulled out by the aid of some such instrument as that which the Greeks call the Dioclean cyathiscus, because invented by Diocles, whom I have said already to have been among the greatest of the ancient medical men. The instrument consists of two iron or even copper blades, one blade has at each angle of its end a hook, turned downwards; the other blade has its sides turned up so that it forms a groove, also its end is turned up somewhat, and perforated by a hole. The latter blade is first passed up to the weapon, and then underneath it, until the point is reached, the blade is then rotated somewhat until the point becomes engaged in the perforation. After the point has entered the perforation, the hooks of the first mentioned blade are fitted by the aid of the fingers over the upturned end of the blade already passed, after which simultaneously the cyathiscus and the weapon are withdrawn. (*De Medicina* VII, 5, 3; trans. W. G. Spencer)

One of these Dioclean scoops was said to have been found with an extensive group of instruments at Ephesus,[49] but recent research has cast doubt on its veracity.

Despite such care and ingenuity, infection followed by gangrene, one of the scourges of early surgery, must often have necessitated limb amputation, and Celsus has a chapter on this. The method he advocated, circular amputation, allowed primary closure and is still considered a sound technique.[50] Galen proudly claimed to have suffered only two deaths during his time as physician to the gladiators at Pergamum, compared to the sixty of his predecessor. The figures may be exaggerated, but his success was probably due to a meticulous treatment of wounds, which would have reduced the occurrence of infection and gangrene.[51]

Celsus' clear step-by-step descriptions must have aided many a raw military doctor, for it is probable that, together with the work of other early medical authorities, his compilation was available to the army in the form of military medical manuals. Marcus, a military doctor in Alexandria in the third century AD, presumably had access to such manuals and did not, therefore, require his own collection of medical texts. These he evidently left at home, and, in a letter to his parents, asks that they 'shake the dust off my medical books, shake it off and remove them from the window, where I left them on my departure'. [52]

The army offered considerable oportunity for a young doctor to broaden his experience. The treatment of wounds in particular gave the chance to learn about internal organs and structure, to gain a fuller understanding of anatomy and physiology than could be achieved in civilian practice. Of necessity a medical corps had evolved, matched in efficiency and success to the fighting arm itself. The systematisation of this army medical service – for such it was – dated from the later first century BC and early first century AD, when the first Roman emperor, Augustus, instituted a series of reforms culminating in the establishment of a professional standing army. Prior to this the health of soldiers and care of the wounded had been on a more *ad hoc*, often haphazard basis, dependent upon the whim of individual generals and therefore variable in effectiveness.

Under Augustus and his successors the Roman army became a deadly efficient force, whose extraordinary achievements were the result of adaptability, constant training and careful organisation. But it was also immensely expensive and, as one of Rome's most precious assets, it is hardly surprising that very considerable measures were taken to ensure and maintain the health of legionary and auxiliary soldiers alike. Commonsense precautions, carefully observed and systematically applied, formed the mainstay of such measures. For the function of the military medical corps was not only to care for soldiers wounded in battle, but, even more importantly, to prevent, control or treat infectious diseases. Much more effective than the enemy in felling an army, disease was feared by all military commanders. Even such things as food-poisoning could have a devastating effect, as another letter home reveals, this time written to his father by Claudius Terentianus, a soldier of the Egyptian Fleet based at Alexandria: 'For it was at that time that so violent and dreadful an attack of fish-poisoning made me ill, and for five days I was unable to drop you a line, not to speak of going up to meet you. Not one of us was even able to pass through the camp gate.'[53] In this case Terentianus recovered as too, perhaps, the others affected, and the outbreak fortunately appears to have occurred when the unit was not involved in hostilities.

To Augustus, the casualties of the Civil War through which he came to power would have been fresh in his memory as he drafted his reforms. In 35 BC over half of the disastrous losses in Parthia of his opponent Mark Antony were suffered through disease, and such a proportion was not unusual in the ancient world.[54] Preventive measures included the avoidance of unhealthy sites for the construction of temporary camps or more permanent bases, careful provision for fresh water and waste disposal, regular and rigorous exercise and a diet as full and as varied as conditions permitted. Added to this, a rigorous selection procedure at recruitment could reduce if not eliminate the occurrence of individual or mass illness.

Health and fitness were ensured from the very beginning of a soldier's career.

At enlistment hopeful recruits were subjected to a series of tests, including a medical examination. The ideal recruit was a young but fully grown adult, normally within the age range 18–23 years old. The Roman writer Vegetius provides much of our information on military recruitment in his *Epitome of Military Matters*. Although written in the later fourth century AD, this was a compilation largely based on writings of the early Empire, and Vegetius' sources include the military regulations of the emperors Augustus, Trajan and Hadrian, as well as the works of Celsus. On the physical requirements of the new recruit Vegetius writes: 'a young man who is to be selected to be a soldier should have lively eyes, carry his head erect, his chest should be broad, his shoulders muscular, his arms strong, have long fingers, a modest belly, thin buttocks, and his feet and calves should be sinewy, not overfat'.[55]

A number of papyrus documents testify to the reality of such selection procedures. Part of one document, relating specifically to the medical examination, records that in AD 52 a weaver named Tryphon was discharged because he failed an eye test.[56] The reason was 'weak eyesight caused by a cataract', a condition which, as we have seen, could nonetheless have been remedied even at this period. The phrase: 'The examination was conducted in Alexandria' repeated three times on Tryphon's discharge has been taken to mean that a panel of three doctors was present at this medical examination.

Once the recruit had been enlisted he was allocated a post and sent to his unit. Here he underwent basic training in such things as arms practice, manoeuvres, route marches and drill. This was a probationary period during which an unsatisfactory performance could still result in discharge. On completion the soldier took up his duties, but physical fitness was monitored and high standards maintained throughout his period of service by regular exercise and work. In military as in civilian affairs there was a keen appreciation of the importance of preventive medicine and of the shortcomings of medical treatment. Vegetius wrote that: 'those who are most knowledgeable in military matters are of the opinion that daily exercise contributes far greater health to the soldiers than do the physicians'.[57]

As important as physical fitness was basic hygiene. Though tactics and strategy largely dictated the general siting of forts and fortresses, other factors also influenced the precise positioning if we are to believe Vegetius: 'As far as situation is concerned, do not keep the troops in an unhealthy region in the vicinity of marshes that bring diseases, on arid plains or hills lacking trees to provide shade ... Do not allow the army to use water that is unwholesome or marshy, as drinking bad water, just like poison, causes illness for the men.'[58] Vegetius is here referring to the marching camps and temporary forts of troops on campaign, but archaeology reveals that just as careful attention was paid to the siting of permanent and semi-permanent forts. They were normally built on well-drained ground, often on a slope or eminence and, wherever possible, adjacent to a river. Water might be drawn direct from the river or, as was very often the case, from wells dug within the fort. Not infrequently, however, a running water system was laid on. In militarily sensitive regions it was clearly undesirable to draw attention to the source of the garrison's water supply, and the normal form of military aqueduct was a simple covered channel, unostentatious, but carefully constructed and often exceedingly accurately levelled.[59]

Latrines, normally either incorporated in the bath-house or set against the back of the rampart, were communal like their civilian counterparts, and they differed widely in their degree of sophistication. At the top end of the scale were stone-built flushing latrines, like those at Housesteads and Caerleon. Their sewers have seldom been traced far beyond the immediate environs of a fort, but although drainage systems usually emptied into the fort ditch, it is likely that sewers would have been extended well beyond the fort defences to terminate in rivers or streams or other natural dispersal points. At one period in the life of the fort at Bearsden on the Antonine Wall, though, the latrine debouched directly into the outer defensive ditch.[60] Vegetius would not have approved! He gave very specific warning against such unsanitary conditions: 'If a large number of troops remains for some considerable amount of time in summer or autumn in the same place, this can cause very unwholesome diseases from the contamination of the waters and the foulness of the smell itself, as the drinking water is tainted and the air infected.'[61] However what Vegetius wrote in the fourth century and what the commander of a small frontier unit in second-century Britain instructed were two different things. It serves as a reminder that aspects of medicine and hygiene were often ill understood and that knowledge was neither universal nor universally applied.

Where an integrated running water supply and drainage system were not possible, a simpler type of latrine was provided. This comprised a timber building above a rectangular plank-lined underground tank. Although the superstructure and seating arrangements would have been similar to that of the stone-built flush latrine, the drawback lay in the need to empty the tank at regular intervals, and *ad stercus* (latrine emptying) was one of many unpleasant fatigues undertaken by Roman soldiers. Latrines have occasionally yielded evidence of another important aspect relating to the health of soldiers, that of diet. Increasingly, microscopic study of latrine deposits is throwing light on the range of food eaten, as well as on some bodily afflictions. Examination of a column of sewage from the latrine at Bearsden revealed food particles of various plants, both cultivated and wild, but no animal products, suggesting the diet was a vegetarian one.[62] It has indeed often been claimed that the Roman army of the late Republic and early Empire was essentially vegetarian and that meat would be eaten only under the direst circumstances. However, although corn was a staple for both civilians and the army in most parts of the Roman world, it would have been supplemented by many other foodstuffs.

The huge quantities of animal bones normally found in the rubbish deposits of forts in Rome's north-western provinces indicate at least the normal scale of meat-eating. Beef, mutton and pork in varying proportions were the most popular, but venison, boar and hare were also consumed in quantity, showing that hunting was no less popular in the Roman army than in more recent times.[63] In the absence of refrigeration, however, particular care had to be taken over the consumption of meat and fish. A case of fish-poisoning in Alexandria has already been mentioned. Further north, at Künzing in Germany, the intestinal parasite *Trichuris trichura*, whipworm, has been detected in deposits in the fort latrine, evidence, perhaps, that the soldiers had eaten contaminated pork[64]

Plant remains are less easily detectable, but increasing awareness amongst excavators is providing an ever fuller picture. In Britain the military diet, in addition to meat and cereals, included beans, cabbage, lentils, plums, cherries and many wild

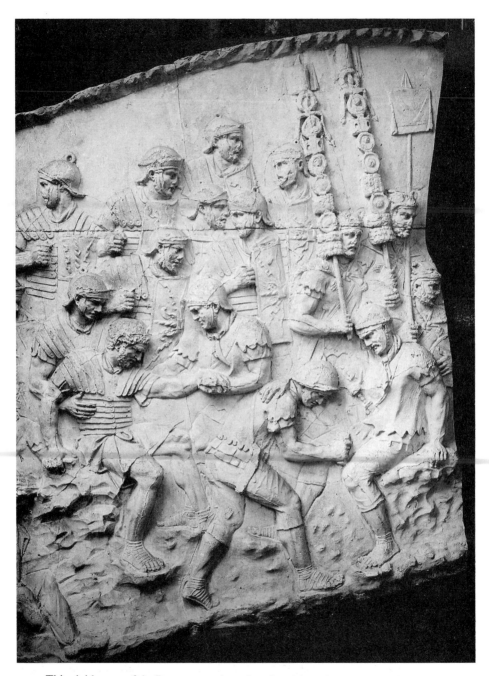

34 This vivid scene of the Roman army in action shows first aid being administered behind the battle front. A medical orderly examines the injured arm of an infantryman, while a cavalry trooper has a thigh-wound bandaged. In the detail of their facial expressions and flexed muscles the sculptor has skilfully captured the agony of both men. From Trajan's Column, Rome, early 2nd century AD.

fruits and nuts, as well as sea-food and dairy products. The importance attached to the sustenance of the armed forces resulted in an elaborate supply network which might include the requisition of food supplies. In times of stress or famine the army was the last to suffer, whilst under normal circumstances their adequate diet might be supplemented by exotic foods carried over long distances. Only on campaign in hostile territory or difficult terrain, where supplies were limited and uncertain, was the soldiers' fare reduced to the basic 'iron rations', a restricted diet of safe commodities – hard tack, bacon fat, cheese and low-quality wine.

One building missing from Roman forts was the canteen, for there was no centralised system of mass catering. In the legions soldiers seem to have eaten their meals in barracks in eight-man units (the *contubernium*), the smallest tactical grouping, of which there were ten to each century. Each *contubernium* possessed a suite of two rooms in the centurial barracks in which they slept and stored their arms and equipment as well as eating their meals. They cooked over small hearths, with bronze boiling pans, iron roasting spits and pottery vessels, and ground their daily grain issue on querns to make simple cereal foods like porridge. Larger mills were used to prepare bread flour for the whole century. This was made into *panis militaris*, a wholemeal bread high in vitamin B$_1$ and recommended by both modern and ancient authorities alike. The loaves were baked in ovens set against the back of the fortress rampart to minimise the risk of fire. To modern eyes this seems a cumbersome system, some-what at odds with the high degree of organisation evident in other areas of the Roman army, although it should be remembered that until comparatively recently the British army, too, had no communal refectory system. One positive though incidental effect would have been to reduce the chances of mass food-poisoning, though to an extent this may have been countered by the use of a centralised food supply system.

If a soldier did fall ill or was wounded, he would have been cared for by the medical corps of his unit. Even on the field of battle he might receive first aid from medical assistants, *milites medici*, or *capsarii*, so named from the bandage box (*capsa*) they carried. Behind the lines in the field hospital, if on campaign, or back at base in the fort hospital (*valetudinarium*), if during peacetime, he would be examined by a more senior man, a *medicus*, who would prescribe treatment or perform surgery.

Within a legion the medical service was one of the areas of responsibility of the camp prefect (*praefectus castrorum*), the second-in command and most experienced soldier of the unit, normally a former chief centurion with around thirty years' service. He deputised the running of the hospital to an *optio valetudinarii*, a junior officer on the H.Q. staff, who was an administrator rather than a doctor.[65] His main concern, in addition to the upkeep and administration of the hospital itself, would have been the provision of medical supplies and special dietary requirements for the sick. The scale of these provisions may be inferred from scraps and snippets of archaeological and literary evidence. Branded stamps on barrels with an estimated capacity of some 678 litres found at the legionary fortress at Aquincum (modern Budapest) record that the barrels and their contents, almost certainly a medicated wine, had passed through a customs zone 'duty-free for the account of the hospital of Legio II Adiutrix',[66] while a government contract of AD 138 for military clothing in Cappadocia reveals the care which was taken to exact the precise form and quality of goods, in this case a single blanket required for a hospital, probably that of Legio II Traiana at

Nicopolis: 'For ... the hospital in the imperial camp ... 1 blanket, plain white, length 6 cubits, width 4 cubits, weight 4 minas ... use ... only wool that is fine, soft, pure white, free of dirt ... produce the clothing well-woven, firm-textured, with finished hems, meeting specifications, without flaws ... '[67] The *optio valetudinarii* would have worked closely with the team of doctors and orderlies from whom he would have received requests for, and advice on, such supplies.

The number and experience of the medical staff will have varied according to the size and prestige of the unit and the part of the world in which it was operating. Thus Cohors IV Praetoria, one of the élite units in Italy, is known to have had medical specialists: Caius Terentius Symphorus, who was a surgeon (*medicus chirurgus*), and Tiberius Claudius Iulianus, a consultant in internal ailments (*medicus clinicus*). Elsewhere a *marsus* was available to provide antidotes and treatment for snake bites or scorpion stings in those parts of the Empire where such hazards were common. Normally, however, the military doctors were described simply as *medici*, men who doubtless were expected and competent to deal with the broad spectrum of injury and illness. The status of these *medici* is far from clear, but there appears to have been a hierarchy, at the top of which were experienced doctors, probably on short-term commission, whose rank approximated to that of senior military officers.[68]

The hospital (*valetudinarium*) was an integral part of Roman fort architecture and many examples have been identified, both in legionary fortresses and auxiliary forts, mostly in Britain and Germany on sites where large-scale excavation has taken place. The first of these were identified on the basis of medical instruments found within them as, for instance, at Neuss (on the Rhine opposite Düsseldorf), where some one hundred medical and pharmaceutical implements were found in one room alone.[69] Detailed examination of plant remains has revealed traces of medicinal plants in some hospitals, while at Chester, in or near the building that is believed to be the legionary hospital, were found two altars dedicated by Greek doctors to Asklepios, Hygieia and other healing deities.[70] Like so many other Roman military buildings, the hospital had a consistent and characteristic design which usually now permits identification from the ground-plan of the building remains alone.

As recommended in a Roman military surveying manual (Pseudo-Hyginus), the legionary hospitals are almost invariably placed in one of the two quiet areas of the fortress, in deference to those convalescing. Often a further buffer against noise was provided in the form of a line of store-rooms along the street frontage. Behind this the hospital proper comprised four wings which enclosed a central open courtyard ensuring air and quiet. This arrangement was inherited from the earlier field hospitals, mentioned as early as Caesar's Gallic Wars, in which the tents were grouped as a hollow rectangle behind a large marquee.[71] They are large, complicated buildings with a systematic layout modified only slightly from one place to another.

The most complete plan is that of the hospital in the double legionary fortress at Vetera (present day Xanten), on the lower Rhine, built of stone in the reign of Nero.[72] Here an entrance hall, flanked by a row of store-rooms, led from the street, via a porter's lodge, to a huge aisled hall. Lit by clerestory windows, this was probably the reception and clearance ward. Opening off beyond was the operating theatre, a smaller though still spacious room, which projected into the courtyard and therefore received light along the entire length of one side. Completing the entrance wing were at one corner a suite of baths with attached latrine and at the other a kitchen. The provision of these facilities meant that the hospital could be almost independent of the main garrison, making life easier for the patients and also minimising the spread of disease.

From each end of the aisled hall a wide circulating corridor extended the length of the three remaining wings. Numerous small wards were arranged in pairs on either side of this corridor, each pair being reached by a short side corridor. Apart from providing greater privacy and keeping the main corridor clear of obstruction, this would have further reduced noise and, intentionally or not, lessened the risk of cross-infection. Other rooms have been identified as a doctor's surgery, a dispensary, a mortuary, isolation wards and two lavatories. At Neuss, which was provided with a very similar hospital, raised hearths found in the operating theatre may have been used for sterilising instruments and dressings, or for heating cauteries. The room with the many instruments may have been a treatment room. The importance accorded to proper sanitation, especially in the hospital, may be gauged by the fact that at Inchtuthil, Scotland, the hospital was the first building of the fortress to receive a stone-lined drainage channel.[73]

Hospitals have also been found in the forts of the auxiliary troops, not just, as was once believed, in those of the larger or more prestigious units, the thousand-strong infantry cohorts and the cavalry *alae*, but also in the smaller infantry and part-mounted cohorts. Medical provision was made for every branch of the armed forces: whatever their status fitness and good health were paramount if they were to function effectively. Like the forts themselves, auxiliary hospitals were simplified and scaled-down versions of their legionary counterparts. Some, like those at House-steads and Benwell on Hadrian's Wall, share the same quadrangular layout with wards and rooms around a central courtyard, into which the operating theatre projected. In an alternative design, found rather more commonly, the hospital seems to have

35 Model reconstruction of the hospital in the double legionary fortress at Vetera (Xanten). 1st century AD.

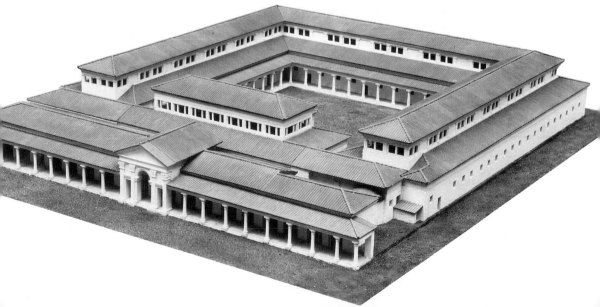

been based upon one wing of a legionary hospital. This arrangement is most clearly seen at the fort of Fendoch in Scotland, built of timber towards the end of the first century AD. A central corridor was flanked by a large operating theatre and ten small wards.[74] Tombstones reveal that *medici* served in both the legions and the auxiliary units, and although we possess less information on the other medical staff of the auxiliaries, it may be presumed that their number was related to the size of the garrison.[75]

Where it has been possible to count, the number of wards in legionary hospitals appears to coincide approximately with the number of centuries, and the evidence from auxiliary hospitals would seem to support this notion. Thus at Neuss there is a ward for each of the sixty centuries of the legion, and at Fendoch ten wards served the needs of the garrison, probably a *cohors milliaria* with ten centuries. It is, however, unlikely that wards were allocated to individual centuries – injury and illness strike neither predictably nor evenly – rather that they represent an attempt to achieve a standard provision for the sick. Calculations suggest that about 5 per cent of the unit's strength could be accommodated in the hospital, but this number could easily be doubled by pressing into service the corridors and ancillary rooms.

After illness a soldier would have required a period of convalescence, which might take the form of an extension of his stay in the fort hospital. It is likely that the sheltered courtyard of many hospitals was used as a garden for those convalescing. It has also been suggested that, as in medieval monastic infirmaries, healing plants and herbs were grown there for use by the medical staff. Certainly, plant remains found in the hospital at Neuss include several species that were recommended by ancient physicians – centaury, for healing wounds and curing eye ailments; henbane, a hypnotic and pain-killer; St John's wort used for various blood ailments; plantain, used against haemorrhage and dysentery; and fenugreek, used as an enema and poultice.[76] Other remains include food traces which may have been part of a convalescent diet prepared in the hospital kitchen, such as oysters, eggs, peas, lentils and figs. Pliny specifically recommended figs for those convalescing, while the other foods were all in Celsus' 'weak' category, those most easily digested and therefore appropriate to the needs of invalids.

Although self-sufficient in most respects, the military hospitals were not geared to longer-term convalescence. After a serious illness or wound, therefore, a soldier might be granted a period of sick leave at home or, as a papyrus document from Egypt records, he might be taken to the coast to recuperate.[77] More often, though, use was made of the facilities at spas, which were widely spread through the provinces. At Bath the curative waters of Sulis Minerva were enjoyed not just by civilians but by the military too, as the many altars and tombstones of serving soldiers testify.[78] However, such arrangements were not always on an official footing. On an inscription set up in AD 238 at another spa, Scaptopara in Thrace (Bulgaria),[79] the inhabitants complained to the emperor that soldiers from two nearby forts made deliberate detours to take advantage of their excellent hot springs. What is more, they demanded food and hospitality and refused to pay for them, despite an order of the governor. Friction between soldier and civilian is clearly nothing new.

If the provincials sometimes had cause for complaint against the army, then they also had reason to be thankful. Many advantages accrued to those who lived in the neighbourhood of military garrisons, not least the opportunity to profit, by trade and services, from the presence of large numbers of well-paid soldiers. Beyond this the army participated in many 'community projects', especially the construction of roads, civic buildings, aqueducts and sewers, undertakings well-suited to the army's combination of expertise and mass labour. This was not sheer altruism, for in peacetime (which might comprise the larger part of a soldier's period of service), the army had to be kept busy with work over and above routine patrolling, exercises and manoeuvres. Many commanders no doubt made a conscious effort to establish and maintain good relations with the local population. They would certainly have worked together with the local aristocracy and town councils, while through common-law marriage of the other ranks (serving soldiers in the earlier Empire were not entitled to legal marriage), we may presume that there was normally a rapid integration of static garrisons.

With the increase in dependents, legal or otherwise, it is easy to imagine that the work of military doctors would not be restricted to the soldiers alone. Either on a formal or, more probably, an informal basis, people from surrounding farms, villages or small towns may often have come to the fort for treatment by the medical staff. In the longer term some of the military doctors, especially those lower in the hierarchy, would have become part of the local community themselves, for on retirement from the army personal ties will have caused many to settle locally. They must frequently have continued to practise, but in a civilian setting.

In this way the army rapidly spread knowledge of Roman medicine throughout each new province of the Empire. As in other matters, this was not a one-way process. At the same time as knowledge and techniques were disseminated, fresh information was collected and new resources exploited, constantly adding to the existing medical and pharmaceutical corpus. Military doctors were able, quite literally, to expand the frontiers of Roman medicine. The mobility that the army provided allowed them to learn of and collect new herbs, a considerable advantage in a world where few drug suppliers were above suspicion of adulterating their wares or substituting a cheaper alternative. A famous and effective styptic, *barbarum*, favoured by Celsus,[80] was discovered, as its name signifies, across the frontiers, probably during military campaigns, while the discovery of the plant *radix britan(n)ica*, successfully used to counter the effect of scurvy during campaigns in the Low Countries, has already been mentioned.

It is probably fair to say that the Roman army was the single most powerful agency in the spread of Graeco-Roman medicine.

Chapter 6

Gods and their magic

October to January 148 AD ... a tumor grew from no apparent cause, at first as it might be for anyone else, and next it increased to an extraordinary size, and my groin was distended, and everything was swollen and terrible pains ensued, and a fever for some days. At this point, the doctors cried out all sorts of things, some said surgery, some said cauterization by drug, or that an infection would arise and I must surely die. But the God gave a contrary opinion and told me to endure and foster the growth. And clearly there was no choice between listening to the doctors or to the God. But the growth increased even more, and there was much dismay. Some of my friends marvelled at my endurance, others criticized me because I acted too much on account of dreams, and some even blamed me for being cowardly, since I neither permitted surgery nor again suffered any cauterizing drugs. But the God held quite firm, and ordered me to bear up with the present circumstances ... Finally the Savior indicated on the same night the same thing to me and my foster father – for Zosimus was then alive – so that I sent to him to tell him what the God had said, but he came to see me to tell me what he had heard from the God. There was a certain drug, whose particulars I do not remember, save that it contained salt. When we applied this, most of the growth quickly disappeared, and at dawn my friends were present, happy and incredulous. From here on, the doctors stopped their criticisms, expressed extraordinary admiration for the providence of the God in each particular, and said that it was some other greater disease, which he secretly cured. (Aelius Aristides, *Hieroi Logoi* I, 61–8; trans. C. A. Behr)

This extract, from the extraordinary 'diaries' of Aelius Aristides, an intelligent and well-educated aristocrat from the Roman province of Asia, demonstrates at once the weaknesses of ancient scientific medicine and the attractive power of the gods, specifically the healer-god Asklepios, Roman Aesculapius. In an uncertain world there was good reason to employ every means available to help ensure good health. The cost, risk, uncertainty, discomfort or sheer pain of ancient medical treatment make it only too easy to understand why people turned to the healing deities for help, but it was not merely a negative response to those shortcomings. The deities were so much part of everyday life that the seeking of divine aid would often have been a first not a last resort. Although there were always those with reservations, like some of Aristides' friends who believed he placed undue faith in the dreams (his 'hot-line' from Asklepios), few people would have considered an appeal to the gods to be an act of despair, as is usually the tendency today. This no doubt explains in large part the otherwise surprising fact that the rise of rational medicine did not eclipse irrational beliefs, and the healing deities flourished alongside scientific medicine in an almost parallel development. Thus the emergence of Hippocratic medicine in early

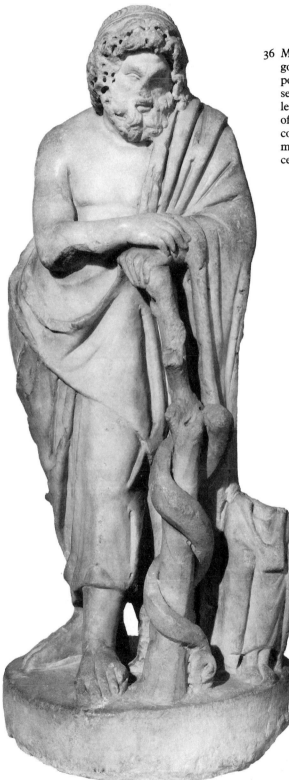

36 Marble statue of the healing
god Asklepios, in characteristic
pose leaning on his knotted,
serpent-entwined staff. At his
left side is the tiny robed figure
of Telesphorus, god of
convalescence, his head now
missing. Roman, probably 3rd
century AD.

fifth-century BC Greece coincided in time and place with the elevation of Asklepios to divine status and the spread of his cult. Indeed, the Hippocratic *Oath* was taken in his name: 'I swear by Apollo the healer, by Asklepios, by Hygieia, by Panakeia and by all the powers of healing, and call to witness all the gods and goddesses that I may keep this Oath and Promise to the best of my ability and judgement.'

Equally, Greek medicine was eased into Roman Italy by the contemporary arrival of the Asklepios cult, itself readily absorbed into a culture which also looked to its gods for preservation of bodily health. The parallel development continued, and at the time when Aristides recorded the miraculous cure of his 'tumour' two events of particular significance were taking place in Pergamum. Construction of a magnificent new temple of Asklepios had just been completed, and the teenage Galen had just embarked on the medical career that was to make him a famous physician and was to influence the course of Western medicine up to the Renaissance. Ironically, it was the appearance of Asklepios in a dream-vision that proved the decisive factor in Galen's choice of a medical career. Later, too, he obtained his first post through the agency of the High Priest of the Pergamene Asklepieion, while it was an instruction received from Asklepios that Galen successfully used as an excuse not to accompany Marcus Aurelius on his military expedition against the Marcomanni.[1]

Galen's links with the cult were not unique, for Asklepios was the patron of physicians, and since the time of Hippocrates there had been frequent contact between physicians and healing cults. Some physicians were sceptical of the healing sanctuaries, others were at least partially in sympathy, and most probably accepted that they had a part to play in the common struggle against disease. At the very least, healing sanctuaries provided doctors with a socially acceptable solution to those cases for whom scientific medicine was to no avail. Thus, while there was no attempt at integration, physicians did not aim to exclude 'temple medicine', and the two healing systems co-existed with little difficulty.

Asklepios was the paramount healing deity, and his cult spanned a period of almost a thousand years. As is so often the case in Greek and Roman mythology, his origins are obscure, and the stories about his birth varied considerably. The generally accepted version was that given in Pindar's 3rd Pythian Ode, composed in the early fifth century BC. Asklepios' father was Apollo, himself the chief healing god of the Greek pantheon who could cast or avert mortal plagues and epidemics, and who healed the wounds and diseases of his fellow Olympian deities. Asklepios' mother was a mortal, Coronis, the daughter of the powerful king Phlegyas of Trikka in Thessaly (northern Greece). While pregnant by Apollo, she took a mortal husband, and in his wrath at her infidelity the god had the couple killed. As their bodies burned on the funeral pyre, the grief-stricken Apollo tore his unborn son, still alive, from the mother's womb and took him to Mount Pelion. There the young Asklepios was raised by the centaur Chiron, who taught him the art of healing. Asklepios became an excellent and renowned physician, and it was as such that he was mentioned in Homer's *Iliad*. A demanding practice in Thessaly kept him from the Trojan War, but he sent instead his two sons, Machaon and Podalirios, who were skilled healers too.[2] Although still a mortal, Asklepios' powers apparently extended to miracles, and it was by reviving the dead (including Hippolytus, the son of Theseus) that he incurred the anger of Zeus. Fearing that resurrections on such a scale might upset

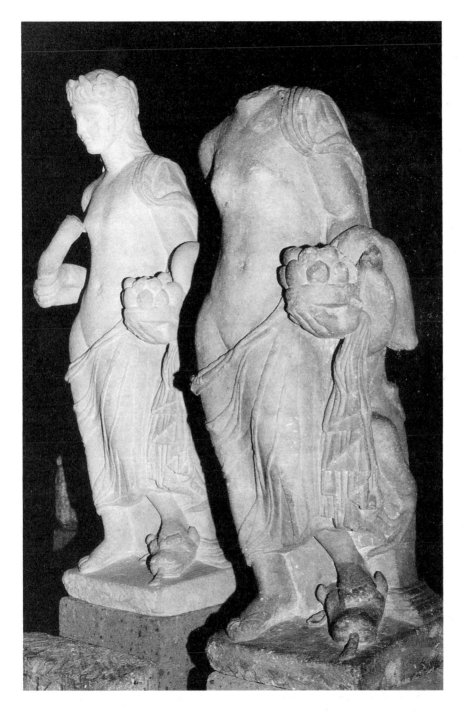

37 Statue of Hygieia, goddess of health, feeding the Asklepian serpents. In the
background is a modern replica with head restored. From Cologne, Roman,
probably 3rd century AD.

the natural order of things, the 'king of the gods' felled Asklepios with a thunderbolt.

In this account, then, Asklepios began as a mortal, an esteemed physician in northern Greece who achieved heroic status, rather like Herakles, and sometime subsequent to his death was raised to the level of a lesser god. Alternatively, he may have originated as a subterranean healing spirit, whose increased popularity required the fabrication of a suitable pedigree – a blood-tie with Apollo. As his cult developed and gathered momentum, so the myths and his family multiplied. The sons Machaon and Podalirius were joined by Asklepios' wife Epione and five daughters, Hygieia, Panakeia, Aceso, Iaso and Aglaea, who embodied particular powers of their father. Only Hygieia, the personification of health, who was sometimes equated with the Roman goddess Salus, rose to prominence, however, and she was often portrayed as Asklepios' partner.

Both in Greek and in Roman art Asklepios was usually depicted in the manner chosen for statues of contemporary physicians, a powerful bearded man of middle or advancing years, with bare or sandalled feet and an ankle-length cloak slung across the left shoulder. His distinctive attribute was a snake-entwined staff, and Hygieia, too, is often shown with the same symbol of healing (36, 37). For amongst other powers and duties she assisted in the temple and fed the snakes that were sacred to her father. The staff probably signified the long walking stick used by Greek travellers. This would have been a natural attribute of Asklepios, who journeyed widely, first as a mortal physician and later as a healing god. It was undoubtedly imbued, too, with symbolic meaning, as a support or relief for the sick.[3] Snakes have many characteristics which are open to symbolic interpretation, and they have a long history in early religions. In the pagan Graeco-Roman world they seldom inspired the fear and horror that is often seen today, nor did they bear the connotation of evil ascribed to them in Christian literature. Instead, they were usually regarded as beneficent, and were not only kept as zoological exhibits or pets, but were also valued for apotropaic and prophetic qualities. Their long association with fertility and healing deities and with the chthonian spirits of the underworld is understandable in view of their tendency to emerge from and disappear into crevices in the ground, Mother Earth, who received the dead but from whom new life sprang. Equally, by reason of the yearly renewal of their skin, snakes became a widespread and powerful symbol of eternal rebirth. Interpreted more widely as a symbol of rejuvenation and restored health, they were particularly appropriate to Asklepios.[4]

At Epidauros, above all other Asklepian sanctuaries, the snake was the typical attribute of the god. There alone, according to the Greek traveller and geographer Pausanias, was found the specific type of snake that was tame with humans and sacred to Asklepios. This Asklepian snake has been identified as *Elaphe longissima longissima*, a harmless yellow species now native to south-east Europe.[5] It was the combination of mystery, power and beneficence that made it such an appropriate attribute of the kindly god of healing. In his cult these snakes also took an active part, for they were sometimes the intermediaries through which the god's cures were wrought. Dogs, too, were believed to be possessed of healing qualities and were sometimes shown as companions to Asklepios and other healing deities.

The beginnings of the cult are no clearer than the myth itself, and when Asklepios emerged as a god in the late sixth century BC his centre was not in Thessaly but in the Peloponnese, notably at a sanctuary in the small city-state of Epidauros. There he gradually gained superiority over the 'resident' deity, his father Apollo with the local epithet Maleatas. As Pausanias recorded in the second century AD, the Epidaurians clearly engaged in a not-so-subtle rewrite of Asklepios' birth to enhance the prestige of their sanctuary:

> When he [Phlegyas] went to the Peloponnesus, he was accompanied by his daughter, who all along had kept hidden from her father that she was with child by Apollo. In the country of the Epidaurians she bore a son, and exposed him on the mountain called Nipple at the present day, but then named Myrtium. As the child lay exposed he was given milk by one of the goats that pastured about the mountain, and was guarded by the watch-dog of the herd. (Pausanias, *Description of Greece* II, xxvi, 3–4; trans. W. H. S. Jones)

The role of the dog in this version of events is doubtless related to its connection with the hunter deity Maleatas and to its subsequent sacred status within the Asklepian cult, while the suckling of the infant Asklepios by a goat probably explains why it was never the custom to sacrifice that animal at Epidauros.

Asklepios was a relative late-comer to the Greek pantheon, but this was more than compensated for by the vigour of his cult, which his priests spread to all corners of the Greek and Roman world. Often they received requests to help establish the cult in new areas. This usually involved not the ousting of a previous incumbent, which was seen as harmful, but the grafting of Asklepios on to an existing sanctuary and his amicable integration with the deities already worshipped there. An inscription[6] records that one Telemachos introduced Asklepios to Athens in 420 BC, very likely as a result of the plague which had ravaged the city some ten years previously, while the Asklepieion established at Cos a few decades later achieved no less renown than its parent foundation at Epidauros. Another off-shoot of the Epidaurian sanctuary was that established at Rome in 292 BC, once more in response to an outbreak of plague. At the request of Roman envoys a sacred Aesculapian snake was despatched there, serving as an embodiment of the god, who was credited with the subsequent abatement of the plague (2).[7]

The most famous Asklepian sanctuaries were those at Epidauros (from which most others stemmed), Cos and Pergamum, but there were numerous others and hundreds of temples, by no means all of which have yet been identified and excavated. By combining the evidence of archaeology, epigraphy and classical literature it is possible to discern some of the rituals and activities that took place at certain of the sanctuaries, as well as to reconstruct the appearance of their buildings and monuments: Pausanias had a particular love of ancient religious sites and his descriptions of the temples and attendant buildings of the Asklepieia he visited flesh out the evidence drawn from standing remains and architectural fragments discovered in archaeological excavations; Aelius Aristides gives an extraordinarily full account of his relationship with Asklepios, together with incidental information on the running of the Pergamene Asklepieion in the mid-second century AD; and the *Iamata*, a series of inscriptions from Epidauros, reveal some of the miraculous cures attributed to Asklepios in the fourth century BC.

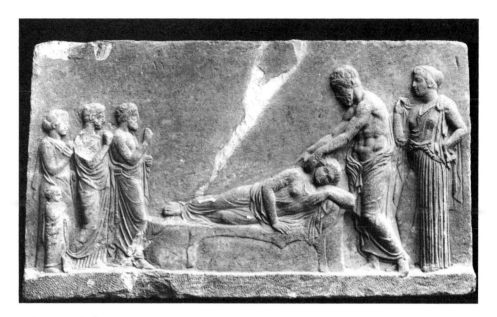

38 Healing by incubation. Asklepios, attended by Hygieia, administers a miraculous
cure to a sleeping woman. Marble votive relief, from the Piraeus Asklepieion,
early 4th century BC.

In common with other ancient religions, the cult of Asklepios was dependent
on a complex set of rituals for both public and private worship. The public occasions
included regular and frequent sacrifices or dedications made by the temple priests
on behalf of local communities. These were of a modest nature compared to the
great festivals which took place annually and which were attended by multitudes
of people from the immediate vicinity and from further afield. At Epidauros a special
festival, the *Asklepieia*, was celebrated once very four years. It took place nine days
after the Isthmian Games, the festival of Poseidon held at the Isthmus of Corinth
in late April. By selecting this date the Epidaurian priests could be assured that
most of the Isthmian Games participants would travel on to Epidauros before returning
home. On the way they sang hymns to Asklepios, and on entering the sanctuary
they were required to carry out a solemn cleansing ritual. This washing had less
to do with hygiene than with spiritual cleansing, as indicated on one of the Epidaurian
inscriptions seen by the writer Porphyry: 'He who enters the fragrant temple must
be pure; purity is to think holy thoughts.' There followed a sequence of rituals before
the start of games and musical contests in honour of Asklepios, and the festival culminated in the performance of a sacrifice at the open-air altar of Asklepios in full view
of the assembled throng. Following this the parts of the sacrificed animals not appor-
tioned to the god were consumed by the participants at a banquet.

These great public ceremonies and the other formal occasions were essentially
similar from one place to another irrespective of the deity involved, and it was in
the private aspect of worship that Asklepieia were radically different to other cults.
Instead of distancing himself as did most of the early-established Greek deities, Asklepios encouraged a close bond between himself and his worshippers. This was achieved

through their physical presence in his sanctuary, his dwelling place. Nonetheless, a formal and set ritual had still to be observed. Each individual, whether attempting to avert illness, giving thanks for continued good health or seeking a cure for some disease or disability, was required to perform the cleansing rite on arrival at the sanctuary. This was normally followed by the offering up of a sacrifice and a further purification by ritual bathing. After these preliminaries, overseen by the priests, those who had come as suppliants were led to the *abaton*, a 'sacred dormitory' adjacent to the temple, in which they passed the night or, occasionally, part of the day. This was 'incubation', the temple sleep, through which Asklepios effected their cure. He generally appeared as a dream-vision and either healed directly or gave instructions which the patient remembered on waking and carried out accordingly. Sometimes the cure was effected by the appearance alone or by the lick of the affected part by a sacred snake or dog. On other occasions the god's dream message was so cryptic that it required the interpretive assistance of the priests, who would then prescribe an appropriate remedy, normally drugs, or a regimen of diet, bathing and exercise.[8] Although it would be naïve to seek an exact modern equivalent, these priests were, broadly speaking, the faith-healers and psychotherapists of the ancient world. Even if they did not directly influence the process of incubation by charlatanry, they undoubtedly heightened the suppliants' expectancy by conversing with them, prior to incubation, on current medical precepts and herbal lore, and by recounting previous miraculous cures. Auto-suggestion, the suppliants' experience and knowledge of medicine, and their subconscious attitude to their own illness must have channelled their dreams into cures of a more or less bizarre nature.

All those who were cured by Asklepios were obliged to dedicate a thank-offering to him. These took many forms, from the sacrifice of an animal, to cakes, money, garlands, cups or plates of precious metal or models of the previously afflicted body parts. Of especial interest today, and no doubt particularly encouraged by the priests, were metal plaques or stone panels on which were depicted or described details of individual cases. Displayed in the sanctuary, these would have advertised the power of Asklepios and the significance of the particular cult centre. Six votive columns inscribed with many 'case-histories' were to be seen at the Epidaurian sanctuary in AD 150 when Pausanias made his visit: 'Within the enclosure stood slabs; in my time six remained, but of old there were more. On them are inscribed the names of both the men and the women who have been healed by Asclepius, the disease also from which each suffered, and the means of cure.'[9] Their importance to the prestige of the sanctuary may be gauged by the length of time they had been preserved, for when Pausanias saw them the inscriptions were already some five centuries old.

Remarkably, four of these columns were found in excavations and two of them are virtually intact. The cures were listed in the form of short narratives, whose terseness highlights their miraculous nature, and there is no differentiation between those that we would regard as wholly incredible and those that would appear to be at least partially explicable. Whatever their basis, they clearly betray the over-zealous desire of the priests to magnify the achievements of their god, and they present a striking contrast to the near-contemporary, sober but scientific Hippocratic case-histories: the case-histories concentrate on symptoms, while the Epidaurian inscriptions focus on cures:

Hermodicus of Lampsacus was paralyzed in body. This one, when he slept in the Temple, the god healed and he ordered him upon coming out to bring to the Temple as large a stone as he could. The man brought the stone which now lies before the Abaton. (Edelstein 1945, I, 232–3, no. 15)

A man with an abscess within his abdomen. When asleep in the Temple he saw a dream. It seemed to him that the god ordered the servants who accompanied him to grip him and hold him tightly so that he could cut open his abdomen. The man tried to get away, but they gripped him and bound him to a door knocker. Thereupon Asclepius cut his belly open, removed the abscess, and, after having stitched him up again, released him from his bonds. Whereupon he walked out sound, but the floor of the Abaton was covered with blood. (Edelstein 1945, I, 235, no. 27)

Some cures were effected in the sanctuary, either waking or sleeping, but without recourse to incubation in the abaton:

A man had his toe healed by a serpent. He, suffering dreadfully from a malignant sore in his toe, during the daytime was taken outside by the servants of the Temple and set upon a seat. When sleep came upon him, then a snake issued from the Abaton and healed the toe with its tongue, and thereafter went back again to the Abaton. When the patient woke up and was healed he said that he had seen a vision; it seemed to him that a youth with a beautiful appearance had put a drug upon his toe. (Edelstein 1945, I, 233, no. 17)

A dog cured a boy from Aegina. He had a growth on the neck. When he had come to the god, one of the sacred dogs healed him – while he was awake – with its tongue and made him well. (Edelstein 1945, I, 234, no. 26)

Incubation by proxy was clearly possible, too:

Arata, a woman of Lacedaemon, dropsical. For her, while she remained in Lacedaemon, her mother slept in the temple and sees a dream. It seemed to her that the god cut off her daughter's head and hung up her body in such a way that her throat was turned downwards. Out of it came a huge quantity of fluid matter. Then he took down the body and fitted the head back on to the neck. After she had seen this dream she went back to Lacedaemon, where she found her daughter in good health; she had seen the same dream. (Edelstein 1945, I, 233, no. 21)

Another similarly bizarre cure may have been intended to demonstrate the pre-eminence of the Epidaurian sanctuary:

Aristagora of Troezen. She had a tapeworm in her belly, and she slept in the Temple of Asclepius at Troezen and saw a dream. It seemed to her that the sons of the god, while he was not present but away in Epidaurus, cut off her head, but, being unable to put it back again, they sent a messenger to Asclepius asking him to come. Meanwhile day breaks and the priest clearly sees her head cut off from the body. When night approached, Aristagora saw a vision. It seemed to her the god had come from Epidaurus and fastened her head on to her neck. Then he cut open her belly, took the tapeworm out, and stitched her up again. And after that she became well. (Edelstein 1945, I, 234, no. 23)

Several cases were phrased as cautionary tales for those who might seek to dupe Asklepios or deprive him of his rightful thank-offerings. The cult certainly had its critics, amongst them Aristophanes, part of whose *Plutus* was a burlesque of temple medicine. Such unbelievers and sceptics were surely to heed the case of Ambrosia:

Ambrosia of Athens, blind of one eye. She came as a suppliant to the god. As she walked about in the Temple she laughed at some of the cures as incredible and impossible, that the lame and the blind should be healed by merely seeing a dream. In her sleep she had a vision. It seemed to her that the god stood by her and said that he would cure her, but that in payment he would ask her to dedicate to the Temple a silver pig as a memorial of her ignorance. After saying this, he cut the diseased eyeball and poured in some drug. When day came she walked out sound. (Edelstein 1945, I, 230, no. 4)

As far as can be gauged from the random but comparatively small remaining sample of these cures, it would appear that the Asklepieia ministered to rich and poor alike and, as Pausanias noted, men, women and, indeed, children, had access to his divine powers. Many of the cures involved childless or pregnant women:

Nicasibula of Messene for offspring slept in the Temple and saw a dream. It seemed to her that the god approached her with a snake which was creeping behind him; and with that snake she had intercourse. Within a year she had two sons. (Edelstein 1945, I, 237, no. 42)

Cleo was with child for five years. After she had been pregnant for five years she came as a suppliant to the god and slept in the Abaton. As soon as she left it and got outside the temple precincts she bore a son who, immediately after birth, washed himself at the fountain and walked about with his mother. (Edelstein 1945, I, 229, no. 1)

Whatever we make of Cleo's extremely precocious infant son and the other extraordinary testimonies, the cult was a potent force in fourth-century BC Greece. At that time Asklepios joined the patron deities of numerous states and cities, and many new Asklepieia were founded. Alexander the Great became a devotee and made dedications at Epidauros, where his patronage no doubt contributed to the international fame of the cult. A major development of the sanctuary brought architectural splendour commensurate with that of the sanctuaries of other Greek deities. Funds were collected from many Greek cities, not only those of mainland Greece and the Aegean Islands, but also some in Thessaly, Macedonia, Thrace, Sicily and southern

Italy. Hardly less remarkable than the votive columns, if more prosaic in their content, are a number of stone inscriptions, the most complete series of their kind to have survived, which record the cost and the legal arrangements involved in the construction of the new buildings.[10] They reveal that some buildings were completed quickly – the temple of Asklepios was finished in just four years and eight months – but others took much longer, and work was still underway a century later. Nevertheless, the functions of the sanctuary were already clearly defined and certain areas were hallowed by use so that the sanctuary ultimately displayed a distinct architectural coherence.[11]

The Asklepieion was approached from the direction of the town of Epidauros by means of a Sacred Way. All pilgrims, whether part of the formal procession of the great festivals or individual suppliants seeking a cure, entered the sanctuary through a gradiose propylon. Like many other of the Epidaurian buildings, the steps more normally encountered in such a structure were replaced with a ramp, which, intentionally or not, would certainly have helped the numerous lame or disabled visitors. It was more than pride that called for a striking entrance to the sanctuary, for the proplyon served to emphasise the threshold, the division of the sacred from the profane, and there were strict rules to be observed by those who entered: 'The sacred grove of Asclepius is surrounded on all sides by boundary marks. No death or birth takes place within the enclosure; the same custom prevails also in the island of Delos. All the offerings, whether the offerer be one of the Epidaurians themselves or a stranger, are entirely consumed within the bounds.'[12] The exclusion of those dying or giving birth has a purely practical explanation, for just as contemporary physicians were advised against treating those patients deemed to be mortally ill, it would have been damaging to the image of Asklepios if his sanctuaries had been strewn with those dying or suffering the pangs of childbirth.

By the third century BC one of the first buildings to be reached after passing through the propylon was a great stoa with internal courtyard and colonnades. Here the pilgrims might rest and discuss among themselves and with the priests their disease or disability, from which, they hoped, Asklepios would free them. The other peripheral structures included fountain houses and water basins, temples to several other divinities, a stadium and gymnasium, and a great banqueting hall for use especially during the festivals. At the heart of the sanctuary were the key cult buildings: the temple of Asklepios confronted by the great altar and flanked on one side by the abaton, on the other by a splendid circular building. Sadly, little of these buildings has survived above foundation level, but from the work of archaeologists and the descriptions of Pausanias the appearance of most can be confidently reconstructed. Within the temple of Asklepios was the cult statue which, according to Pausanias, was 'half as big as the Olympian Zeus at Athens, and is made of ivory and gold. An inscription tells us that the artist was Thrasymedes, a Parian, son of Arignotus. The god is sitting on a seat grasping a staff; the other hand he is holding above the head of the serpent; there is also a figure of a dog lying by his side.'[13] Although the statue has long since perished, the correctness of Pausanias' description is evident from the fact that it coincides exactly with an illustration shown on coins struck at the city of Epidauros in the mid-fourth century BC.

The abaton was a simple rectangular portico in close proximity to the temple. At some stage an extension was constructed, doubling its capacity, an indication

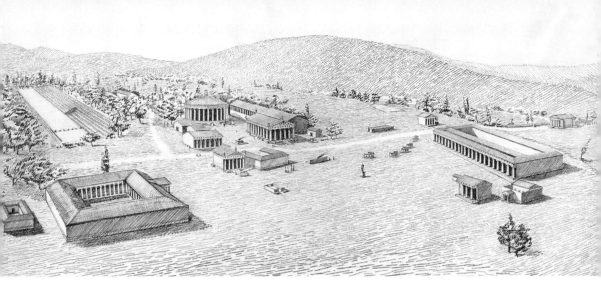

39 Artist's reconstruction of the sanctuary at Epidauros. The temple of Asklepios, abaton and Thymele are in the centre background.

of the increased fame and popularity of the sanctuary. The large circular building or Thymele is architecturally the most striking and sophisticated building in the sanctuary, but it is also one of the most enigmatic. There are no inscriptions that betray its function and Pausanias, though he mentioned it, devoted most of his brief account to an appraisal of the paintings displayed inside. It was made of white marble with a conical roof and with elaborate decoration throughout, and it had a curious arrangement of concentric subterranean passages. Despite attempts to identify it as a treatment centre employing snakes in some form of shock therapy, it is more likely to have been a cenotaph or symbolic tomb of Asklepios who, the Epidaurians claimed, was buried in their lands.[14]

A short distance away from the sanctuary is a theatre, which Pausanias considered to be unrivalled in symmetry and beauty. Built into a hillside, it is now the best surviving structure. Here would have taken place the dramatic and musical events in praise of Asklepios, and the seating capacity of about 13,000–14,000 gives an impression of the numbers that attended the festivals. Many of these would have required accommodation, and in the early third century BC a huge hostel was constructed between the theatre and the sanctuary. For the rest of the year it would also have housed those whose divine prescription required a lengthy stay at the sanctuary.

Over the next few centuries the fortunes of the sanctuary waxed and waned according to the political and economic climate of Greece. Bathing, for reasons both of hygiene and of therapy, became an increasingly important aspect at Epidauros, as at other Asklepieia, and in response suites of baths for communal hot and cold water bathing and individual immersion were constructed. Other buildings were replaced, but some became derelict, and by the end of the Roman civil wars, when there was a renewed interest in Asklepios, the Epidaurian Asklepieion may have been in some decay. Augustus was the first of a succession of Roman emperors to assist in its revival, while shortly before Pausanias visited a 'Roman senator named Antoninus' funded an extensive redevelopment of the sanctuary. This included the restoration of some dilapidated buildings, the dedication of a new temple to Hygieia, Asklepios and Apollo, and the construction of a baths complex. Furthermore: 'As the Epidaurians about the sanctuary were in great distress, because their women had no shelter in which to be delivered and the sick breathed their last in the open, he provided a dwelling, so that these grievances also were redressed. Here at last was a place in which without sin a human being could die and a woman be delivered.'[15]

The Epidaurian Asklepieion, because of its pre-eminence and its comparatively remote location, had an extensive and complex layout. Elsewhere, though still incorporating those architectural components vital to the cult, Asklepieia were often simpler and more compact. At those within or near towns, for example, the ancillary buildings like hostels, baths, gymnasium and theatre could often be dispensed with. Thus the Asklepieion that Telemachos founded on the southern slope of the Athenian Acropolis comprised a small propylon, a temple, altar, abaton and sacred spring, as well as a pit for keeping the sacred snakes or for pouring libations to the chthonic deities.[16] Similarly, at Corinth the fourth-century BC Asklepieion was situated on a salubrious terrace, formerly occupied by a shrine of Apollo, just inside the city wall, where there was ready access to recreational facilities including a theatre and a gymnasium.[17] Immediately adjacent to the Asklepieion, but an adjunct to it rather than an integral part, was a colonnaded court enclosing Lerna, a spring which yielded a steady supply of water. The sanctuary itself comprised simply the altar and temple of Asklepios, the abaton and, just inside the entrance, a basin for ritual purification. Pausanias' description is brief in the extreme,[18] but extensive excavation has revealed much of the detail. On entry the suppliant would have performed the purificatory washing of hands and then proceeded to the altar to make a sacrifice. Following a visit to the temple he would have made his way past the votive offerings displayed in the precinct to the lustral room in the abaton, where he would have undergone the preliminaries to 'incubation'. After his temple sleep in the abaton he may have made his way down to Lerna to eat in one of the adjacent dining rooms or carry out the regimen or therapy advised by Asklepios in his dream-vision.[19]

On a much grander scale was the Asklepieion on the island of Cos, which in its fully developed form rivalled Epidauros in size and architectural splendour. Cos, the birthplace of Hippocrates, was famous throughout the classical world from the fifth century BC onwards as a centre of medical science and healing, but the healing cult of Asklepios may already have asserted itself by the end of the sixth century BC. Certainly, Hippocrates was closely connected with the cult, for he belonged to its hereditary priesthood, the so-called 'family' or guild of Asklepiads. Unfortunately, little other evidence can be mustered to demonstrate such early beginnings, and excavations at the great sanctuary reveal that its main construction dates no earlier than the fourth century BC.[20] The site chosen was a hill-slope above the newly refounded (366 BC) capital city on the north-eastern tip of the island. As at Corinth and Epidauros, Asklepios joined and quickly superseded his mythical father Apollo as the island's healing deity.

Like many other Asklepieia, the Coan precinct was at first architecturally unsophisticated and all activity was focused upon an altar, the most essential component of all ancient Greek religions. The initial development of the sanctuary about the middle of the fourth century BC involved the erection of timber buildings, but within a century these were being progressively replaced and supplemented by stone structures. Completion and embellishment were long drawn out, but by the end of the second century BC the sanctuary had acquired monumental proportions together with a spectacular architectural symmetry that had never been possible at Epidauros. The layout was based on three main terraces, cut one above the other into the hill-slope and commanding a fine view across the sea to neighbouring islands and the coast of Asia Minor. Entering the vast colonnaded court of the lowest terrace through a propylon, the pilgrim would have gazed up to the altar and temples on the terraces above. Before ascending, however, he would have consulted the priests and taken rest or found accommodation in one of the many rooms behind the colonnade. Here too, on his return from incubation, he would have received the treatment prescribed by the god. By Roman times he would also have been able to take advantage of the facilities of a heated baths complex and a flushing latrine. Already he would have seen everywhere the evidence of previous grateful visitors, statues, inscriptions, decorative seats and basins, all given in thanks to Asklepios.

On the second terrace stood the earliest and the key buildings of the precinct, the altar decorated by the sons of Praxiteles, the temple of Asklepios containing a statue of the god and of his daughter Hygieia, another temple, probably of Apollo, the abaton and the priests' house. Finally, climbing two flights of marble steps, the pilgrim would have reached the uppermost terrace, at the centre of which rose a huge temple of Asklepios. A fitting monument in itself to the popularity of the cult, there was doubtless a practical reason behind the construction of a second temple. For, in combination with its extensive flanking colonnades, which served the same role as the abaton of the second terrace, it would have permitted many times the number of suppliants to participate in the 'temple sleep' than had been possible before.

The traditional view that Hippocrates' medicine was a product of his direct involvement with the Coan Asklepieion, taken together with the comment of the geographer Strabo that votive pillars were to be seen not just at Epidauros but also in the sanctuaries at Cos and Trikka,[21] raised considerable expectations when excavations began at the sanctuary in 1901. Unfortunately, these remained unfulfilled, for nothing like the Epidaurian *Iamata* was found. Nonetheless, there is no doubting the close connection between secular and temple medicine, especially at Cos. As if

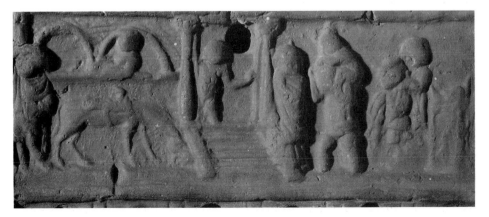

40 Visit to a healing shrine. A group of people assemble in front of a temple. One is carried on the back of a fellow and may be seeking a cure for a leg injury or disability. Detail from a terracotta lamp, 1st century AD.

to underline the continuing link are the benefactions to the sanctuary made by C. Stertinius Xenophon, court physician to the emperor Claudius and himself a member of the Asklepiad family of Cos. His therapeutic use of medicinal waters reflected a similar predilection in the Asklepian sanctuaries, and at Cos there was a plentiful supply of fresh water from a spring on the lowest terrace.

Our best evidence for the functioning of an Asklepieion belongs to the Roman period, when the cult enjoyed a renewed vitality. At Rome itself in the second century AD priests of the Tiber Island Asklepieion recorded miraculous cures not dissimilar to those inscribed at Epidauros some five centuries earlier:

> To Lucius who suffered from pleurisy and had been despaired of by all men the god revealed that he should go and from the threefold altar lift ashes and mix them thoroughly with wine and lay them on his side. And he was saved and publicly offered thanks to the god, and the people rejoiced with him.

> To Julian who was spitting up blood and had been despaired of by all men the god revealed that he should go and from the threefold altar take the seeds of a pine cone and eat them with honey for three days. And he was saved and went and publicly offered thanks before the people. (*IG* XIV, no. 966; trans. in Edelstein 1945, I, 251)

Difficult as it is to accept such cures at face value, they cannot be dismissed as mere fiction perpetrated by dishonest priests. For rational sources, like Galen and Rufus of Ephesus, give their support to Asklepios' wondrous cures. Dreams, whether predictive or non-predictive, were thought to have considerable medical significance, and Galen was not alone in valuing them as a means of prognosis and diagnosis in mental and in physical illness. He accepted as equally valid both patient-inspired and divine-inspired dreams, and he himself occasionally acted on divine instructions.[22]

An intriguing description of temple medicine has been left by Aelius Aristides, who wrote a detailed if idiosyncratic account of his experiences at the Asklepieion of Pergamum, where he spent many years as a patient and devotee. Born in AD 118 into a wealthy land-owning family in Mysia, Asia Minor, Aristides received a full and liberal education from some of the most respected teachers of the time. Alexander, his tutor in Greek literature, went on to teach the young Marcus Aurelius, while in Athens Aristides studied rhetoric under the eminent Herodes Atticus. After completing his formal education he travelled to Greece and Egypt, sightseeing and exploring as well as making his first public speeches. Then at the age of twenty-six he made the journey to Rome, where he was presented at court. He seemed poised to start an illustrious career in oratory, but serious and persistent ill health frustrated his plans. The symptoms, which included respiratory difficulties, fever, swollen stomach, chest troubles, deafness and toothache, eventually forced him to depart Rome within the year. His home-coming, far from being a celebration of newly won success, seemed to spell the end of a promising career before it had truly begun. The best doctors were consulted, but to no avail, and his faith in Serapis, an Egyptian healing deity, brought little relief either.

Thus it was, in the depths of despair and depression, while at the Warm Springs, a famous resort near Smyrna, that Aristides received his first revelation from Asklepios: 'He ordered me to go forth unshod. And I cried out in my dream, as if in a waking state and after the accomplishment of the dream: "Great is Asclepius! The order is accomplished."'[23] The command was trivial enough, but it marked the point of 'conversion' to Asklepios that was to lead to much more bizarre treatments. Although subsequently he still occasionally consulted physicians and made obeisance to Serapis and Isis, he considered himself thenceforth to be entirely in the service of Asklepios. Through a constant stream of visions and dreams, both within and outside temple precincts, the god guided his life in every respect. One of his first orders was that Aristides should write down his dreams, instructions and cures and one day make them public for the benefit of the cult, and it is in their edited form, as the *Hieroi Logoi*, that Aristides bequeathed his voluminous notes to posterity. They constitute a unique record of Graeco-Roman paganism, the first religious autobiography.

Despite his new-found allegiance to Asklepios, Aristides remained in ill health and despondent until the summer of AD 145, when he received a dream-summons to visit the Pergamene Asklepieion. There he was destined to remain as an incubant for the next two years. The sanctuary, which lay in a little valley outside the city, was founded in the fourth century BC from the parent temple at Epidauros. It reached its zenith in the second century AD, and in Aristides' day the sick and ailing flocked there from far and wide. It is to this period, when the sanctuary was numbered amongst the 'wonders of the world', that the major surviving buildings belong. They were ranged along the east side of a large rectangular plaza closed on the other three sides by colonnades. A small Sacred Theatre was joined to the outside of the north colonnade at its west end, while at the south-west corner a luxurious suite of flushing latrines was built. The earlier structures within the plaza which were spared demolition in the Roman redevelopment included altars, wells and springs, as well as the temple and altar of Asklepios and temples of Apollo, Hygieia and Telesphorus.

Access to the principal new buildings was from the plaza via a grandiose marble propylon at which terminated the Sacred Way linking the city to the sanctuary. To one side of the propylon stood a library, within which was a statue of the deified Hadrian, the emperor under whom most of the rebuilding had been initiated. To the other side was the temple of Asklepios Soter (Zeus Asklepios), an imposing circular building whose interior walls were richly veneered with marble and whose domed roof was covered by a cupola decorated with mosaics. Opposite the entrance, in the principal of seven wall-niches, would have stood the cult statue. Like the Pantheon in Rome, of which it was a smaller version, the temple was probably lit through a central aperture in the dome. Adjacent to the temple but at a lower level was another circular building, an immense and singular structure on two stories, connected with the plaza by an underground passage. Six large apses radiated from the upper storey, while the undercroft incorporated stone baths and was served by an intricate water supply system, channelled from the principal spring at the centre of the sanctuary. The exact function of this enormous rotunda is uncertain, but medicinal bathing must have been at least a part of the activities that took place there.

We know that the temple of Asklepios Soter was funded by L. Cuspius Pactumeius Rufinus, a friend of Aristides who had been consul in AD 142, and its completion cannot have occurred long, if at all, before Aristides' arrival.[24] The adjacent rotunda was erected after the temple and so would not have been operative during Aristides' first visit. Certainly he made no mention of it, but then neither he nor Galen, who was also well acquainted with the sanctuary, were concerned to give a description of the buildings. They shed no direct light, for example, on the place of incubation and as the archaeological evidence for an abaton is also uncertain, some have assumed that incubation took place both in the porticoes and in the temple buildings. As far as Aristides was concerned, the buildings were incidental and were important only in as much as they enabled him to commune with Asklepios and carry out the god's instructions.

Aristides owned no property in Pergamum, and there was no suitable accommodation near the sanctuary, but through his family connections he was invited to stay at the house of one of the two temple wardens, Asclepiacus. The wardens assisted the temple priest, who was responsible for the maintenance and running of the sanctuary, the performance of sacrifices and the accounting of money and gifts. The priesthood was a prestigious post, a hereditary life-time office open only to those who were descendants of the 'Asklepiad families'. There were probably, too, a number of honorary positions held by the social élite of Pergamum. Of lower status than the wardens were a variety of other temple functionaries attested on inscriptions from Pergamum and other Asklepieia. They include a herald, a door-keeper, a custodian of keys and a bath attendant, as well as the chorus who sang the ritual hymns.[25]

The religious calendar at the Pergamene Asklepieion was marked by three great annual festivals, during which poetic contests and nightly vigils took place in honour of the god. As at Epidauros, these festivals also included games with athletic and gymnastic events, a fitting tribute to the god of health and physique. Throughout the year there was a constant traffic of those individually or corporately seeking to ensure continued good health. The normal services were held morning and evening, when the temple was open to worshippers and incubants; white garments were worn for their symbolic significance in the purification ceremonies, which also involved ritual washing at the Sacred Well. Prayers and choral hymns were an integral part of the liturgy, and honorific speeches, composed by literary devotees such as Aristides, were declaimed in the theatre.

There is no evidence that physicians were formally a part of the temple staff. However, they were occasionally to be found in sanctuaries,[26] though whether as visitors or in a professional capacity is not clear. During his stay at Pergamum Aristides regularly consulted the physician Theodotus, who was in sympathy with the cult, even if at times a little reluctant to assist in the god's more bizarre prescriptions. Indeed, Theodotus and Asclepiacus became close confidants of Aristides and, together with Asklepios, they played a large part in his physical and spiritual recovery: 'After these things had been seen, when it was dawn, I summoned the doctor Theodotus. And when he came, I recounted my dreams to him. He marvelled at how divine they were, and was at a loss as to what he should do, since he feared the excessive weakness of my body in winter time. For I lay indoors during many successive months. Therefore we thought that it was no worse to send also for the temple warden Asclepiacus. At that time I was living in his house, and besides I was accustomed to share many of my dreams with him.'[27]

At Pergamum Aristides was no ordinary incubant. He moved in a restricted circle of wealthy, leisured and distinguished men, cultivated, like himself, and all of them passionate and impressionable devotees of Asklepios. While servants and retainers attended to their daily needs and whims they indulged in literary discussions, talked about their illnesses, shared the experiences of their dreams and visions and compared notes on treatment: 'We had been left alone in the Temple, two of the more distinguished worshippers, I and a Nicean, a man of praetorian rank, called Sedatius, but originally Theophilus. Therefore we were sitting in the Temple of Hygieia, where the statue of Telesphorus is, and we were asking one another, as we were accustomed, whether the God had prescribed anything new. For some of our diseases were also the same.'[28] This ambience of refined hypochondria has justifiably been compared to that of the spas and sanatoria of nineteenth-century Europe.

Aristides' other close and trusted friend was Zosimus, his foster-father, who accompanied him to Pergamum and through whose dream on the very first night of incubation Asklepios inaugurated Aristides' regimen. Over the years this proved to comprise principally walking barefoot, riding on horseback, taking cold baths, and submitting to purging, blood-letting and sweating under piles of blankets. All of these methods were known to, and employed by, the physicians of Aristides' day but, as Galen ruefully observed, it was the context, not the technique from which the god drew his power: 'Thus at any rate even among ourselves in Pergamum we see that those who are being treated by the god obey him when on many occasions he bids them not to drink at all for fifteen days, while they obey none of the physicians who give this prescription. For it has great influence on the patient's doing all which is prescribed if he has been firmly persuaded that a remarkable benefit to himself will ensue.'[29] Even the eminent Satyros, one of Galen's medical teachers, made little headway against Asklepios:

> I [Aristides] was so weak that I could not even endure in bed at home. And the doctor Satyrus, a sophist, as was said, of no mean rank, was at this time in Pergamum. This man visited me while I was lying in bed, and felt my chest and abdomen. When during the course of the conversation, he heard how many purges of blood I had had, he ordered me to stop them and not to undermine my body. 'But I,' he said, 'shall give you a very light and simple ointment, which you should put on your stomach and abdomen, and you will see how much it will help.' He advised these things. And as regards my blood, I denied that I had the authority to do one or the other, but that while the God commanded the letting of my blood, I would obey whether willing or not, and moreover never unwillingly. Still I did not ignore Satyrus' prescription, but took and kept it. It was no cornucopia. (*Hieroi Logoi* III, 7–9; trans. C. A. Behr)

However, in addition to the comparatively normal prescriptions, even those applied in excess, Aristides received a series of quite irrational commands from Asklepios, many of which involved such extreme measures that the physicians frequently doubted his ability to survive them. To a great extent it was the very uniqueness of the commands that made them effective. For Aristides, and doubtless too his fellow incubants, received a considerable psychological boost from the knowledge that Asklepios had devised a treatment specific to their illness, and this could also have triggered an improvement in their physical health:

> And these things happened in Pergamum, in the house of the temple warden Asclepiacus. First he commanded that I have blood drawn from my elbow, and he added, as far as I remember, 'sixty pints.' This was to show that there would be need of not a few phlebotomies, but that appeared from later things. For the temple wardens, being of such years, and all who were worshippers of the God and who served him, confessed that they knew of no one at all who had been operated on so much, except Ischuron, and that his case was among the strange ones, but even so that mine surpassed it. (*Hieroi Logoi* II, 46–7; trans. C. A. Behr)

This was personal devotion to a personal saviour, and healing the physical symptoms of illness was only a part of the process. Spiritual guidance and fulfilment were equally significant. The same symptoms often recurred or new ones followed hard on the heels of those that had been cured, and Aristides' miracles were of a quite different nature to the earlier ones recorded at Epidauros. Of those he wrote that he had read and heard but never witnessed anything of the kind. Nevertheless, as we have seen, such miracles were still being recorded at Rome in Aristides' day. In fact, healing centres dependent on faith could be sustained with only a tiny percentage of miraculous cures. For the remainder of the devotees a daily round of mundane and often sound therapeutic measures, interspersed with occasional extreme or bizarre features, sufficed to maintain allegiance to Asklepios and to create the illusion of success, however short-lived the results.

When he left Pergamum after two years of divine treatment Aristides was still a sick man, despite his 'miraculous' treatments, but, far from being disillusioned, he had reached an equilibrium. Through Asklepios he had learnt to live with his afflictions and, furthermore, he now possessed both a firm faith and a renewed confidence in his ability to win personal glory:

> During approximately the first year of my sickness, I gave up the study of rhetoric, since I was in such great physical discomfort. And at the same time, I became despondent. While I now rested in Pergamum because of a divine summons and my supplication, I received from the God a command and exhortation not to abandon rhetoric ... And he commanded me to go to the Temple Stoa, which is at the Theater, and to offer to him the very first fruits of these improvised and competitive orations. And so it happened ... It was often my experience that when I received my problems and stood ready for the contest, I was in difficulty and scarcely recovered from the failure of my breath; but as I proceeded in my introduction, I now became more comfortable and was able to breathe; and as my speech proceeded further, I was filled with strength and lightness ... And once that famous Pardalas, who, I would say, was the greatest expert of the Greeks of our time in the knowledge of rhetoric, dared to say and affirm to me that I had become ill through some divine good fortune, so that by my association with the God, I might make this improvement. (*Hieroi Logoi* IV, 14–27; trans. C. A. Behr)

In the decades that followed his sojourn at Pergamum Aristides travelled widely, declaiming in the cities of Greece and Asia Minor and in Rome to the emperor himself, and on these tours he found the glory that had earlier eluded him. Always a neurotic hypochondriac, illness continued to trouble him intermittently for the rest of his life. However, Asklepios remained his salvation and he continued to receive divine guidance and medical prescriptions through his dreams. On several occasions he returned to the Pergamum sanctuary for a short period, and in AD 155 he visited the great sanctuary at Epidauros. Until AD 165 his symptoms were mostly of a respiratory nature, many of them psychosomatic in origin. In that year, however, he was one of those who contracted the plague, probably smallpox,[30] which swept across the Roman Empire from the east and which, incidentally, caused Galen's precipitate departure from Rome. Although the physicians gave Aristides up for dead, he survived that and a subsequent epidemic, but he suffered many after-effects, mostly intestinal disturbances.

Galen, who may or may not have known Aristides personally, diagnosed him as a consumptive:

> I have seen many people whose body was naturally strong and whose soul was weak, inert and useless. Thus their sicknesses have arisen from a sort of insomnia and apoplexy and enervation and sicknesses of the sort of epilepsy . . . And as to them, whose souls are naturally strong and whose bodies are weak, I have only seen a few of them. One of them was Aristides, one of the inhabitants of Mysia. And this man belonged to the most prominent rank of orators. Thus it happened to him, since he was active in teaching and speaking throughout his life, that his whole body wasted away. (*CMG* Suppl. I, 1934, 33, trans. in Behr 1968, 162)

Despite everything, Aristides reached the respectable, if not advanced, age of sixty-three when, finally, even Asklepios was powerless against his 'consumption'. He had frequently alluded to honour and reputation as the rewards of a great orator, and they were undoubtedly the most powerful motivating forces in his life. It is somewhat ironic, therefore, that the compositions that above all ensured his lasting fame were not his polished orations, admired by his contemporaries for the purity of their Attic diction, but the *Hieroi Logoi*, his disordered and rambling discourses in praise of Asklepios.

Whatever else Aristides may have dedicated to Asklepios, his greatest thank-offering was the *Hieroi Logoi*. Less literary but no less grateful devotees left evocative testimony in votive reliefs and anatomical ex-votos. A series of sculptured marble panels dedicated in Athens and Piraeus in the fourth century BC depict Asklepios receiving patients and administering his miraculous cures to sleeping incubants, sometimes accompanied by Hygieia or the sacred snakes.[31] Less costly were the anatomical ex-votos, stone carvings or bronze plaques which showed ears, eyes, limbs and other parts of the body, including internal organs. Some of the ear and eye votives were consecrated to Asklepios in the hope that he would listen to the suppliants' prayer or observe their illness, while others were probably given in gratitude at having received divine attention by these means. Still others must have been dedicated for the relief of specific aural and ocular disorders, but the exact nature of the disorder is very

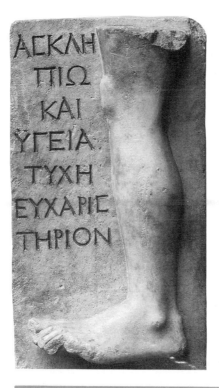

ΑCΚΛΗ
ΠΙΩ
ΚΑΙ
ΫΓΕΙΑ
ΤΥΧΗ
ΕΥΧΑΡΙC
ΤΗΡΙΟΝ

41 Marble votive relief showing the lower part of a left leg. The inscription states that a certain Tyche dedicated it as a thank-offering to Asklepios and Hygieia, who had presumably wrought a cure to some affliction of his leg or foot. From the Greek island of Melos.

42 *Below* Terracotta votives – here a foot, hand, male genitalia, ears, eye and breast – were offered up to healing deities in the hope of a divine cure or in thanks for one already effected. Roman, 3rd–1st century BC.

43 *Below right* Temple scene, with two votive legs and a hand suspended in the background. Vase-painting, 5th century BC.

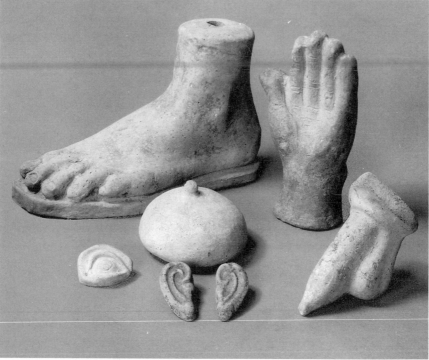

rarely depicted on any of the anatomical ex-votos. An interesting exception is the leg with enlarged varicose vein shown on a fourth-century BC stone relief from Athens.[32]

Legs and feet were common ex-votos and they serve as a reminder that of all diseases and disorders those affecting mobility, and therefore livelihood, were amongst the most feared. At the Corinthian Asklepieion numerous legs and feet were included among several hundred votive offerings which date to the century between about 400 and about 300 BC.[33] Unlike most other Greek anatomical votives of this period, which were made of stone or metal, those from Corinth are almost exclusively terracottas, probably because Corinth had a long tradition of expertise in that medium and no local source of suitable stone. The models of heads and chests had flattened bases so that they could be stood on shelves or ledges, but most of the other anatomical votives were perforated so that they could be fixed to walls or posts or suspended from the ceilings of the temple buildings, as indicated on contemporary vase-paintings. In common with other terracottas, the Corinthian votives were painted, which enables differentiation of the sexes: female parts were coloured white, male parts red. However, in only one case is there a definite indication of the disease, a growth on the back of a hand.[34]

Concurrently with their adoption at Corinth, terracotta anatomical ex-votos also became widespread in Republican Italy. It is uncertain whether the rite had a common origin, but the distribution of Italian sites with anatomical ex-votos does not coincide with those parts of Italy which had long seen Greek settlement. Instead, such shrines appear to have been especially popular in central Italy west of the Apennines, the

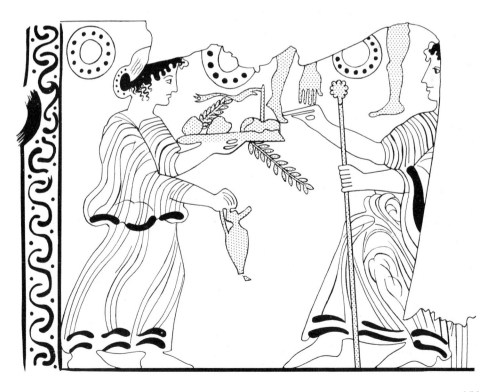

regions of Etruria and Latium.[35] The Italian sanctuaries have seldom yielded evidence of the identity of their healing deity, and although many of the votives found in the River Tiber at Rome had probably been dedicated at the island sanctuary of Asklepios, it is clear that, as in Greek lands, there were many other regional healing deities in addition to Asklepios.

The range and quantity of the votives is sometimes astonishing. Probably made at kilns nearby and sold to visiting suppliants from stalls at the shrine, they include some finely modelled examples, but most were mass-produced and of rather indifferent or poor quality (42). Large quantities of these inexpensive offerings would soon have accumulated and periodically the temple buildings had to be cleared. As the ex-votos were part of the sacred property of the deity and could not be destroyed or re-cycled, they were packed into small buildings or rooms or buried in sacred pits; because they were of no value as loot and do not easily deteriorate in the ground, many have survived the passage of time.

'Specialisation', which has been inferred from the preponderance of particular types or groups of anatomical ex-votos, may well have begun at Greek Asklepieia in the fourth century BC. For while the Corinth votives comprised mainly legs, feet, arms, hands, breasts and genitals, the inventory lists of the Athenian Asklepieion[36] indicate a preference there for eye votives, and at another Greek healing sanctuary, the Amphiareion, chests predominated. Certainly, the relative frequency of different anatomical ex-votos at shrines in Italy has been interpreted as evidence that particular classes of disease were catered for at some shrines. At the Republican healing sanctuary of Ponte di Nona, for example, statistical and medical studies of over 8,000 terracotta votives have led to the tentative conclusion that foot and hand disorders were the special concern of the healing deity there.[37] The shrine was established in the later fourth or early third century BC on a small ridge alongside the Via Praenestina fifteen kilometres to the east of Rome. The ancillary structures of the temple included what was probably a circular pool, a small hostel building or *mansio* with a suite of baths, and a cave-like *nymphaeum*, which may have enclosed the mineral spring that issued at the site. Although there was a direct road connection with Rome, the shrine served a rural population and it is in an agricultural context that the votives should be regarded. Two out of three are feet, hands or limbs, a concentration which perhaps reflects the physical stresses to which farm labourers were subject, and the long distances that they would have travelled on foot each day. Feet were four times as common as hands, and such a marked disparity is probably to be explained both by the lower incidence of spontaneous healing in feet and their less adaptable nature. The foot votives could have been dedicated by those either supplicating or giving thanks for a cure to one of many disorders, such as fallen arches, ingrowing toenails, torn ligaments, wounds and ulcerations, or deformities such as club foot and, most frequently, arthritic joints.[38]

The few votives from Ponte di Nona which show male and female sexual organs might be taken to suggest that sexual disorders were seldom 'treated' there. Certainly, sexually transmitted diseases were more rapidly spread in an urban environment, and it is interesting to note that the healing sanctuary of Campetti in the Etrurian city of Veii has a marked preponderance of votives which depict male and female sexual organs, and a correspondingly small number of hand and foot votives.[39] The symptoms of gonococcal disease include urethritis, cystitis and urethral stricture, while other diseases such as phimosis, hydrocele, scrotal varix, testicular tumours and urethral stricture, all recorded in the medical literature of the day, must have occasioned the dedication of many of the male genital votives. Not all necessarily indicate the cure of an ailment, and some of the male genitals as well as many of the female breast and womb votives were probably offered in gratitude for the birth of a child.

To judge by the large number of terracotta heads at Ponte di Nona, headache may have been another common complaint of the surrounding community. Often it would have been a painful symptom of malaria,[40] which was a scourge of the low-lying coastal regions of Greece, Italy and the other Mediterranean countries until recent times. However, a few of the head votives portray one side only and these may have been dedicated by sufferers from *hemikrania*, literally 'half-head'. This Greek term, itself derived from Egyptian medicine, has given rise to our word migraine, and it accurately characterises the localisation of pain in this all too common ailment.

Eye complaints were universal, and eye votives comprise a significant proportion of the deposit at Ponte di Nona. Most depict the eye complete with eyelids and periocular tissue, but some portray just the eyeball. This may represent a deliberate distinction between those afflictions like trachoma and chronic conjunctivitis, which affected the eyelids as well as the eye, and those like myopia, cataract and squint that involved the eyeball alone.

The anatomical votives are an intriguing class of evidence, for they offer a tantalising glimpse of personal reactions to disease in antiquity. However, they are also perplexing, for they are open to many interpretations. Attention has already been drawn to the fact that in the case of most we are unable to tell whether they were given in supplication or in gratitude, and also to the uncertainty as to the type of affliction intended. Those maladies already mentioned are but a brief selection from many hundreds of possibilities, and the potential frequency of skin diseases, in particular, should not be forgotten.[41] In the absence of disinfecting cleansing, these were many and varied, and exceedingly troublesome, as Pliny, Celsus and other medical writers made clear.[42] At Ponte di Nona, although there is no evidence that they did so, sufferers from certain skin complaints could have gained relief through use of the shrine's magnesium-rich spring water, a tonic also for bowel disorders.

The choice of hot or cold mineral springs as a focus for Asklepieia and other healing shrines became increasingly common in Hellenistic Greece and later Republican Italy, a reflection of the contemporary medical predilection for hydropathic treatment. It would appear also, from Vitruvius' advice on their siting, that healing shrines were commonly used as a safe, if temporary, haven from plagues and epidemics, such as typhus and malaria:

> There will be a natural decor: first, if for all temples there shall be chosen the most healthy sites with suitable springs in those places in which shrines are to be set up; secondly and especially for Aesculapius and Salus; and generally for those gods by whose medical power sick persons are manifestly healed. For when sick persons are moved from a pestilent to a healthy place and the water supply is from wholesome fountains, they will more quickly recover. So will it happen that the divinity (from the nature of

the site) will gain a greater and higher reputation and authority. (Vitruvius, *De Architectura* I, ii, 7; trans. F. Grainger)

In another section Vitruvius described some of the more remarkable curative springs of his day: sulphur springs which had the power to 'refresh muscular weakness by heating and burning poisonous humours from the body'; alum springs which were beneficial to those suffering from paralysis; bitumen springs which purged and healed 'interior defects'; alkaline springs which lessened 'scrofulous tumours'; and acid springs whose waters were drunk to dissolve bladder stones.[43] In Pliny a more extensive list includes: a hot spring near Puteoli (Pozzuoli) which was 'very beneficial for eye complaints'; the waters of Sinuessa in Campania which were 'said to cure barrenness in women and insanity in men'; several sources which cured bladder stone; and the waters of Albula, near Rome, which healed wounds.[44] Most revered of all were the thermal springs and sulphurous sweat-baths of Baiae, which, by the first century BC had become the Roman fashionable resort *par excellence*. The rich, invalids and healthy alike, visited in droves to take the waters and to socialise, and Baiae became as renowned for licentious living as for its thermal facilities.[45] Pliny the Younger described the arrangements and captured the atmosphere of a much smaller spring site in Umbria:

> The banks are clothed with ash trees and poplars, whose green reflections can be counted in the clear stream as if they were planted there. The water is as cold and as sparkling as snow. Close by is a holy temple of great antiquity in which is a standing image of the god Clitumnus himself clad in a magistrate's bordered robe; the written oracles lying there prove the presence and prophetic powers of his divinity. All round are a number of small shrines, each containing its god and having its own name and cult, and some of them also their own springs, for as well as the parent stream there are smaller ones which have separate sources but afterwards join the river. The bridge which spans it marks the sacred water off from the ordinary stream: above the bridge boats only are allowed, while below bathing is also permitted. The people of Hispellum, to whom the deified Emperor Augustus presented the site, maintain a bathing place at the town's expense and also provide an inn; and there are several houses picturesquely situated along the river bank. Everything in fact will delight you, and you can also find something to read: you can study the numerous inscriptions in honour of the spring and the god which many hands have written on every pillar and wall. Most of them you will admire, but some will make you laugh – though I know you are really too charitable to laugh at any of them. (*Letters* 8, 8; trans. B. Radice)

The Romans systematically developed mineral springs as they encountered them in newly conquered provinces, as at Aix-en-Provence (Aquae Sextiae), Vichy (Aquis Calidis), Baden (Aquae Helveticae), Baden-Baden (Aquae), Wiesbaden (Aquae Mattiacae), and Aachen (Aquae Granni). Although not all were directly associated with healing cults, the majority were already presided over by a native deity or spirit, for the phenomenon, especially, of hot water bubbling up from the depths of the earth must always have inspired a sense of wonder and a belief in the limitless powers of the divine spirits. Under Roman rule these native deities, whether of purely local or of wider significance, were usually conflated with a Graeco-Roman divine counterpart chosen for the broad similarity of their powers and spheres of influence. The Gallic and Germanic healing deities were frequently identified with Apollo the Healer, as at Essarois near Dijon, where an inscription records Apollo Vindonnus, or at Aachen where Apollo joined the native deity Grannus to preside over the thermal springs. Apollo Grannus was an especially popular healing deity of springs in the Rhine/Moselle region. Sometimes he had a divine partner, the goddess Sirona, who fulfilled the same role as Hygieia. Thus on a statue from the shrine of Apollo and Sirona at Hochscheid, near Trier, Sirona is depicted in the guise of Hygieia feeding a sacred snake which is entwined around her forearm.[46]

Compared to the many roles of the god Apollo, Aesculapius' very specific and characteristic powers may have been more difficult to match with those of Celtic deities, and unlike Apollo he was seldom identified with them. Nevertheless, the influence of his cult was widespread, and there were temples to Aesculapius in many of the larger Gallic towns. He was also worshipped at the temples and shrines of other healing deities, as at Augst, Switzerland, where an altar to Aesculapius was found in the precinct of the double temple of Apollo and Sirona, and at Bath where a stone block with carvings thought to illustrate the Asklepios legend was found in the cistern of one of the thermal springs.[47]

The custom of dedicating anatomical votives, which had almost died out in Italy by the first century BC, continued for several more centuries in the provinces of Gaul and Britain. Those that survive are mainly of metal or stone, and eyes are particularly common. The many stone votives from a shrine at Halatte, near Paris, include heads, torsos, limbs, feet and genitals. Several temples may have specialised in problems of childbirth and fertility, as at Massigny-les-Vitteaux, near Dijon, where numerous stone votives of children and pregnant women were found, and at Essarois, where the votives included swaddled babies and male and female figurines with pronounced genitals.[48] One of the most extraordinary discoveries, however, was made in excavations at the source of the River Seine, some thirty-five kilometres north-west of Dijon. There, in the early first century AD, the Gallo-Roman sanctuary of the goddess Sequana was established. The architectural setting of the shrine and water source, which was unsophisticated at the outset, became increasingly elaborate, and it is probably to one of the structural changes that we owe the survival of the several hundred wooden carvings that have given the site its exceptional importance.[49] The carvings, which until then had probably stood or hung in buildings within the temple precinct, were ritually buried as a single deposit in the ground which has remained below the water-table ever since. Similarly, at Chamalières (Clermont-Ferrand, France) an even greater number of wooden votives, dedicated in the early first century AD, were preserved in the waterlogged ground surrounding another spring, the 'Sources des Roches'.[50]

Most of the wooden carvings from the Seine source are offerings dedicated to Sequana in her capacity as a goddess of healing. Many are anatomical ex-votos whose large number, in comparison with those examples of stone or metal, indicates that there, at least, wood was their normal medium, and we may infer that the position was often the same elsewhere. Together with a few other rare instances, they are a forcible reminder of the huge volume of such evidence that has been lost at those sanctuaries where less favourable conditions prevailed. The carvings, all worked in oak heart-wood, include representations of animals, male and female figurines, heads, arms, legs, torsos, male and female sexual organs and plaques showing internal organs. Like their counterparts in stone, they display a variety of styles reflecting both native traditions and Roman influence. Even in their present condition some still reveal the masterly skill and sensitivity of their makers.

The anatomical ex-votos which show the torso and internal organs are perhaps the most interesting carvings, although they are artistically less pleasing than the figurines and heads. As with the Italian terracottas, it is sometimes difficult to tell which organs are depicted. Most of the 'thorax plaques' are stylised carvings with schematic representations of the oesophagus or trachea together with lungs and stomach, but occasionally it is possible to identify the ribs and additional organs like the heart and the kidneys.[51] Their variable and schematic nature was probably a fair reflection of contemporary anatomical knowledge. Many of those plaques which show the torso, the female breasts or male or female genitals were probably related to fertility and childbirth. However, the protruberance adjacent to the genitals on a few of them appears to be an indication of hernia.[52] Common enough today, hernia must have been an occupational hazard of most working people in antiquity.[53] For they endured harsh living conditions and, with few labour-saving devices, they often had to submit their bodies to excessive physical stress. Among the afflictions apparently shown on the stone votives are goitre, breast cancer and eye troubles.[54] Blindness is depicted on one of the wooden votives from Chamalières, the head of a young man with one empty eye socket,[55] but otherwise ailments and diseases are unspecified. Some were probably painted on – one plaque from Chamalières still retains traces of painting – but it is unlikely that such vulnerable evidence will ever prove to be more than a tantalising possibility.

Roughly contemporary with the ritual activity at Chamalières and the Seine source was the development of the thermal springs at Bath. There, despite difficulties similar to those encountered at most of the other major hot and mineral springs, where continuing popularity has resulted in the sealing or destruction of the Roman installations, archaeologists have gradually and painstakingly revealed the remains and pieced together the appearance of the central structures of the Roman spa.[56] The presiding deity was Sulis Minerva, as demonstrated by numerous inscriptions and the life-size gilded bronze head of Minerva, probably from the cult statue. Minerva, whom the Romans identified with the Greek Athena, was a goddess of learning, sometimes of war, but she also had a healing role. In this latter capacity, as Minerva Medica, temples were dedicated to her in several cities, including Rome, while it was to Athena that Aelius Aristides attributed his recovery from the plague in AD 165. Sulis, or Sul, was a native Celtic deity of whom, unfortunately, little is known. Conflated with Minerva she (or he) controlled one of the principal Roman thermal springs of the Western Empire.

The King's Bath spring, the most powerful of the three springs which surface at the centre of Bath, delivers in excess of a quarter of a million gallons of hot mineral water a day at a temperature of 46°C (120°F). With consummate skill, the Roman engineers enclosed the spring-head in a reservoir, drained the surrounding area, and constructed a temple precinct and monumental range of baths around the spring. This massive and carefully integrated complex of classical buildings, constructed only two or three decades after the Roman conquest of Britain, must have been an awesome sight to Roman and native Briton alike. The spring itself was incorporated in the south-east corner of the temple precinct where the baths abutted, and it was the unifying link between the two. Watched over by Sulis Minerva, its steaming waters were channelled into the Great Bath where people could immerse themselves to gain the full effect of its curative properties (47). Devotees and grateful suppliants could approach the spring from the temple or the baths to contemplate the holy waters and throw in their votive offerings.

By the later second century AD the spring was enclosed in a huge vaulted chamber and was embellished by the addition of several statues supported at water level on pedestals erected within the reservoir. The dank and humid atmosphere, and luxuriant growth of mosses and ferns on the walls, the statues shrouded in steam in the eerie half-light, all must have combined to create the conditions which triggered mystic experiences not dissimilar to those of the Asklepian incubants. At least one visitor

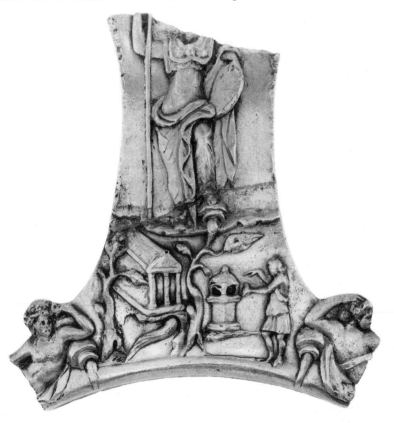

44 A Roman spa. Minerva presides over a sacred spring, here symbolised by the water gushing from an upturned pot beneath her foot. Below, a figure takes a draught of the healing water from a fountain in front of a classical temple. Silver and gilt patera handle, Capheaton hoard, England, 2nd–3rd century AD. Length 8 cm.

to Bath was prompted to make a fulsome dedication as the result of a vision.[57] Offerings were normally of a more modest nature, metal vessels, trinkets and, above all, coins, of which the spring has yielded many thousands. Sadly, it was evidently not customary to dedicate anatomical ex-votos at Bath, food offerings and coins doubtless taking their place, and there is only one possible example, an amulet of breasts carved in elephant ivory.[58]

The temple of Sulis Minerva, a compact prostyle building with fine Corinthian columns, stood in a spacious paved precinct. Its pediment sculpture included two thoroughly classical winged victories and the famous 'Gorgon-head' centrepiece, a classical motif carved in uncompromisingly Celtic style. Intentionally or not, this conjunction of different traditions aptly mirrored the twinning of Minerva and Sulis. Furthermore, the Gorgon sculpture possesses characteristics reminiscent of both sun and water deity, and may have been an intentional expression of the combined power of both gods, logically regarded as the creators of hot springs.[59] In front of the temple stood the altar, the focus of religious activity, which was positioned so that it was visible both through the entrance of the temple precinct and across the spring from the baths. Here the sacrificial animals were ritually slaughtered under the auspices of an augurer (*haruspex*), who foretold future events from omens observed in the entrails. We know the name of one of these men, Lucius Marcius Memor, for he dedicated a gift, probably a statue, to Sulis Minerva.[60]

The baths, which were constructed initially as a curative adjunct to the temple rather than an independent healing facility, comprised pools served by the thermal spring and artificially heated suites of rooms. Like the temple precinct, they underwent elaboration and change during some four centuries of use. Sauna-type facilities were added, and curative immersion was formalised by the provision of sunken baths with underwater stone benches on which the patients sat up to their necks in the healing water. The bathers probably sought cures for a wide range of diseases and symptoms, and, as in more recent times, many must have found relief from gout, rheumatism and arthritis. For other complaints the powers of the goddess and her spring would have been supplemented by the remedies of an assortment of quacks and physicians. These men were always to be found where the sick and ailing congregated, whether at town baths, healing sanctuaries or spas; a *collyrium* stamp marked with the eye prescriptions of Titus Junianus was lost by one of them in the region of the baths.[61]

A *collyrium* stamp was also found at the rather remarkable Romano-British temple site at Lydney Park fifteen kilometres north-east of Chepstow.[62] There, on a spur overlooking the Forest of Dean and the Severn Estuary, was the cult-centre of the Romano-Celtic god Nodens, a sort of British Epidauros (45). On two votive plaques from the site Nodens is identified with Mars, a conflation also seen in the inscription on the base of two statuettes found near Lancaster.[63] Mars was one of the most popular Roman gods in the Celtic provinces, but like Minerva his martial image was supplemented by several other roles, including one of healing. Assimilated to the Gallic god Lenus, for example, as Lenus Mars, he was the principal healing deity of the Treveran tribal region of Gaul with a cult-centre at Trier. There is good reason for believing that Mars Nodens was a healer-god too.

The Lydney temple, an unusual basilican building, lay in a spacious precinct. To the north stood a huge guest-house of normal quadrangular plan with suites of rooms grouped around an internal colonnaded garden court. Adjacent to it was an equally grandiose range of heated baths, while further south, hard against the temple itself, was a long narrow building with a veranda that faced the temple. This has been identified as an abaton, for in plan and position it compares closely to that at Epidauros. The combination of temple, abaton, guest-house and baths as a discrete and coherent complex is also matched at other Asklepieia, and there seems little doubt that the Nodens cult at Lydney had a healing function. Among the offerings, mostly coins and trinkets, are two anatomical votives, a miniature bronze arm and an engraved bone plaque which depicts a naked woman.[64] The woman's hands are pressed against her belly, and the plaque was probably a childbirth votive.

Dogs were clearly of importance in the Nodens cult, for the votives include several stone carvings and seven bronze models of canines, one of which had been ritually buried in the floor of the temple. A dog also figured on an inscribed bronze plaque which had been dedicated to Mars Nodens by one Pectillus.[65] As we have seen, dogs were of especial significance in the Asklepian cult, and they were also included in the iconography at other healing shrines.[66] Perhaps the Lydney hounds, like those of Asklepios, assisted the god with his divine cures.

Lydney was an isolated sanctuary, and overnight accommodation would probably have been required by all but the most local worshippers. Those seeking cures may have stayed for several days or weeks, and the comparatively sumptuous facilities of the guest-house and baths would have afforded them some comfort. The prosperity of the cult must have depended upon the popular appeal of healing deities and upon the benefactions of a small number of wealthy devotees. Funds were available to commission a splendid mosaic for the floor of the temple. This was dedicated by Titus Flavius Senilis, who seems to have been an aristocratic priest of the cult with responsibility for the temple treasury: in an inscription worked into the border of the mosaic he recorded that it had been financed 'out of offerings'.[67] The same inscription reveals that a certain Victorinus, who oversaw the laying of the mosaic, was an *interpres*. He, too, must surely have been a priest, a specialist in interpreting the dreams of incubants.

Victorinus and Senilis officiated over the Lydney shrine in the later fourth century AD. Mars Nodens' healing cult was evidently flourishing there, despite the general demise of pagan religions in the face of increasing pressures from Christianity. Its period of prosperity approximately coincided with the accession of the emperor Julian (AD 360), and the cult may have owed a part of its vitality to his policy of restoring pagan worship throughout the Empire. The shrine's rural location probably also helped to preserve it from destruction by zealous Christians, but above all it must have been the strong appeal of healer gods, which the Christians found so difficult to break, that ensured its survival.

Elsewhere at this time the fortunes of healing shrines were variable. At Pergamum the Asklepieion was destroyed and not rebuilt after an earthquake sometime between AD 253 and 260. At Epidauros, on the other hand, new altars were dedicated, and the sanctuary continued to function down to the time of Julian. Thereafter, however, decline was rapid and may have been accelerated by deliberate destruction at the hands of Christians. Certainly, the Asklepieion at Aigai, Cilicia, was razed to the ground at the command of the newly converted emperor Constantine and

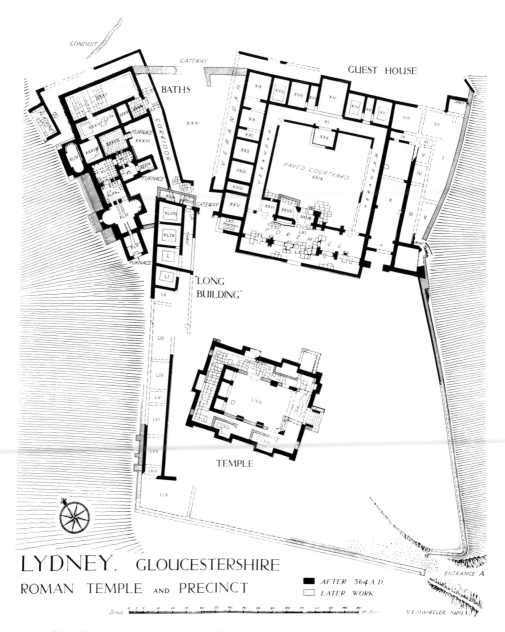

45 Plan of the precinct and temple of Nodens at Lydney Park, England. 4th century AD.

remained a ruin despite Julian's efforts to have it rebuilt.[68] Ironically, it was the very similarity between certain aspects of Christianity and the Asklepios cult that put the two faiths in direct conflict and resulted, ultimately, in the eradication of Asklepios. Despite the fact that many of the Asklepian rituals and precepts ante-dated their adoption by Christian groups, they were nonetheless considered as blasphemous parodies. Most notable among them, and the cause of the greatest rancour, was the role of Asklepios as a physician and wondrous healer of diseases, a saviour, as he was often addressed, for here, superficially at least, the deeds of Christ were especially closely paralleled. Even though Christians sought to discredit Asklepios by claiming that he was an evil spirit, 'who does not cure souls but destroys them', they found that people were loath to forego his emotive powers. A saviour of souls was all very well, but a saviour of the body had a more tangible reward on offer. Thus Eusebius, describing the destruction of the Aigai sanctuary, complained that Asklepios was attracting many people away from 'the true saviour'.[69] It was the attractive power of Asklepios, not just blasphemy, that occasioned the fear and hostility of Christians.

Although 'exterminated' by the authorities, Asklepios and some other healing deities survived in restricted areas of the Roman Empire where their worshippers, if hardly tolerated, were at least not persecuted. Some Christians must have sensed that a pragmatic approach to these mild pagan deities was more likely to succeed than methods of violence and destruction. In the end they were right, but Asklepios, the founder of medicine, divine healer and patron of doctors, had survived as long as any other of the pagan divinities of Greece and Rome. Furthermore, his influence, as that of other divine healers, was not entirely eclipsed. Churches rose from the ruins of many Asklepieia, including Epidauros, Corinth and Rome, and some assumed the healing mantle left by their pagan precursor. At Athens, for example, a large Christian basilica, built in the fifth or sixth century AD on the foundations of the demolished Asklepieion, was dedicated to the memory of the doctor saints.[70] Certainly, people still had the desire to ward off or seek relief from disease, only now invocation was made to patron saints instead of pagan deities. Just as the pagan medical writings were not entirely excluded by Christian physicians, the powers of the Greek and Roman healing deities were assimilated to saints of the Christian church. Similarly, the dedication of anatomical ex-votos fulfilled a very basic and deep-seated human need, and the Greek and Roman examples have their counterpart in the miniature metal plaques and wax models of afflicted body parts still to be found in churches in Greece, Italy and other Mediterranean countries.

Chapter 7

Dying and death

At the feet of the god Asklepios was sometimes shown a curious dwarf- or child-like figure enveloped in a hooded cloak. This was Telesphorus, god of convalescence, whose powers complemented and logically extended those of the other Asklepian healer deities. Convalescence was considered an integral and important aspect of healing, especially by the Methodists, and, as already seen, this was reflected in the regimens recommended by Asclepiades and Soranus. Celsus, who admired Asclepiades' methods, also underlined the importance of convalescence, no matter how slight the disease.[1] He stipulated that residence and climate as well as diet should be changed often, a requirement that would have caused little hardship for the wealthy, who frequently owned properties in several different regions. The Younger Pliny, attentive to the needs of his wife, despatched her to Campania to recuperate from illness, while on several occasions he rested at his country estates to regain health himself.[2] The rich and moderately wealthy also convalesced at famous healing shrines and mineral springs, the sanatoria and health resorts of antiquity, but the poor were unlikely to have travelled further afield than their local shrine or town baths.

Comparatively few diseases were curable, however, and many people suffered debilitating and painful afflictions, even those like the emperor Marcus Aurelius, who commanded the services of the top physicians of his day. He suffered from chest pains which he tried to conquer through Stoicism:

> pain is neither unbearable nor unending, so long as you remember its limitations and don't add to it with your imagination . . . what we cannot bear takes us away [from life]; what lasts can be borne . . . Pain in the hand or foot is not against nature, provided that the foot and hand are fulfilling their own tasks. (Marcus Aurelius, *Meditations* 7, 64; 7, 33; 6, 33, trans. in Birley 1966, 295)

Nevertheless, any drug that would alleviate pain was readily accepted, and Marcus Aurelius found some relief in the *theriac* that Galen prescribed for him. This was the universal antidote, similar in composition to *mithridatium*, whose most powerful but addictive ingredient was opium. More drastic was the treatment resorted to by a wealthy Roman, Servius Clodius, who 'owing to the severe pain of gout, was forced to rub his legs all over with a poison, after which that part of his body was as free from sensation as it was from pain.'[3] Pain and despair drove some to suicide, especially those suffering from diseases of the head, stomach or bladder,[4] telling evidence, indeed, for the many shortcomings of medical treatment. The prevalence of suicide as a means of resolving disease is evident from one of the letters of the Younger Pliny, in which he noted as unusual not suicide on account of incurable illness, but the case of a man, Titius Aristo, who determined to endure his suffering:

His patience throughout this illness, if you could only see it, would fill you with admiration; he fights against pain, resists thirst, and endures the unbelievable heat of his fever without moving or throwing off his coverings. A few days ago he sent for me and some of his intimate friends, and told us to ask the doctors what the outcome of his illness would be, so that if it was to be fatal he could deliberately put an end to his life, though he would carry on with the struggle if it was only to be long and painful; he owed it to his wife's prayers and his daughter's tears, and to us, his friends, not to betray our hopes by a self-inflicted death

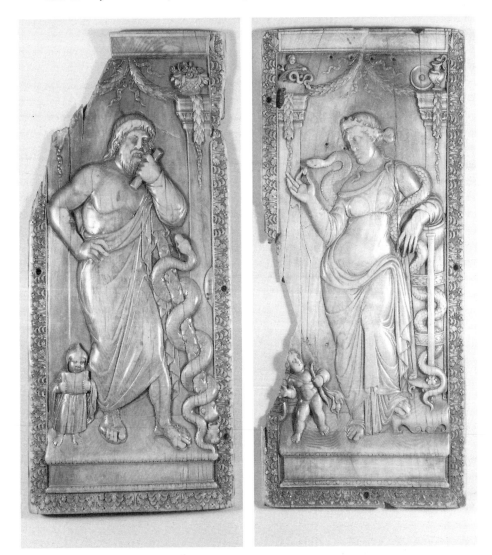

46 Asklepios and Hygieia carved in late Roman style on a ceremonial ivory *diptych*. The tiny god of convalescence, Telesphorus, stands at the foot of Asklepios reading from a scroll. From Rome, *c*. AD 400. Height 31.4 cm.

so long as these hopes were not vain. This I think was a particularly difficult decision to make, which merits the highest praise. Many people have his impulse and urge to forestall death, but the ability to examine critically the arguments for dying, and to accept or reject the idea of living or not, is the mark of a truly great mind. (*Letters* 1, 22; trans. B. Radice)

As indicated by the provision at Epidauros of a building specifically to accommodate the dying, some of those with chronic or terminal illnesses sought the relative tranquillity of healing shrines to end their days. Others were attracted to the enervating atmosphere of spas, like Julius Vitalis and Gaius Murrius Modestus, two legionary soldiers who died at Bath aged just twenty-nine and twenty-five years respectively.[5] They were probably casualties of wounds or infection which even the curative powers of Sulis Minerva and her springs could not heal.

Vitruvius specifically recommended the choice of salubrious sites for healing shrines, remarking that a healthy atmosphere and hygienic facilities would assist the recovery of the sick and hence glorify the deity.[6] At times of epidemic disease both spas and healing sanctuaries must have been especially popular, for a natural reaction to 'pestilence' was to get away from the centre of the outbreak. Celsus, for example, in describing the 'observances necessary for a healthy man to employ during a pestilence',[7] recommended a voyage or a trip abroad. This was not considered vital, however, and most of his precautions concerned regimen which was to be especially carefully monitored. For it was generally believed that infections were spread by 'bad air' and could be avoided by those who maintained a healthy state.

As we have seen, Greek and Roman medical researchers had little concept of diseases as separate and active entities. Although it had been observed that certain diseases, like phthisis (pulmonary tuberculosis), psora (scabies), and lippitudo (ophthalmia) were communicable, this effect was normally attributed to the transmission of exhaled putrid air, of exuded substances or of *pneuma* charged with noxious rays. However, some medical writers, including Galen, experimented with the hypothesis of 'seeds of disease', a slightly more tangible concept of contagion than 'bad air'.[8] The theory harks back to the doctrine of Anaxagoras (p. 18), who used 'seeds' as a metaphor for the substance of creation. Minute 'seeds', both good and bad, were thought to circulate freely in the atmosphere, where their conjunction occasionally caused the air to putrefy. Illness was caused by the 'bad seeds' themselves, by exposure to the putrid air, or by the consumption of food or water contaminated by it, and those at greatest risk were the undernourished or the over-indulged, whose bodily equilibrium was out of balance. Galen also suggested that 'bad seeds' could enter the body and lie dormant until some outside stimulus activated them. In these ways the uneven susceptibility of individuals to disease could be explained.

Although this was potentially a more sophisticated disease theory than 'putrid air' it was no more capable of proof, for each depended on causative matter that was effectively invisible. Galen himself was generally reluctant to indulge in theoretical investigations that could not be substantiated by practical research, and he seems never to have wholeheartedly espoused the 'seeds of disease' theory. Nor, too, did it have much relevance to the practising physician, who had no chance of eliminating agents of disease that he could not even see.

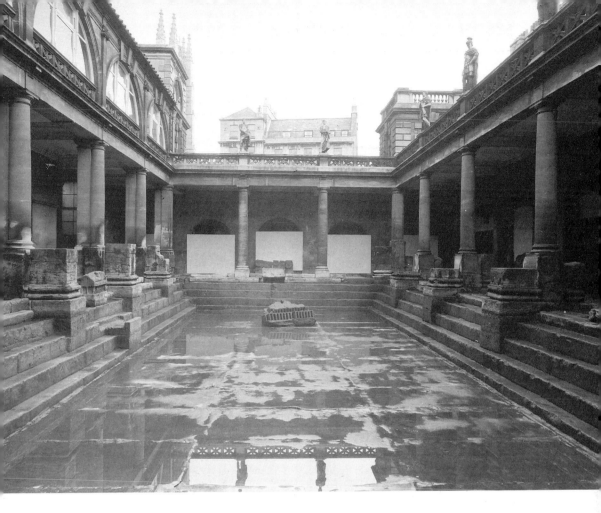

47 The Great Bath at Bath. In Roman times the bath was enclosed, and the bases
of the piers which supported the massive roof are visible beneath and next to
the modern columns. Temporarily drained of its hot spring water, the stepped
seating around the edges of the pool is fully revealed.

Galen would certainly have had some incentive to consider contagion and its
causes, for at the time that he was speculating on 'seeds of disease' one of the most
severe epidemics of antiquity was ravaging the countries around the Mediterranean.
It arrived in AD 165/6; Aelius Aristides seems to have contracted it in that year but
recovered; Galen left Rome hurriedly the following year and avoided it; and Marcus
Aurelius, over most of whose reign it cast its shadow, was still troubled by it on
his death bed in AD 180. Although by ancient standards it was well documented,
the descriptions are still insufficient to identify it certainly with any modern disease,
and, indeed, it may well have comprised several different infections including smallpox, or a disease ancestral to it.[9] This was by no means the first Roman epidemic
– Livy records many outbreaks of pestilence in Republican times. Nor was it necessarily
the most virulent: 30,000 people were said to have died in an epidemic in Rome
in the autumn of AD 65, while the pestilence that broke out around AD 189 commonly
took the lives of 2,000 people a day in Rome.[10] It was, however, unusually protracted
and widespread, and had considerable repercussions. It was first caught by the Roman

army involved in the Parthian Wars in Mesopotamia, and Lucius Verus' return with the infected troops spread the disease widely and brought it to the very heart of the Empire. The death rate was high, especially in army barracks and the crowded quarters of Rome, and it is not difficult to imagine the fear and hysteria it caused.

The plague was rumoured to have started when a soldier broke open a casket in the temple of Apollo at Seleuceia, unwittingly releasing the dread vapour that it contained, a story with an obvious affinity to the legend of Pandora's Box. Many people believed it to be divine retribution for the sack of Seleuceia in violation of an agreement. To try to allay the fears engendered by such stories Marcus Aurelius instituted in AD 167 in Rome a succession of religious ceremonies comprising both traditional Roman and foreign purificatory rites. The plague continued unabated, however. Such was the scale of mortality that space ran short in cemeteries, and new edicts were issued to prevent the unlawful appropriation of existing graves.[11]

The disease remained epidemic for at least fifteen years, breaking out afresh as it was transmitted from one part of the Empire to another, and even returning to places that had already suffered it. 'From the frontiers of the Persians as far as to the Rhine and Gaul the foul touch of plague polluted everything with contagion and death,' wrote the historian Ammianus Marcellinus,[12] while Orosius chronicled its effect still more graphically: 'Such great pestilence devastated all Italy that everywhere estates, fields, and towns were left deserted, without cultivators or inhabitants, and relapsed into ruins and woodland.'[13]

Both accounts have to be used with caution, however, for their authors were recording an event that had taken place several centuries before their time, and, as a Christian, Orosius may have had cause to exaggerate this pagan catastrophe. Neither the disease itself nor its demographic consequences are known with any degree of precision, for the contemporary sources are not sufficiently specific. If, as seems likely, the disease was new to the Mediterranean region, then by analogy with more recent and better recorded examples of the effect of epidemic diseases on 'virgin' populations it may be assumed that mortality was high, though not even. Some communities would have survived relatively unscathed, but others, especially those concentrated in towns or dependent upon them, may have suffered losses of 25 per cent or more.[14]

More surprising than the deficient descriptions of lay writers is Galen's sparing and disappointingly uninformative account. Although he refers to it as a great plague and one which persisted for a long time, his references to it are scattered and brief.[15] Shortly after his departure from Rome he was recalled to serve as court physician, and Marcus Aurelius persuaded him to join the imperial staff at Aquileia, where an army had been assembled for the launch of an offensive in the following spring. The concentration of soldiers in this already populous coastal city had proved to be particularly fertile ground for the ever-present plague. Yet Galen's descriptions of the epidemic and its victims lack precision and they have defied attempts at a conclusive modern diagnosis. Although he noted epidemic outbreaks of fever together with pustules, his humoral system rendered such symptoms of secondary importance and they received scant attention. Indeed, far from concentrating on the skin rash, Galen was more concerned with the spitting of blood from which he diagnosed the disease as an abscess of the lungs.[16]

This, the so-called 'Antonine plague', is but one of the more celebrated of ancient epidemics. Just as many others preceded it, there were many others, too, that followed, including another protracted outbreak, seemingly still more devastating, in AD 251–66. At the height of that epidemic it was reported that 5,000 people a day were dying in Rome alone. Rural communities were not unaffected, but towns must have fared particularly badly, above all the cosmopolitan centres of the Empire, with their close-packed and often unsanitary housing. Still more at risk were the Mediterranean ports and coastal towns, which probably bore the brunt of another epidemic in AD 542–3. Known as the 'plague of Justinian', this has been identified as bubonic plague, *Pasteurella pestis*, spread in the main by the black rat.[17] If this diagnosis is correct, it may have been the first appearance of the disease in the Mediterranean region. At all events, it was of lethal effect and catastrophic proportions, and it ushered in a succession of pestilences and epidemics which raged intermittently for the next two centuries. Justinian himself caught the disease and was fortunate to recover, for in Constantinople, where it lasted four months, it is reported that in its early stages it claimed the lives of 10,000 people daily.[18]

As the causes of these epidemics were unknown there was no effective protection, even for those wealthy enough to retain a bevy of physicians, and the casualties included people from all walks of life, slaves and free, soldiers and officers, artisans and town councillors, farm-workers and government officials alike. Depopulation, whatever the real scale, together with the instability created by fear of the disease and the diversion of resources into coping with its consequences, must have been a contributory factor to the gradual economic decay of towns and of the Roman administrative system of which they were a key component.

The epidemic diseases, however, that had such a dramatic and obvious effect, were only a part, and probably a small part, of the range of human suffering in antiquity. Other acute conditions, together with the majority of chronic diseases, like osteoarthrosis (often known as osteoarthritis), were seldom of sufficient interest to non-medical writers to merit attention. Even the descriptions in medical works seldom provide the quantity and quality of information desired, yet these were painful, debilitating, often crippling diseases, which were far more significant than plagues to the majority of the population. Fortunately, chronic diseases, wounds and injuries can frequently be diagnosed from observed skeletal changes. Medical historians have therefore turned to the human remains, most commonly cremations and inhumations, in their quest for further evidence of ancient diseases. When subjected to the scrutiny of osteo-archaeologists, radiographers, radiologists, physical anthropologists and other specialists, such remains can shed light on the individual's sex, age, stature, racial origins and health: in a curious inversion the bodies of the dead can provide invaluable information on the health of the living.

The studies of early populations (palaeodemography) and ancient diseases (palaeopathology) are still in their infancy, and existing techniques are constantly being improved and new ones developed. Osteo-archaeology especially is time-consuming, labour-intensive and costly, but as an investigation of the primary evidence it is a vital component of the study of disease in antiquity. Only by combining its results with those of microbiologists, epidemiologists, palaeodemographers, physical anthropologists and classical philologists will significant progress be made.

Although comparatively few large Roman cemeteries have yet been subjected to systematic and comprehensive study, the results are already intriguing for the light they shed both on the prevalence and spread of certain diseases and on the health and social conditions of ordinary people, the 'background noise' to historical accounts. Nevertheless, it should not be forgotten that while the bones are 'facts', the diseases extrapolated from them are seldom diagnosed with certainty, for they are normally arrived at by means of a series of inferences and conjectures which are open to specialist debate. Thus, for example, unequivocal evidence of congenital disease is seldom found, partly no doubt because gross abnormalities of the foetus would normally have resulted in spontaneous abortion, still birth or infanticide, but also because there is difficulty in interpreting skeletal defects of apparent congenital origin. Spina bifida is one malformation that has occasionally been identified, though only in its lesser form, spina bifida occulta. Unlike gross spina bifida, which is normally associated with a severe defect of the central nervous system, exposure of the spinal cord and consequent infection, spina bifida occulta is comparatively insignificant. It involves a defect in the bony spinal canal whereby the vertebrae do not fully encircle the spinal cord, although protection is still afforded by cartilage or membrane; twelve individuals from the cemeteries at York and Cirencester who had spina bifida vertebral defects were probably neither incapacitated by their condition, nor even aware of it.[19]

Achondroplasia, dwarfism, an inherited condition characterised by arrested growth of the long bones, probably had a rather higher incidence than today because of the intermarriage of closely related males and females in remote villages and small towns. Although few achondroplastic skeletons have been found, dwarfism was commonly shown in the art of the period, and Tiberius is but one of a number of Roman emperors known to have retained dwarfs in his entourage.[20]

Far more significant numerically were the degenerative diseases of advancing age. Given the tough and physically demanding life-styles of most working people and a mean age at death normally within the bracket 35–50 years, these affected most people from their thirties onwards. In fourth-century AD Roman Cirencester, for example, it appears that over 80 per cent of the adults would have suffered from osteoarthrosis, one of the most common identifiable diseases of the Roman world.[21] Often described as a 'wear and tear' disease, osteoarthrosis involves a progressive deterioration of the articular surfaces of the synovial (free-moving) joints through repeated trauma and over-use. A common result is the development of a flange of newly formed bone round the margin of the joint. Though not a direct cause of death, the most advanced stages can involve intense pain, gross deformity and, ultimately, immobility. Those worst affected could then have taken little active role in the life of the community, on whom they would have become an increasing burden. Pliny the Younger described the pitiful state of Domitius Tullus, an elderly invalid of his day:

> Crippled and deformed in every limb, he could only enjoy his vast wealth by contemplating it and could not even turn in bed without assistance. He also had to have his teeth cleaned and brushed for him – a squalid and pitiful detail – and when complaining about the humiliations of his infirmity was often heard to say that every day he licked the fingers of his slaves. (*Letters* 8, 18; trans. B. Radice)

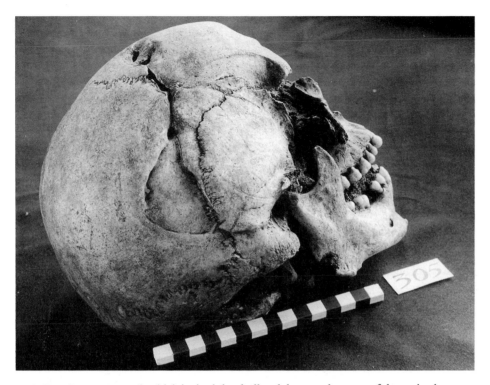

48 Despite a severe gash which incised the skull and depressed an area of the parietal
bone this man survived his injuries. However, the depressed bone probably caused
pressure on the brain, and an elliptical hole at the top of the skull may be a
trephination performed to relieve the symptoms of this pressure. Inhumation 305,
Bath Gate Romano-British cemetery, Cirencester, 4th century AD.

For the family of the wealthy Tullus this was distressing, but for those at subsistence
level such disability could have caused severe, perhaps intolerable hardship.

The occurrence of osteoarthrosis in particular joints reflects the uneven stresses
and strains to which the body was subject, and these in turn may reveal the activities
and occupations undertaken by different individuals. Thus at Cirencester, where spinal
arthrosis was both common and almost undifferentiated by sex, it would seem that
women as well as men commonly undertook 'back-breaking' work such as digging,
hoeing or carrying heavy burdens.[22] Another common arthrotic site is the temporoman-
dibular joint, reflecting both the toughness of the diet and the common use of the
teeth as a 'third hand' or as a substitute for an injured or diseased hand.

Osteoarthrosis was not restricted to any one region of the Empire, and it may
have been responsible for many of the hand and foot votives dedicated at healing
shrines. Certainly, joint disorders and pains were commonly referred to by medical
writers,[23] although some of these descriptions were of a more specific joint disease:
gout. Although this condition was apparently known to physicians at least as early
as the first century AD,[24] it was not always differentiated in the medical literature.
Thus Celsus seems to have used the terms *podagra* and *cheiragra* to describe any

177

pain in the feet and hands and their joints. True gout is due to a metabolic disorder caused by an excess of uric acid in the blood. This results in the deposition of urate crystals in the joint tissues, which gradually degenerate with consequent destruction of the joint surfaces. The victim experiences swelling, inflammation, pain and, frequently, restricted use of the hands and feet.

The traditional association of gout with the regular and excessive consumption of port has some foundation, for it seems to have been one of a range of diseases caused by the ingestion of lead-adulterated wines. Both in the Roman period and the more recent past concentrated wine syrups (*sapa*) prepared in lead containers were used to preserve and improve the flavour of wines, and their toxicity would often have been sufficient to cause kidney failure, leading to an increase in the level of uric acid in the blood.[25] Pliny and Galen described a new form of *podagra* which had become prevalent in their time and which they believed was inheritable and attributable to the consumption of luxury food and drink.[26] Lucian, too, considered gout one of the curses of the rich who had no self-discipline,[27] while the Younger Pliny more sympathetically recorded the case of a friend, Corellius Rufus, who suffered from gout for many years:

> At the age of thirty-two, I have heard him say, he developed gout in the feet, just as his father had done; for like other characteristics, most diseases are hereditary. As long as he was young and active he could keep it under control by temperate living and strict continence, and latterly when he grew worse with advancing age, he bore up through sheer strength of mind, even when cruelly tortured by unbelievable agony; for the disease was now no longer confined to his feet as before, but was spreading through all his limbs. (*Letters* 1, 12; trans. B. Radice)

The doctors who attended him were clearly unable to provide effective treatment and, eventually, unwilling to endure the pain any longer, Rufus starved himself to death. If we are to believe the account of Diophantus, a temple attendant, he fared rather better by seeking divine aid:

> I, a beloved temple attendant, say these things to you, Asclepius, son of Leto's child. How shall I come to your golden abode, O blessed longed-for, divine head, since I do not have the feet with which I formerly came to the shrine, unless by healing me you graciously wish to lead me there again so that I may look upon you, my god, brighter than the earth in springtime.
>
> So I, Diophantus, pray you, save me, most powerful and blessed one, by healing my painful gout: in the name of your father, to whom I offer earnest prayer. For no mortal man may give release from such sufferings. Only you, blessed divine one, have the power. For the gods who are eminent above all gave you to mortal men as a great gift, the compassionate one, the deliverance from sufferings.
>
> Thrice-blessed Paeon Asclepius, by your skill Diophantus was healed of his painful incurable ailment; no longer does he appear crab-footed nor as if walking on cruel thorns, but sound of foot, just as you promised. (*IG* II[2], 4514; trans. in Edelstein 1945, I, 241–2)

More prosaic was Celsus' treatment, which included blood-letting, diuretics, emetics, hot fomentations, refrigerants and repressants. In periods of remission he recommended gentle exercise and spare diet, and he also observed, significantly, that 'some have obtained lifelong security by refraining from wine, mead and venery for a whole year'.[28]

Although gout or gout-like afflictions feature prominently in the classical literature, few indisputable cases have been discerned by palaeopathologists. The most celebrated example is an Egyptian mummy of an elderly man of the Coptic period, from Philae on the Nile.[29] Recently, however, three more cases were identified in male skeletons from the Cirencester cemetery. One of these men must have been sorely troubled, for the lesions were widespread and advanced, affecting most of the bones and joints in the feet and others in the hands, ulnae, radii, patellae and tibiae.[30]

The degenerative diseases were common and troublesome, and the epidemics terrifying though sporadic, but the real killers of antiquity were the infectious diseases. Most viruses and bacteria affect primarily the soft tissues of the body, and if such infections as appendicitis, meningitis and pneumonia are not rapidly and effectively treated, death will usually occur before the infection spreads to the bone. These and other acute infections, therefore, pass completely undetected in the skeletal remains. They are an invisible and practically unquantifiable component of ancient mortality. Diphtheria, for example, which may equate with a disease described by Aretaeus of Cappadocia, has never been discerned osteologically, and its early history remains obscure. A similar uncertainty surrounds the origins and prevalence of typhus, an acute disease of war, famine and catastrophe, whose infecting organism is spread by fleas, lice or ticks. Typhus must have been a frequent and unwelcome visitor, and it may have caused the plague that struck Piraeus and Athens in the second

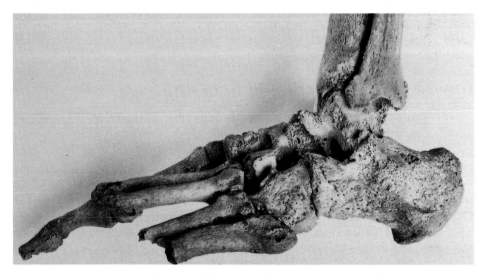

49 Gout in Roman Britain. The left foot of inhumation 42 from the Romano-British cemetery at Bath Gate, Cirencester, showing the extensive destruction of joint surfaces characteristic of gout. 4th century AD.

year of the Peloponnesian War (430–429 BC) and destroyed about a quarter of the Athenian land army.[31]

Of more restricted significance but horrifying in its effect was tetanus. Although osteologically invisible, its symptoms are so extreme that the disease has been recognised in a number of written accounts. In the Hippocratic Corpus the references to fatal convulsions after wounds and injuries probably signify tetanus, while an unequivocal account was given by Aretaeus of Cappadocia. He graphically characterised the convulsions which 'arch the patient's back like a drawn bow and drag his head between his shoulder blades. An inhuman calamity! a spectacle agonising even to the beholder; a malady beyond all cure!'[32]

Some infections, however, have a less speedy resolution and may leave their mark on bones. One such is poliomyelitis, a virus infection of the central nervous system, most commonly contracted in childhood. The clinical manifestation is usually paralysis of one or more muscle groups, resulting in muscle-wasting and limb atrophy, and retrospective diagnoses on ancient skeletons tend to be made on the evidence of unequal bone growth of opposite limbs. This type of deformity has several other potential causes, including difficult delivery, and certainty is seldom possible. However, four skeletons from the Cirencester cemetery which display unilateral atrophy of the arm bones are thought to have been polio victims,[33] while a built-up shoe found at Vindonissa may have been made for another sufferer.

Those bacterial infections of bone that cannot be differentiated by the traces they have left on skeletons, the non-specific infections, are normally termed periostitis, osteitis or osteomyelitis, according to their severity. There are many potential causes including secondary infection, via the blood, from septicaemia in another part of the body. Such diseases, especially prevalent in poor living conditions, would have been extremely serious, and few would have recovered from the accompanying fever. Another mode of infection is through serious injuries or wounds which, without proper treatment, may ultimately erode underlying tissue and bone, and there are several examples of such chronic lesions on skeletons from the York and Cirencester cemeteries.[34] While some of the York burials may have been those of soldiers, the great majority of burials at Cirencester must have been of civilians, and the surprisingly large number of weapon wounds and fractures of aggression are an indicator of the violence and danger that were often faced (48).

A few specific chronic infections can occasionally be discerned in the skeletal remains, including pulmonary tuberculosis and leprosy. Pulmonary infections are a particular hazard of towns or other population aggregates if there is a high proportion of densely occupied, poorly ventilated and unhygienic housing. Thus phthisis, pulmonary tuberculosis, was one of the scourges of the poorer sections of the urban societies of Greece and Rome.[35] As it is a lingering disease with a long infectious phase, it can remain highly endemic even in dispersed groups who have only occasional contact with population centres. The bacilli are transmitted directly from one person to another, either exhaled in coughing or excreted in sputum, and the primary site of infection is the lung. It is often contracted in childhood, and many of those who did not develop an immunity would have suffered chronic ill health, a distressing cough, pain and emaciation. Celsus described phthisis as the most dangerous of the 'wasting diseases':

The malady usually arises in the head, thence it drips into the lung; there ulceration supervenes, from this a slight feverishness is produced, which even after it has become quiescent nevertheless returns; there is frequent cough, pus is expectorated, sometimes blood-stained. When the sputum is thrown upon a fire, there is a bad odour, hence those who are in doubt as to the disease employ this as a test. (*De Medicina* III, 22, 3; trans. W. G. Spencer)

More comprehensive descriptions were given by Soranus and by Aretaeus of Cappadocia, and most other Hellenistic and Roman medical writers made mention of it as a universally known, common and serious, though not necessarily mortal disease.[36]

Few famous figures are known to have died from tuberculosis, partly, perhaps, because mortality would have been highest amongst the young, but possibly, too, because the disease was to an extent class specific. Tuberculosis has been tentatively diagnosed as the cause of death of L. Minikios Anthimianos, a four-year-old child from Smyrna. The sad account of the course of his disease, given in the inscription on his tombstone, describes the vain attempts made by his father, apparently a physician, and his father's friends to save him.[37] Not surprisingly, it was one of the afflictions that Asklepios was called upon to heal, and one thankful devotee, Thersandrus of Halieis, left record of his miraculous cure at Epidauros.[38] In fact a salubrious climate and carefully chosen diet, which could often have been provided at healing sanctuaries, would probably have comprised the best available treatment. Alternatively, many medical writers recommended the change of air that a sea voyage could bring. Celsus especially favoured the voyage from Italy to Alexandria, where the climate was 'denser',[39] and it was to Egypt that the Younger Pliny sent his freedman reader Zosimus:

Some years ago he was exerting himself during a passionate performance when he began to spit blood. I then sent him to Egypt, and after a long stay there he recently returned with his health restored. Now after demanding too much of his voice for several days on end he has had a slight return of his cough as a reminder of the old trouble, and once again has brought up blood. I think the thing to do is to send him to your place at Forum Julii, for I have often heard you say that the air is healthy there and the milk excellent for treating this kind of case. (*Letters* 5, 19; trans. B. Radice)

Tuberculosis commonly affects the lungs, liver, spleen and lymph nodes, but seldom spreads to the bones, and the disease must have been many times more destructive than might appear from the osteo-archaeological record alone. Where bone infection does occur it is often at the knee- or hip-joint, but the most common location is the upper part of the vertebral column, and the angular distortion of the spine typical of this stage of the disease was probably the stimulus for some of the Egyptian and Graeco-Roman hunch-backed figurines (50). This tuberculous osteomyelitis of the spine, known as Potts' disease, can be difficult to differentiate from changes wrought by other infectious organisms, and although the disease can sometimes be identified with certainty, as in a skeleton from the Roman cemetery at Poundbury Camp, Dorchester, the diagnosis is often only tentative, as in the single possible occurrences at York and Cirencester. In any case it seems apparent that even systematic and detailed osteo-archaeological study will reveal 'only the tip of the tuberculosis iceberg of antiquity'.[40]

Of the same genus of bacteria as tuberculosis, *Mycobacterium*, is another chronic infective disease, leprosy, whose hideous mutilations have always inspired horror and fear. This reaction led to the shunning of those afflicted and their segregation into leper colonies and lazar houses. Yet it has been found that, unlike tuberculosis, leprosy has a low pathogenicity: although the bacterium is highly infective, it is often present in subclinical form and seldom induces clinical disease, even in those in close contact with lepers. The modern consensus is that it is probably a comparatively recent disease in man, perhaps going back no further than the Neolithic period. From literary references it has been inferred that leprosy was present in China in the first millennium BC, and it has been suggested that Alexander's returning armies carried it from the Indo-Gangetic Basin to the Mediterranean region in 327–326 BC.[41] However, the earliest osteological evidence comprises four leprous skulls from a Ptolemaic cemetery at the Dakhleh Oasis, Egypt, of the second century BC.[42] Certainly, leprosy, though not unknown, appears to have been still of limited extent in the first century AD.

The disease normally identified as leprosy in the classical medical literature

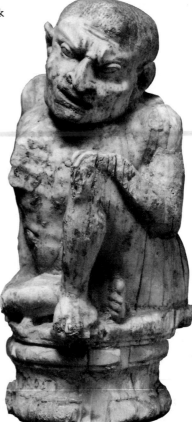

50 Ivory figurine showing a negro man with Pott's disease. The hunch-back deformity, the asymmetric 'pigeon-chest' and the careworn expression are all skilfully captured. Greek, possibly from Italy, 1st century AD.

is elephantiasis, but this term may sometimes also have been used less specifically to describe a number of other serious disfiguring skin complaints, such as psoriasis. Pliny remarked that elephantiasis was native to Egypt, that it did not occur in Italy before the time of Pompey, and that it 'quickly died out in Italy'.[43] Celsus also believed it to be almost unknown in Italy:

> The disease which the Greeks call elephantiasis, whilst almost unknown in Italy, is of very frequent occurrence in certain regions; it is counted among chronic affections; in this the whole body becomes so affected that even the bones are said to become diseased. The surface of the body presents a multiplicity of spots and swellings, which, at first red, are gradually changed to be black in colour. The skin is thickened and thinned in an irregular way, hardened and softened, roughened in some places with a kind of scales; the trunk wastes, the face, calves and feet swell. When the disease is of long standing, the fingers and toes are sunk under the swelling. (Celsus, *De Medicina* III, 25, 1–2; trans. W. G. Spencer)

Celsus' description is probably of the most severe form of leprosy, which afflicts people with a low disease resistance and causes nerve impairment, skin change and bone erosion. Bacterial invasion of the nerves beneath the skin and small blood vessels causes skin irregularities, localised loss of sensation, and disturbed blood circulation; the tissues of the face, nose and eyes are commonly affected, resulting in loss of facial hair, inflammation, ulceration, erosion of bone in and around the nose, loss of the upper central teeth, and even blindness; infection of the larynx causes a characteristically hoarse voice; ulcers form on the hands and feet, and the fingers and toes are progressively lost through gangrene.[44]

Despite its low pathogenicity leprosy may be spread widely because of its long period of incubation. After contracting the disease it can take as long as ten years for the characteristic symptoms and physical features to develop. Meanwhile the victim, unaware of his condition, might introduce the infection to many new communities. The increased mobility that became possible under the Roman Empire gave considerable potential for the spread of leprosy, and it was probably at this time that the disease reached northern Europe, where the earliest evidence to date has been found in the Poundbury Camp cemetery.[45] There it has been diagnosed in the remains of a mature adult, buried at the very end of the period of Roman rule, around the year AD 400. Unfortunately, the upper part of the skeleton was missing, but the tibiae, fibulae and feet all display pathological changes characteristic of the disease. Destruction of the toes and bones of the feet was advanced, and deformity must also have extended to the face, especially the upper jaw, palate and nose. There can be little doubt that well before death the individual and those with whom he came into contact would have been only too aware of his affliction, even if they did not know what it was. It is interesting to note, therefore, that the body was buried alongside many hundreds of other apparently non-leprous skeletons in a Christian cemetery. The status and origins of this person are unknown, but the implication is that ostracism of lepers, the barbaric custom that became so prevalent in medieval Europe, had not taken effect in late Roman Britain, or, at least, that segregation in life was not extended to death.

Leprosy, which appears to have had a fairly restricted effect in the Roman period, spread rapidly and widely in the medieval period only to decline just as rapidly in many parts of Western Europe in the later Middle Ages. This phenomenon cannot be explained as a result of effective treatment, for none existed. Instead, it appears that in some complex manner its fluctuations are connected with those of tuberculosis. There is a degree of cross-immunity between these two diseases, and it has been suggested that the tuberculosis bacillus might normally take precedence over that of leprosy.[46] If so, then an explanation is offered for the low level of leprosy in the urban societies of Greece and Rome and its virtual elimination from the growing towns of later medieval Europe, in which pulmonary tuberculosis was such a significant disease. The related socio-economic implications are evident: urbanisation fostered the rise of tuberculosis, which largely excluded leprosy. Such a crude simplification, however, belies the complexities involved, and there are few certainties in the study of evolutionary epidemiology. Bacterial and viral diseases in particular are subject to change over time, and it is seldom possible to make a simple equation between an ancient disease and a modern one.

A particularly vexed question is that concerning the origin and spread of syphilis. Venereal syphilis is but one of a number of diseases caused by bacteria of the genus *Treponema*, the others being pinta, yaws and endemic syphilis.[47] All are exclusively human diseases transmitted directly from one person to another, and all except pinta may ultimately cause bone changes which are very similar in appearance. However, while pinta, yaws and endemic syphilis are usually contracted in childhood by bodily contact which need not involve the sexual organs, venereal syphilis is specifically a disease of adulthood acquired through sexual intercourse with an infected person. Venereal syphilis is the most severe of the four 'species', and it is the only one which can be passed from a mother to her unborn child. By the nature of its mode of transmission many saw venereal syphilis as retribution for those who indulged in 'pleasures of the flesh'. It has generally been regarded as a socially unacceptable disease and it has often provoked self-righteous condemnation. Inevitably, such views have influenced interpretations of the evidence for its extent and prevalence in the past. In fact, the osteological evidence is extremely sparse before the sixteenth century AD, and written accounts of all periods are tantalising and confused.[48] Genital ulcers, mentioned not infrequently in Greek and Roman lay and medical texts, may sometimes suggest the final stage of syphilis, but the cases are never described in sufficient detail to permit a sound diagnosis:

> I was sailing on our Lake Como with an elderly friend when he pointed out a house with a bedroom built out over the lake. 'From there,' he said, 'a woman of our town once threw herself with her husband.' I asked why. The husband had long been suffering from ulcers in the private parts, and his wife insisted on seeing them, promising that no one would give him a more candid opinion whether the disease was curable. She saw that there was no hope and urged him to take his life; she went with him, even led him to his death herself, and forced him to follow her example by roping herself to him and jumping into the lake. (Pliny the Younger, *Letters* 6, 24; trans. B. Radice)

The Younger Pliny related this poignant episode as an example of female courage, and the medical condition, peripheral to his story, received scant attention. Although some have diagnosed syphilis, uro-genital tuberculosis is perhaps more likely, but neither is capable of proof.[49]

Despite such imprecise literary sources and the negative evidence from the examination of many thousands of skeletons,[50] it is likely, according to modern pathological theory, that venereal syphilis, as well as certain other venereal diseases, was present in the populations of Greece and Rome, though not necessarily in the form that it takes today. However, until definite osteological evidence is found the question must remain open.

This brief survey of palaeopathology provides some indication of the wide range of ailments and abnormalities that beset the people of the ancient world. In their unequal struggle against disease the Roman physician and his patients faced thousands of potential killers, and they had to come to terms with the fact that it was quite outside their scope to prevent or contain many of them. The fervent prayers for divine intervention, and the dedication of votives at healing temples were a natural response. Tombstones, literary sources and the skeletons themselves, however, demonstrate how frequently such hope was in vain, and from the very outset of his career the physician must quickly have become accustomed to attending those in the throes of death.[51] Celsus succinctly summarised the facial signs that presaged imminent death:

> that the last stage has now been reached is indicated by the nose becoming pointed, the temples sunken, the eyes hollowed, the ears cold and flaccid with the tips drooping slightly, the skin of the forehead hard and tight: the aspect is dusky or very pallid, and much more so when there has been no preceding insomnia, nor diarrhoea, nor loss of appetite. From which causes these appearances at times arise, but only last one day: and so when they last longer death is indicated. (*De Medicina* II, 6, 1–3; trans. W. G. Spencer)

This syndrome of symptoms had long been recognised, and Celsus' description was derived from the account at the beginning of the Hippocratic treatise *Prognosis*. Still today the description of the signs of approaching death is known as the 'Hippocratic facies'.

Plagues and accidents apart, there is no doubt that socio-economic factors affected not just the quality of life but also its longevity. Thus in the wealthy circles, which included most of the classical authors, people not uncommonly attained the biblical 'three score years and ten', despite the 'diseases of luxury', while all the evidence from cemeteries serving 'working class' communities points to the rarity of people over the age of fifty years. Somewhere between these two social groupings were those who had sufficient means to leave provision for the erection of a tombstone, and analysis of the funerary inscriptions from the Roman province of Africa, for example, indicates that there of those who survived childhood, 28 per cent of women and 38 per cent of men reached the age of 62 years.[52]

Such approximate or restricted mortality figures should not obscure the fact that many of these people, whether long- or short-lived, suffered chronic and acute diseases which had a constant and direct effect upon their lives. The diseases of deficiency, which weakened the body and increased its susceptibility to other diseases, were the bane of the poor. Hunger, which was never far away, must have been a powerful determining factor in the course of their lives, while diseases which affected mobility, vision and, to a lesser extent, hearing must often have had disastrous consequences if they afflicted the main breadwinner of the family. While the rich, whose wealth was not dependent upon their health, might readily survive such personal crises, they were not immune to disease, and pain, with its reactions of anger, despair and distraction, must often have dictated their behaviour too. Upsetting at family level, this would have had much more serious implications for those in positions of power: reduced concentration and impaired judgement caused by pain and disease must often have resulted in hasty, flawed decisions by military officers, top officials, even the emperor himself.

In many instances physicians, even the most eminent, were unable to effect a cure or even ease suffering, especially in cases of mental illness, epidemic disease or serious internal injury. However, as we have seen, there were also signal achievements, notably in dietetics and surgery, and all was not gloom, at least not for those who received treatment of the kind advocated by writers like Galen, Soranus, Dioscorides and Celsus. In their works we find a sensible and sympathetic approach which was often truly scientific; we see a well-balanced attitude towards illness based on an awareness of the limitations of medical knowledge; and we note a genuine concern for the welfare of the patient. Certain general principles were to be followed, but the need is stressed for careful observation of each case so that the treatment could be adapted to new conditions or circumstances. A conscious effort was made to employ first the form of treatment which involved the patient in the least discomfort, and a cure was preferably to be sought by diet and regimen. Where drugs or surgery were necessary they were to be employed sparingly and precisely.

With these guiding principles Roman doctors could inspire hope and provide some relief for their patients, whether emperors or artisans, and there is little doubt that doctors as well as diseases had a very real influence on the course of Roman history.

Abbreviations and notes

Abbreviations

BHM	*Bulletin of the History of Medicine*
CIG	*Corpus inscriptionum Graecarum*
CIL	*Corpus inscriptionum Latinarum*
CMG	*Corpus medicorum Graecorum*
IG	*Inscriptiones Graecae*
JHM	*Journal of the History of Medicine and Allied Sciences*
K (e.g. IX 464K)	Kühn, C. G., ed., *Claudii Galeni Opera omnia* (Leipzig 1821–33; repr. Hildesheim 1964–5)

LCL	Loeb Classical Library
Med. Hist.	*Medical History*
RE	Pauly-Wissowa *Realencyclopädie der klassischen Altertumswissenschaft* (Stuttgart 1894 ff)
RIB	Collingwood, R. G. and Wright, R. P. *Roman Inscriptions in Britain* (Oxford 1965)
SHA	*Scriptores historiae Augustae*

1 Origins

1. Pliny, *Natural History* XXIX, viii, 18–21, trans. in N. Lewis and M. Reinhold (eds), *Roman civilization* (New York 1966), 314. Anti-medical sentiments were not exclusively Roman. Kudlien (1970, 99ff.) has noted similar attitudes in Greek literature. Furthermore, it is difficult to determine how typical was either Pliny's or Celsus' regard for medicine. At all events, as has been observed elsewhere (V. Nutton, 'Ammianus and Alexandria', *Clio Medica* 7 (1972), 173), it would be incautious to accept the views of any classical author as those of the entire educated class.
2. Pliny, *Nat. Hist.* XXIX, 7, 14, trans. in Rackham *et al.*; Plutarch, *Parallel Lives*, Cato Maior XXIII, 3–4; Kudlien 1970, 98ff.
3. Cato, *De Agri Cultura* ii, 7, trans. Hooper and Ash.
4. e.g. Cato, *De Agri Cultura* cxxvii. Spells and incantations also played a part in early Greek pharmacy. See e.g. H. D. Betz (ed.), *The Greek magical papyri in translation. Vol. 1: Texts* (Chicago 1986).
5. Homer, *Odyssey* XVII, 382–4.
6. Homer, *Iliad* XI, 514–15. On Homeric wounds see Majno 1975, 142ff.
7. Warren 1970, 372–5; R. Janko, 'Herbal remedies at Pylos', *Minos* 17 (1981), 30–34; Tzavella-Evjen 1983.
8. Homer, *Odyssey* IV, 219–34, trans. in Warren 1970, 373. For Egyptian medicinal substances see e.g. Ghalioungui 1973, esp. 139ff.
9. G. E. Smith, 'The most ancient splints', *British Medical Journal* 1 (1908), 732–7; Majno 1975, 73–5.
10. J. H. Breasted, *The Edwin Smith surgical papyrus* (Chicago 1930); Dawson 1953; Majno 1975, 72ff.; Ghalioungui 1973, 38–45.
11. B. Ebbell, *The Papyrus Ebers. The greatest Egyptian medical document* (Copenhagen 1937);

Dawson 1953; Majno 1975, 72ff.; Ghalioungui 1973, 33–5.
12. Herodotus II, 84, trans. A. D. Godley.
13. *Ibid.* II, 77. On disease theories see Ghalioungui 1973, 52ff.
14. Thivel 1981, 317ff.; Ghalioungui 1973, chapters 7–10.
15. Herodotus III, 125 and 129–37, trans. A. D. Godley.
16. 'Portraits' of Hippocrates: Barrow 1972. 'Biographies' of Hippocrates: J. R. Pinault, 'How Hippocrates cured the plague', *JHM* 41 (1986), 52–75.
17. Smith 1979.
18. Jones 1947; V. Langholf, 'Kallimachos, Komödie und hippokratische Frage', *Medizinhistorisches Journal* 21 (1986), 1–30.
19. Galen, *CMG* V 10, 2, 1, trans. in Smith 1979, 200.
20. Smith 1973; Lonie 1978; Thivel 1981, esp. 275–85 and 385–6; Di Benedetto 1986.
21. Grmek 1983, 150, 478.
22. Hippocrates, *Aphorisms* VII, 87, trans. Chadwick and Mann.
23. Hippocrates, *On Fractures* XIII, 39–52; *On Joints* LXXII; *Hippocrates*, trans. Jones and Withington, vol. III, 129, 373, 453; Majno 1975, Fig. 4.20; Di Benedetto 1986. On Hippocratic treatment and surgery: Majno 1975, 147ff.
24. Hippocrates, *The Oath*, trans. Chadwick and Mann.
25. Pliny, *Nat. Hist.* XXVI, 10.
26. F. Kudlien, 'Probleme um Diokles von Karystos', *Sudhoffs Archiv* 47 (1963), 456ff; W. Jaeger, *Diokles von Karystos* (Berlin 1938): Letter to Antigonus 70–113.
27. Michler 1968; Fraser 1972, chapter 7; Harris 1973, chapter 4; Lloyd 1973; 1975b; Potter 1976; Longrigg 1981; Smith 1982; Scarborough 1985a; von Staden 1975; and forthcoming.

28. Galen IX 464K. Praxagoras defined the pulse as a movement of the arteries. These, he believed, served as channels for *pneuma*, not blood. The *pneuma* was pumped into the arteries via the heart in the form of bubbles derived from blood in the veins. A rhythmic pulsation signified a healthy state, while an irregular pulse signified an interrupted flow of *pneuma* bubbles, caused by a contamination of the blood by morbid humours, hence ill health. *RE* XXII 2 (1954), 1735–43; F. Steckerl, 'The fragments of Praxagoras of Cos and his school', *Philosophia Antiqua VIII* (Leiden 1958), esp. 19–36; J. Longrigg, 'Praxagoras', *Dictionary of scientific biography* 11 (New York 1975), 127–8.

29. Celsus, *De Med.* Prooemium, 74, trans. W. G. Spencer; von Staden 1975, 178ff; Scarborough 1976; G. B. Ferngren, 'A Roman declamation on vivisection', *Transactions and Studies of the College of Physicians of Philadelphia* new series 4 (1982), 272–90.

30. Tertullian, *De Anima* 10 and 25. However Tertullian's testimony has to be treated with caution, for he was vehemently opposed to any scientific investigation by pagan researchers: Lloyd 1973, 75ff. Opinion is divided on the issue of whether or not human vivisection was actually practised by Erasistratus or Herophilus, for the evidence is inconclusive. See, e.g. Longrigg 1981, 160ff.

31. Celsus, *De Med.* VII, Prooemium 3, trans. W. G. Spencer; Michler 1968.

32. For the meaning of 'schools' in ancient medicine see e.g. H. von Staden, 'Hairesis and heresy: the case of the *hairesis iatrikai*', *in* B. F. Meyer and E. P. Sanders (eds), *Jewish and Christian self-definition in the Graeco-Roman world* (London 1982), 76–100.

33. Archagathus: Pliny, *Nat. Hist.* XXIX, vi. As Nutton has pointed out (Nutton 1981a, 18), Archagathus was not the first Greek doctor in Rome but the first there to be appointed as a civic doctor in the Hellenistic tradition. Asclepiades: E. D. Rawson ('The life and death of Asclepiades of Bithynia', *Classical Quarterly* 32 (1982), 358–70) has demonstrated that Asclepiades' career in Rome must be centred on the date *c.* 120 BC, not *c.* 90–60 BC as was formerly believed.

34. *Anonymus Londinensis* XXIV, 30; Pliny, *Nat. Hist.* XXVI, vii-viii.

35. Celsus, *De Med.* Prooemium, 11.

2 Fitness, food and hygiene

1. *De Med.* Prooemium, 9.
2. *Nat. Hist.* XXVI, vii, 13, trans. Rackham *et al.*
3. *Ibid.*
4. *De Med.* I, 1, 1, trans. W. G. Spencer.
5. *Ibid.* I, 2, 1–3.
6. *Ibid.* I, 2, 5–7.
7. *Ibid.* I, 2, 9.
8. For example Pliny the Younger, *Letters* 9, 36.
9. *Nutriment* XXXIV, trans. Jones and Withington; *De Med.* I, 1, 3, trans. W. G. Spencer.
10. V 899–910K.

11. Celsus, *De Med.* II, 14, 2, trans. W. G. Spencer.
12. *Epistulae Morales* LVI.
13. *De Med.* II, 15, 1; IV, 32, 1; IV, 26, 5, trans. W. G. Spencer.
14. *Ibid.* II, 18, 1.
15. *Ibid.* II, 18, 13.
16. Apicius III, ii, 1–5; I, xx, 1–2.
17. *De Sanitate Tuenda* VI, 412.
18. e.g. Seneca, *Epistulae Morales* XCV, 14–23. However, fish sauces and dried fish were also recommended as medical ingredients by writers like Galen: R. I. Curtis, 'Salted fish products in ancient medicine', *JHM* 39 (1984), 430–45.
19. *Letters* I, 15, trans. B. Radice.
20. The additive sulphur dioxide is now used in most wines to prevent oxidation, a measure that is particularly necessary for the sweeter white varieties. Dr V. Nutton and G. L. Varndell, pers. comms.
21. Waldron 1973, 391–9; Eisinger 1982, 279–302.
22. Apicius I, viii; I, ix, 1–2; I, vii, 1, trans. Flower and Rosenbaum.
23. e.g. Juvenal, *Satires* XI, 82–5.
24. e.g. parasites from the fort latrines at Künzing, Bavaria: W. Specht, 'Eine interessante Erdprobe aus einer Abortgrube im Römerkastell Künzing', *Saalburg Jahrbuch* 21 (1963/4), 90ff.
25. e.g. Davies 1971; A. King, 'Animal bones and the dietary identity of military and civilian groups in Roman Britain, Germany, and Gaul', *in* T. F. C. Blagg and A. C. King (eds), 'Military and Civilian in Roman Britain', *British Archaeological Reports* 136 (1984), 187–217.
26. Brothwell 1969, 179–81.
27. Soranus, *Gynaecology* II, 43–5.
28. Manchester 1983, 77ff.
29. White 1984, 63ff; F. G. Simpson, *Watermills and military works on Hadrian's Wall* (Kendal 1976); Jones 1973, 1047ff.
30. Horace, *Satires* I, 5, 86–91.
31. Petronius, *Satyricon* lxvi, 2.
32. Pliny, *Nat. Hist.* XVIII, 67.
33. Jones 1973, 696ff; Garnsey and Whittaker 1983, esp. 56–65; G. E. Rickman, *The corn supply of ancient Rome* (Oxford 1980).
34. Dio Cassius, LXXVI 1, 1; Carcopino 1941, 16 fn. 31.
35. e.g. *CIL* X, 6328: an inscription commemorating Caelia Macrina, a benefactress to two hundred children of Tarracina.
36. Pliny, *Letters* 7, 18; *CIL* V, 5262.
37. Seneca, *Epistulae Morales* XCV; Plutarch, *Table Talk* VII, 9.
38. Local or widespread famines, caused by climatic fluctuations, crop disease and war, were common. In Britain, for example, some two hundred were recorded between AD 10 and 1850. Aristotle knew of rust as a serious disease of cereal crops, and Pliny and Theophrastus related its frequency to land and climate: Brothwell 1969, 176ff. See also E. Lieber, 'Galen on contaminated cereals as a cause of epidemics', *BHM* 44 (1970), 332ff.
39. *Nat. Hist.* XXVI, i, trans. Rackham *et al.*
40. *Ibid.* XXVI, iii, 3.
41. *Letters* 2, 8, trans. B. Radice.

42. *Ibid.* 5, 6; 2, 17.
43. *Ibid.* 5, 6.
44. Juvenal, *Satires* III, 190–6; *Digest* XIX, 2, 3; Plutarch, *Parallel Lives*, Crassus 2, 5.
45. Ashby 1935, 298ff; Frontinus, *Aqueducts* II, 65–73.
46. *Aqueducts* II, 65; II, 69; II, 75; II, 87, trans. C. E. Bennett.
47. *Ibid.* II, 88; I, 16.
48. *Ibid.* I, 19.
49. Howe, 1972.
50. Vitruvius, *De Architectura* VIII, vi, 2, trans. F. Grainger.
51. *Nat. Hist.* XXXIII, xl, 122, trans. Rackham *et al.*
52. Vitruvius, *De Arch.* VIII, iv, 2, trans. F. Grainger.
53. Pliny, *Nat. Hist.* XXXI, xxiii, 39, trans. Rackham *et al.*; Vitruvius, *De Arch.* VIII, iii, 17–18, trans. F. Grainger.
54. Pliny, *Nat. Hist.* XXXI, i–xxxii.
55. *De Arch.* VIII, ii, 1, trans. F. Grainger.
56. Celsus, *De Med.* II, 18, 11–13.
57. For eye-salves, e.g. Celsus, *De Med.* VI, 6, 10; Galen, XII 786K; for diarrhoea, e.g. Celsus, *De Med.* IV, 26, 3–4.
58. *Nat. Hist.* XXXI, xxi, 32–4, trans. Rackham *et al.*
59. *Ibid.*
60. Vitruvius, *De Arch.* VIII, vi, 15, trans. F. Grainger.
61. e.g. *Ibid.* VIII, iii, 6.
62. Juvenal, *Satires* II, 152; VI, 446; Seneca, *Epistulae Morales* LXXXVI, 9.
63. Künzl 1986, 491ff.
64. Celsus, *De Med.* III, 22; II, 17, 2–3, trans. W. G. Spencer. On the importance of baths in classical medicine see, e.g., M-T. Fontanille, 'Les bains dans la médecine Greco-Romaine' *in* Pelletier (ed.) 1985.
65. *Letters* 2, 17, trans. B. Radice.
66. G. C. Boon, *Silchester: the Roman town of Calleva* (Newton Abbot 1974), 86ff.
67. *Epigrams* VI, xciii, trans. W. C. A. Ker.
68. Pliny, *Nat. Hist.* XXVI, viii, 14; CIL II, 5181: regulations of the baths of the imperial mines at Vipasca, Portugal.
69. Juvenal, *Satires* III, 38; S. Frere, *Verulamium excavations* II (London 1983), 246ff.
70. Martial, *Epigrams* XI, lxxvii, 1–3.
71. Carcopino 1941, 41.
72. Toilet sponges: e.g. Seneca, *Epistulae Morales* LXX, 20; Martial, *Epigrams* XII, xlviii; at York: P. C. Buckland, *The environmental evidence from the Church Street sewer* (London 1976) 14ff. Moss: 'The Roman Fort on the Antonine Wall at Bearsden' *in* D. J. Breeze (ed.) *Studies in Scottish antiquity* (Edinburgh 1984), 33ff.
73. *Letters* 10, 98, trans. B. Radice; CIL V, 5262–3, 5667.
74. *Aqueducts* II, 111, trans. C. E. Bennett.
75. Galen, VI 722–3K. I am grateful to Dr V. Nutton for this reference.
76. Martial, *Epigrams* XI, xi, 5; XIV, cxix.
77. *Ibid.* VI, xciii; Pompeii: *Fullonica Stephani*, Reg. I, Ins. 6, n. 7.
78. Pots: e.g. Pompeii: Reg. IX, Ins. 13; Martial, *Epigrams* VI, xciii. Tax: Suetonius, *Divus Vespasianus* 23, 3; Dio Cassius, LXV, 14.
79. Reg. I, Ins. 6, n. 15; Reg. III, Ins. 2, n. 1.
80. e.g. Celsus, *De Med.* II, 8, 30–33.
81. Martial *Epigrams* VII, lxxxiii; XI, lxxxiv. Pliny, *Nat. Hist.* XXIX, 36.
82. Martial, *Epigrams* VI, lvii, trans. W. C. A. Ker.
83. *Ibid.* III, xliii; XIV, xxvi, xxvii.
84. Depilatories: e.g. Seneca, *Epistulae Morales* LVI, 1–2; Juvenal, *Satires* XI, 156–8; Pliny, *Nat. Hist.* XXIX, viii, 26–7; XXVIII, 250; XXX, 132; XXXII, 136. Lice: e.g. H. Keil, 'The louse in Greek antiquity', *BHM* 25 (1951), 305–23.
85. Martial, *Epigrams* IX, xxxvii, trans. W. C. A. Ker.
86. *De Arch.* VIII, vi, 10–11; *De Med.* V, 27, 12.
87. Martial, *Epigrams* XIV, lx, trans. W. C. A. Ker; cf. also III, xlii; VI, xciii.
88. *De Med.* V, 18, 24; II, 33, 5.
89. e.g. Martial, *Epigrams* VI, lv; VI, xciii; Juvenal, *Satires* VI, 460–7.
90. Martial, *Epigrams* I, lxxxvii, trans. W. C. A. Ker; cf. also XIV, cx; Pliny, *Nat. Hist.* XXIII, iii; Juvenal, *Satires* VI, 303.
91. e.g. Juvenal, *Satires* VI, 457–73.
92. Seneca, *Epistulae Morales* CVIII, 16, trans. R. M. Gummere; Martial, *Epigrams* VI, lv; Plautus, *Mostellaria* 273.

3 Physicians and their medicine

1. Suetonius, *Julius Caesar* 42; D. Knibbe, 'Neue Inschriften aus Ephesos VIII', *Jahreshefte des Österreichischen Archäologischen Institutes in Wien* 53 (1981/2), 147D, 136–40; Kudlien 1986.
2. Nutton 1986, 37.
3. See, for example, Seneca's testimony, *On Benefits* VI, 16, 1–4.
4. Suetonius, *Augustus* 59, 81; Dio Cassius LIII, 30, 3.
5. Tacitus, *Annals* XII, 61; XII, 67.
6. Exemptions: Nutton 1971; 1981a; Jones 1973, 1405 fn. 57; Fischer 1979, 166. Difficulty in obtaining exemption: M. Valerius Gemellus, physician, petition to the prefect of Egypt, *c.* AD 140, *in* A. S. Hunt and C. C. Edgar, *Select Papyri* (London 1934), 270–1, no. 283.
7. Pliny, *Nat. Hist.* XXIX, vi, 12–13. However, this is the only certain instance.
8. e.g. Pliny, *Nat. Hist.* XXIX, i, 2; iii; v, 7–9; viii, 17, 22. Kudlien 1976.
9. J. Benedum, 'Titos Statilios Kriton', *Clio Medica* 7 (1972), 249–58; Galen, XIV 641–7K; Smith 1979, 84; Nutton 1986, 35–6. For poor physicians see Galen, XII 916–17K.
10. Galen, V 751K; Nutton 1971; 1977; 1981a; *Codex Theodosianus* 13, 3, 9, 370; Hopkins 1965, 129.
11. *Letters* 3, 21, trans. B. Radice; for the physician as victim of the satirist, epigrammatist, etc., see further Martial, *Epigrams* I, xxx; II, xv; V, ix; VIII, lxxiv; X, lxxvii; XI, lxxi; Juvenal, *Satires* III, 58ff; XIII, 120ff; Babrius, *Fables* 75; 120; *Greek Anthology* XI, 112–126.

12. Phaedrus (c. 15 BC–AD 50), *Fables* I, 14; cf. also Galen, IX 804K. On the character of ancient medical education see e.g. Drabkin 1944; Kollesch 1979.
13. *Epigrams* V, ix, trans. W. C. A. Ker.
14. Turin: *CIL* V, 6970. Beneventum: *CIL* IX, 1618. Aventicum: *CIL* XIII, 5079. F. Staehelin, *Die Schweiz in römischer Zeit* (Basel 1948), 483–5. Regarding literacy, Galen's comment that most physicians of his day could not read (XIX 9K) was probably an exaggeration.
15. Nutton 1971, 55 fn. 37.
16. *De Med.* Prooemium, 39, trans. W. G. Spencer.
17. *That the Best Physician is also a Philosopher*; A. J. Brock, *Galen, on the Natural Faculties* (London 1916), xxxvi.
18. e.g. Martial, *Epigrams* VI, xxxi. Kudlien (1970, 99ff) has highlighted the invidious position of the doctor, who risked accusations of murder whether he administered or withheld drugs. On physicians and the law see, e.g., Amundsen 1977.
19. *Annals* XII, 67, 2, trans. M. Grant.
20. *SHA, vita Marci* 15, 5.
21. *Letters* 8, 1; 10, 5; 7, 1; 8, 24; 1, 22, trans. B. Radice.
22. Sarton 1954, 19. For the best biography of Galen see Moraux 1985.
23. Galen XIV 647–7K; *CMG* V 8, 1, 110–16.
24. Smith 1979, 64. For a concise account of Galen's complex, often brilliant, but sometimes inconsistent practice of medicine see V. Nutton's commentary on *Galen: On Prognosis, CMG* V 8, 1 (Berlin 1979).
25. *On the Natural Faculties* I, xiii, 34, trans. A. J. Brock. Galen often stressed the need to temper theory with practical considerations. See, e.g., his suggestions for several valid reasons for the study of anatomy in *On Anatomical Procedures*: Singer 1956; Lloyd 1973, 150ff.
26. Galen's proof came from a brilliantly simple experiment on a live animal: he ligated an artery in two places and cut open the section between (IV 724K). For his theories on blood flow see, e.g., Lloyd 1973, 147ff. For Galen on the use of animals in dissection see, e.g., *On Anatomical Procedures* II, 220; Sarton 1954, 41–2; Lloyd 1973, 143ff.
27. *On the Usefulness of the Parts of the Body* I, 412–25.
28. XIV 627K. For Galen's vivisections to investigate the nervous system see e.g. Lloyd 1973, 146ff. See also E. S. Smith, 'Galen's account of the cranial nerves and the autonomic nervous system', *Clio Medica* 6 (1971), 77–98 and 173–94.
29. Toledo-Pereyra 1973, 357–75.
30. Galen's fame: Galen's claim that his work was known in all corners of the Roman Empire gains some support from a recently discovered fragmentary papyrus leaf; see Nutton 1984 and Hanson 1985. Galen's death: AD 199 or 200 was for long the accepted probable date, but a rather better case may be made for the year AD 210 or a little later; see e.g. Nutton 1984, 323–4. Physicians' memorials: see e.g. C. Foss, *Ephesus after Antiquity* (Cambridge 1979), 21–2, fig. 3, a statue of the doctor Alexander, erected on the main street of Ephesus in the late antique period.
31. Nutton 1971; Smith 1979, 100.
32. e.g. Galen, XIV 622–4K. In fact, those who sought the services of a doctor had at their disposal few other means of determining his competence than those of reputation and personal recommendation. However, according to Scribonius Largus, few people ever checked the reputation of a doctor before placing themselves and their families under his care; see Hamilton 1986, 211, 215.
33. *CMG* V 10, 1, 401ff.
34. e.g. Celsus, *De Med.* V, 26.
35. *Ibid.* Prooemium, 65; Harig 1971, 189ff.
36. Suetonius, *Claudius* 25; Harig 1971; Miller 1985.
37. Eschebach 1984; Harig 1971, 187; M. Della Corte, *Case ed abitanti di Pompei* (2nd edn, Rome 1954), 191–2, nos 459, 463; Krug 1985, 71.
38. Hippocrates, *In the Surgery* VI, trans. Jones and Withington.
39. Bliquez 1983, 25ff; Pliny, *Nat. Hist.* VI, xxviii, 105.
40. *In the Surgery* III, 17–21, trans. Jones and Withington.
41. Nutton 1986, 36.
42. *De Med.* III, 6, 6, trans. W. G. Spencer.
43. *Ibid.* V, 25, 3. Dioscorides, Pliny and Galen recommended juice from the seeds of the plant *Cannabis sativa* (hemp, marijuana) as an analgesic especially effective in the relief of ear-ache. Though Galen noted that 'The seed creates a feeling of warmth, and – if consumed in large amounts – affects the head by sending to it a warm and toxic vapour', there is no evidence to suggest the use of marijuana as an intoxicant in the classical world. See T. F. Brunner, 'Marijuana in ancient Greece and Rome?', *BHM* 47 (1973), 344–55.
44. *De Med.* II, 10, 14, trans. W. G. Spencer.
45. E. Berger, *Das Basler Arztrelief* (Basle 1970), 12ff, figs 9–17; Phillips 1973, pl. 8.
46. Künzl 1982a.
47. e.g. Soranus, *Gyn.* III, 11; III, 23.
48. e.g. Milne 1907, pl. IV; Berger 1970.
49. G. Calza, *La necropoli del porto di Roma nell'isola sacra* (Rome 1940), 250 no. 39 fig. 149; Tabanelli 1958 pl. XV; Rostovtzeff 1966, pl. XXXI, 1.
50. A. M. McCann, *Roman sarcophagi in the Metropolitan Museum of Art* (New York 1978), 138–40 no. 24.
51. Rectangular boxes: F. Beck, 'Objets gallo-romains découverts à Échevronne', *Antiquités Nationales* 9 (1977), 50–65. Cylindrical boxes: e.g. D. Michaelides, 'A Roman surgeon's tomb from Nea Paphos', *Report of the Dept of Antiquities Cyprus 1984* (Nicosia 1984), 315–32. Stacking box: Jackson 1986, 158–9.
52. Nielsen 1974; A. Oxé and W. von Stokar, 'Von römischen Augenärzten', *Germania* 25 (1941), 23–30; W. G. Spencer, *Celsus De Medicina* vol. II (London 1935–8), vii–lx.
53. Scarborough 1986, 59. For Pliny's drugs see e.g. J. Stannard, 'Medical plants and folk remedies in Pliny, *Historia naturalis*', *History and Philosophy of the Life Sciences* 4 (1982), 3–23.

54. Riddle 1985.
55. On drug fraud see e.g. Nutton 1985a.
56. W. G. Spencer, *Celsus De Medicina* vol. II (London 1935–8), xxii.
57. Pliny, *Nat. Hist.* xxv, iii, 6, trans. Rackham *et al.*
58. *De Med.* V, 23A, trans. W. G. Spencer.
59. W. G. Spencer, *Celsus De Medicina* vol. II (London 1935–8), xl–xli.
60. Scribonius Largus, *Compositiones* XIX. Scribonius Largus, probably a Greek freedman, wrote his great pharmacological work, the *Compositiones*, between AD 43 and 48. He is believed to have served as a military doctor and went to Britain with the emperor Claudius. See Hamilton 1986.
61. Boon 1983, 9.
62. *Nat. Hist.* XXVI, lxxxvii, 140.
63. Boon 1983, 9; Krug 1985, 110; F. F. Troisi, *Archeologia Classica* 33 (1981), 329–31; Majno 1975, 375–7.
64. *Germania* 12 (1928), 70, fig. 1.
65. Davies 1970a, 104ff; 1970b, 92.
66. Nutton 1986, 55–6 fn. 67.
67. See, e.g., E. A. E. Raymond, *A medical book from Crocodilopolis* (Vienna 1976), a second-century AD Demotic papyrus probably copied from a Ptolemaic book of the third to second centuries BC.
68. G. C. Boon, *Silchester: the Roman town of Calleva* (Newton Abbot 1974), 137; Celsus, *De Med.* V, 5; 9; 22, 2, 5, 6.
69. *De Med.* IV, 16, 3.
70. Davies 1970a, 101–3.
71. *Journal of Roman Studies* 53 (1963), 166, no. 51; Davies 1970b, 94 fig. 10.
72. *Journal of Roman Studies* 56 (1966), 224, no. 51; Davies 1970b, 95 fig. 11.
73. *De Med.* IV, 5, 2; IV, 26, 3, 9, trans. W. G. Spencer.
74. Nielsen 1974, 9–10.
75. G. R. Watson, *The Roman soldier* (London 1969), 41, 168 fn. 84; Pliny, *Letters* 7, 21; J. Benedum, 'Die Augenanomalie an einem römischen Bildnis', *Medizinhistorisches Journal* 16 (1981), 446ff; T. Meyer-Steineg, 'Darstellungen normaler und krankhaft veränderter Körperteile an antiken Weihgaben', *Jenaer medizinhistorische Beiträge* 2 (1912), 14ff, pl. I, 1–2.
76. Galen, XII 749K; Nielsen 1974, 81–92.
77. Nielsen 1974, 19–58, 105–6.
78. XII 786K.
79. *CIL* XI, 5400. On the question of 'specialists' see, e.g., Baader 1967, and Mudry 1985.
80. *L'Année Épigraphique* 1924, 106; 1953, 59.
81. *Greek anthology* IV, 112, trans. W. R. Paton.
82. Künzl 1982b, 61–7.
83. Nielsen 1974, 11–18, 62–7.
84. Voinot 1984; Künzl *in* Feugère, Künzl and Weisser 1985, 479–81.
85. G. C. Dunning, *Antiquaries Journal* 12 (1932), 437ff.
86. Künzl *in* Feugère, Künzl and Weisser 1985, 476–7, figs 18–19.
87. *Digest* xxvii, 1, 6. 1; Nutton 1972.
88. *CIL* XIII, 5079.

4 Women's diseases, birth and contraception

1. *Nat. Hist.* xxv, v, 9–10.
2. E. Kalinka (ed.), *Tituli Asiae Minores* II², 223, no. 595; *RE* Suppl. XIV, 1974, 48–9.
3. XIII 250 and 341K.
4. e.g. *CIL* II, 497; V, 3461; VI, 6851, 7581, 8711, 8926, 9614–7, 9619; VIII, 24679; IX, 5861; XIII, 2019, 3343, 4334. Galen, VIII 414, 7ff. K.
5. Tacitus, *Annals* I, 69; Juvenal, *Satires* II, 141; Martial, *Epigrams* XI, lx; XI, lxxi.
6. e.g. Flavia Hedone of Nîmes: *CIL* XII, 3343, Rémy (1984), 126 no. 5. For female doctors in Greece see, e.g., S. B. Pomeroy, 'Plato and the female physician (*Republic* 454 d2)', *American Journal of Philology* 99 (1978), 496–500.
7. Slaves: e.g. Melitine, *CIL* XII, 6851. Freedwomen: e.g. Minucia Asste and Venuleia Sosis, *CIL* VI, 9615, 9617. Lefkowitz and Fant 1982, 162 no. 174.
8. Cf. also Scribonia Attice, from Ostia, whose husband was a physician-surgeon: Rostovtzeff 1966, pl. XXXI, 1–2; and Pantheia, a lady doctor from Pergamum, whose husband and father-in-law were also doctors: H. W. Pleket, 'Texts on the social history of the Greek World', *Epigraphica* II (Textus Minores vol. XLI. Leiden 1969), 32–3, no. 20.
9. Wealthy *medicae*: e.g. Metilia Donata, of Lyons, *CIL* XIII, 2019; Rémy 1984, 138–9, no. 18. Specialists: e.g. Aspasia, a gynaecologist and obstetrician, praised by the sixth-century AD medical authority Aetius of Amida; and Metrodora, who wrote a treatise on diseases of the uterus, stomach and kidneys. Both were active in the second century AD. Ricci 1949. See also Baader 1967, 233; and Hurd-Mead 1938, 56–9 and 63–6.
10. Iulia Saturnina: *CIL* II, 497. Victoria: Theodorus Priscianus, *Euporista* 3, 1. 13.
11. Galen, for instance, refers to women doctors for women's diseases: XII 250, 3ff; XIII 341, 2ff. K.
12. Soranus, *Gyn.* III, 3, trans. O. Temkin. The role of the *medica* and *obstetrix* and the distinction between them is unclear, but a considerable overlap should be envisaged. On this problem of roles see, e.g., Nickel 1979, and King 1986, 55 and 59–60.
13. Galen, *On Prognosis* 8, *CMG* V 8, 1, 110–16 (XIV 641–7K).
14. Smith 1979, 74.
15. *Gyn.* I, 3; Temkin 1956, xxxvii.
16. *Gyn.* III, 14–16; Drabkin 1951; Frede 1982.
17. e.g. *Gyn.* I, 39; II, 10; Lloyd 1983, 168ff.; Gourevitch 1984b.
18. *Gyn.* III, 42, trans. O. Temkin. Such humanity and shrewd sense are recurrent features of Soranus' work, as, most strikingly, in his notably modern-sounding advice on the treatment of insanity, preserved in Caelius Aurelianus, *On Chronic Diseases* I, 155; Drabkin 1951, 512ff.
19. *Gyn.* I, 17.
20. *Gyn.* IV, 5. However, Soranus may have derived this information from an author he calls

'Demetrius the Herophilean'. Galen (II 220K) recommended Alexandria as the only place where dissection was practised in his day.

21. *Timaeus* 91c; Herophilus, as quoted by Soranus (*Gyn.* III, 3), was at pains to demonstrate the normality of the uterus, probably in a conscious attempt to discredit this 'animal-in-animal' theory.

22. Aretaeus, *On the Causes and Symptoms of Acute Diseases* 2, trans. in Lefkowitz and Fant 1982, 225, no. 215.

23. Galen, *On Prognosis* 6, Lefkowitz and Fant 1982, 232–4, no. 219. The ability to recognise lovesickness was popularly regarded as a measure of a physician's skill: see, e.g. Amundsen 1974, 320–37. On the history of hysteria see, e.g., I. Veith, *Hysteria* (Chicago 1965).

24. *Gyn.* III, 26, trans. O. Temkin.

25. *Ibid.* I, 55; II, 7; III, 10.

26. Baader 1967, 233 fn. 62.

27. Celsus, *De Med.* V, 28, 2.

28. Pliny, *Nat. Hist.* XXVI, xc; Celsus, *De Med.* IV, 27.

29. *Gyn.* IV, 14–15.

30. *Ibid.* IV, 7.

31. Milne 1907, 107.

32. Naples, Museo Nazionale, inv. no. 78, 235; Milne 1907, pl. XXXVIII no. 1.

33. Soranus, *Gyn.* III, 41, 44; IV, 7; II, 56.

34. *De Med.* V, 21, 1, trans. W. G. Spencer.

35. Pliny, *Nat. Hist.* XXVI, xc, 152–8.

36. *De Med.* V, 21, 7.

37. Soranus, *Gyn.* IV, 38; IV, 36.

38. Hippocrates, *Aphorisms* V, xlvii; Soranus, *Gyn.* III, 41.

39. *De Med.* VII, 28, 2, trans. W. G. Spencer.

40. *Gyn.* III, 40, trans. O. Temkin.

41. Longfield-Jones 1986.

42. Only seven are known: Longfield-Jones 1986.

43. *Gyn.* I, 29, trans. O. Temkin. Cf. Aristotle, who believed that generation occurred through a combination of menstrual fluid and the male semen (*De generatione animalium* 729a 20–33; Blayney 1986, 234).

44. *Gyn.* I, 30.

45. *Ibid.* I, 34.

46. e.g. Hippocrates, *Aphorisms* V, xli; Galen, *On the Natural Faculties* III, iii. On Graeco-Roman theories of the process of conception see Blayney 1986. Galen believed that the female seed was less substantial than the male seed which it supplied with nourishment after fusion; and that the determination of gender depended on heat – the right side of the womb and seeds from the right testes (male and female) were warm and yielded boys, while the left side of the womb and seeds from the left testes were cold and yielded girls.

47. *Gyn.* I, 36; trans. O. Temkin; Hopkins 1965, 140 fn. 47.

48. *Gyn.* I, 47; trans. O. Temkin. On mental illness see, e.g., J. Pigeaud, *La maladie de l'âme* (Paris 1981); and Simon, 1978.

49. *Gyn.* I, 48, 49, 53, 56.

50. Miscarriage: *Ibid.* I, 59; III, 17, 26, 47–8; Balsdon 1962, 195ff. Caesar's daughter suffered a miscarriage four years after her marriage to Pompey. She recovered but died in childbirth a year later. Nero's wife Poppaea also perished in childbirth.

51. Paulus, *Opinions* 2, 24, 7–8, trans. S. P. Scott in Lefkowitz and Fant 1982, 196. Cf. *Digest* XXV, 4, 1; Amundsen and Ferngren 1979, 39–56, esp. 40–41 and 47.

52. e.g. Sotira: Pliny, *Nat. Hist.* XXVIII, xxiii, 83.

53. e.g. *CIL* VI, 6325, 8947, 9721, 9723.

54. *CIL* VI, 9720, 9723.

55. *Nat. Hist.* XXVIII, vii, 38.

56. *Gyn.* II, 2, trans. O. Temkin.

57. *Ibid.* II, 3.

58. Another very similar childbirth scene is depicted on a carved ivory plaque in the Museo Nazionale, Naples. As on the Ostia relief, a birthing chair is in use and the midwife appears to have only a single female assistant who is restraining the labouring woman from behind: Gourevitch 1984b, facing page 265.

59. *Gyn.* II, 6, trans. O. Temkin.

60. *Ibid.* II, 12.

61. *Ibid.* II, 45.

62. *Ibid.* II, 18. Plutarch considered it noteworthy that Cato's wife Licinia had breast-fed her own son (*Cato the Elder* 20.3), perhaps implying that this was the exception rather than the rule. On Roman attitudes to maternal nursing see Bradley 1986.

63. On free and slave wet-nurses see Bradley 1980; 1986.

64. Prima: *CIL* VI, 4352.

65. *Gyn* II, 19, trans. O. Temkin.

66. *Oxyrhyncus Papyrus* 91, trans. in A. S. Hunt and C. C. Edgar *Select Papyri* (London 1932), 228–231, no. 79.

67. *Gyn.* II, 47, trans. O. Temkin. For nursing periods attested on other papyrus documents see Bradley 1980, 322 fn. 5. On the formation of bladder stones in infants prematurely weaned see P. T. Makler, 'Nutrition in ancient Greece', *Klio* 62 (2), (1980), 317–19.

68. *Nat. Hist.* XXVIII, xxi.

69. e.g. Twenty-seven infant skeletons at Portchester: B. Hooper, 'The human bones' *in* B. Cunliffe, *Excavations at Portchester Castle Vol. I: Roman* (London 1975), 375–7.

70. *De Med.* II, 8, 30–31, trans. W. G. Spencer.

71. *Historia Animalium* vii.

72. G. F. Still, *The history of paediatrics* (London 1931), 454–5.

73. Soranus, *Gyn.* IV, 7, trans. O. Temkin.

74. *Ibid.* IV, 8.

75. Celsus, *De Med.* VII, 29, 7.

76. *Gyn.* IV, 2.

77. Meyer-Steineg 1912, 6ff. pl. VI, 1; Künzl 1982b, 49–52 pl. 20, no. 29.

78. Milne 1907, pl. L, 1.

79. *Gyn.* IV, 12, trans. O. Temkin.

80. e.g. Pliny, *Letters* 4, 21; Soranus, *Gyn.* III, 17; III, 40.

81. B. M. Willmott Dobbie, *Med. Hist.* 26 (1982), 79–90. For nineteenth- and twentieth-century statistics on mortality from post-partum sepsis see Shorter 1983, 297–317.

82. e.g. Pliny, *Nat. Hist.* XXVIII, ix, 42. Dioscorides, *Mat. Med.* V, 159–61.
83. *Journal of Roman Studies* 54 (1964), 180–1, pl. 15, 3–4.
84. *De Uteri Dissectione*, IX 280K.
85. Wells 1982, 192–4.
86. Jones 1973, 1044.
87. Balsdon 1962, 193ff.
88. *Satires* VI, 602–9.
89. e.g. Brough-on-Humber, Yorkshire: R. Powers and D. Brothwell, 'Human remains' *in* J. S. Wacher, *Excavations at Brough-on-Humber 1958–61* (London 1969), 233–7.
90. Soranus, *Gyn.* I, 60, trans. O. Temkin.
91. *Ibid.* I, 65.
92. Trans. in Wells 1967a, 140–1.
93. Wells 1967a, 139–41, pl. 17b.
94. Hopkins 1966, 134–5.
95. *Nat. Hist.* XXIX, xxvii, 85, trans. Rackham *et al.*
96. Hopkins 1966, 141 fn. 51.
97. Lefkowitz and Fant 1982, 99 no. 104; Hopkins 1966, 143 fn. 60.
98. Hopkins 1966, 139–41; Bradley 1980, 323ff.

5 The surgeon and the army

1. *Nat. Hist.* XXV, xciv, 150, trans. Rackham *et al.*
2. Wangensteen 1978, 36–8; E. Bennion, *Antique medical instruments* (London 1979), 55.
3. e.g. Celsus, *De Med.* V, 19, 1–28. For the antiseptic and antibiotic powers of wine, vinegar, pitch, resins and metallic compounds see Majno 1975, 186–8, 215–21 and 369–70.
4. Milne 1907; Künzl 1982b; Jackson 1986; Tabanelli 1958.
5. Galen, II 682K.
6. *Adversus indoctum* 3.29.
7. R. Meiggs, *Roman Ostia* (Oxford 1960), pl. XXVIIa.
8. Tabanelli 1958, pls X–XV.
9. Møller-Christensen 1938; Jackson 1986, 137ff.
10. Jackson 1986, 154–6.
11. Künzl 1982b, 12–15; Hippocrates, *Decorum*, viii, 10–13.
12. Milne 1907, pl. XLIII; Künzl 1982b, fig. 85, 2.
13. *Nat. Hist.* XXV, vii, 23, trans. Rackham *et al.* Trephination was also performed to treat epilepsy, though Soranus censured the practice: Caelius Aurelianus, *On Chronic Diseases* I, 118.
14. Manchester 1983, 62–3. For treatment of a potential skull fracture in Hippocratic times see *Epidemics* V, 16; Majno 1975, 166–9.
15. J. Como, *Germania* 9 (1925), 152–62; Künzl 1982b, 80–85.
16. D. R. Brothwell, 'Osteological evidence of the use of a surgical modiolus in a Romano-British population', *Journal of Archaeological Science* I (1974), 209–11.
17. *Epigrams* X, lvi, trans. W. C. A. Ker.
18. Künzl 1982b, figs 11, 1; 45; 46, 1; 85, 10; Jackson 1986, fig. 1, 12.
19. R. Lanciani *Pagan and Christian Rome* (New York 1892), 353.
20. *De Med.* VI, 9, 5, trans. W. G. Spencer.
21. *Ibid.* VII, 12.
22. Cicero, *De Legibus* II, 24.
23. Tabanelli 1963, pl. L.
24. *Epigrams* V, xliii, trans. W. C. A. Ker.
25. Wells 1982, 146–51.
26. Manchester 1983, 51–3.
27. Martial, *Epigrams* XIV, xxii, trans. W. C. A. Ker; Dioscorides, *Mat. Med.* V, 166.
28. *Ars Armatoria* III, 279.
29. Celsus, *De Med.* VI, 9, 1–2, trans. W. G. Spencer; Dioscorides, *Mat. Med.* IV, 69; Pliny, *Nat. Hist.* XXV, 105; Scribonius Largus, *Compositiones* X. The idea of worms as the cause of tooth decay was a long-lived, widespread and persistent theory that has been identified in many societies, from the days of ancient Egypt down to recent times. See, for example, B. R. Townend, 'The story of the tooth-worm', *BHM* 15 (1944), 37–58.
30. Künzl 1982b, 61ff.
31. *Ibid.*, 12–15.
32. Feugère, Künzl and Weisser 1985.
33. e.g. Galen and Antyllos: Feugère, Künzl and Weisser 1985, 463–4, 496ff; Pliny: *Nat. Hist.* XXIX, viii, 21.
34. Nutton 1972, 16–29.
35. *Epigrams* VIII, lxxiv, trans. W. C. A. Ker.
36. *Ibid.* X, lvi.
37. e.g. Celsus, *De Med.* VII, 9, 1; see also J. Rubin, 'Celsus' decircumcision operation', *Urology* 16 (1980), 121–4.
38. Milne 1907, pls XXX–XXXII; Møller-Christensen 1938, 136ff. Extraction of the uvula was no novelty: Praxagoras performed the operation in the fourth century BC.
39. *De Agri Cultura* CLIX, trans. Hooper and Ash.
40. Milne 1907, pl. XLVI, 1; L. J. Bliquez *BHM* 56 (1982), fig. 8; Jackson 1986, 145ff. fig. 2, 19, pl. XII, A.
41. Caelius Aurelianus, *On Chronic Diseases* II, 1, 13.
42. *De Med.* VII, 26, 1; Jackson 1986, 147–51, fig. 3, 20–22.
43. *Nat. Hist.* XXV, vii, 23, trans. Rackham *et al.* W. G. Spencer, *Celsus, De Medicina* vol. III (London 1935–8), 426 fn. b. On the formation of bladder stones in young children see P. T. Makler, 'Nutrition in ancient Greece', *Klio* 62 (2), (1980), 317–19.
44. Hippocrates, *Oath*, 22ff. trans. Chadwick and Mann.
45. Künzl 1983.
46. Dio Cassius, LXVIII 14, 2, trans. in Davies 1970b, 94.
47. Plutarch, *Cato Minor* 70, 6. Stitching: for fine work Celsus recommended the hair of a woman (*De Med.* VII, 7, 8c); for deep, gaping wounds metal pins, *fibulae*, were to be used in place of sutures (*De Med.* V, 26, 23).
48. *De Med.* VII, 16, trans. W. G. Spencer.
49. Künzl 1982b, fig. 18, 10; Majno 1975, fig. 9.15.
50. Wangensteen 1978, 40–41.
51. Nutton 1973, 163; Toledo-Pereyra 1973, 361ff.
52. *P. Ross-Georg.*, III, 1, 1–7, trans. in Davies 1969, 93–4.
53. *P. Mich.* 478, 1–18, trans. in Davies 1970b, 101.

54. Plutarch, *Mark Antony* 50. Cf. also Septimius Severus' siege at Hatra in AD 198: Herodian, *Histories* III, 9, 6.

55. Vegetius, *Epitoma rei militaris* I, 6, trans. in Davies 1970b, 99.

56. *P. Oxy.* I, 39, trans. in G. R. Watson, *The Roman soldier* (London 1969), 41.

57. *Epitoma rei militaris* III, 2.

58. *Ibid.* I, 22, trans. in Davies 1970b, 85.

59. G. R. Stephens, 'Military aqueducts in Roman Britain', *Archaeological Journal* 142 (1985), 216–36.

60. D. J. Breeze (ed.), *Studies in Scottish antiquity* (Edinburgh 1984), 56.

61. *Epitoma rei militaris* I, 22, trans. in Davies 1970b, 85.

62. B. A. Knights *et al.*, *Journal of Archaeological Science* 10 (1983), 139–52.

63. W. Specht, *Saalburg Jahrbuch* 21 (1963/4), 90–94.

64. Davies 1971, 122–42; A. K. Bowman and J. D. Thomas, *Vindolanda: the Latin writing-tablets* (London 1983), 83–96. For epigraphic evidence of game hunting by military officers see, e.g., *RIB* 1041.

65. Vegetius, *Epitoma rei militaris* II, 10; *Digest* L, 6, 7; *CIL* IX, 16.

66. *Germania* 17 (1933), 237.

67. Davies 1970b, 101–2.

68. Davies 1969.

69. R. Waterman, *Ärztliche Instrumente aus Novaesium* (Cologne 1970).

70. V. Nutton, *Journal of the Chester Archaeological Society* 55 (1968), 7–13; D. F. Petch, 'The Legionary Fortress' *in* B. E. Harris and A. T. Thacker (eds), *Victoria County History: Chester* I (Oxford 1987), 141ff.

71. *De Bello Gallico* VI, 38; I. A. Richmond, 'The Roman Army medical service', *Univ. of Durham Medical Gazette* 46 (3), (1952), 2–6.

72. *Bonner Jahrbücher* 136/7 (1932), 273ff.

73. L. F. Pitts and J. K. St Joseph, *Inchtuthil* (London 1985), 100.

74. Davies 1970b, 96–8.

75. Davies 1969, 83ff.

76. Davies 1970a, 101ff.; Majno 1975, 384–8.

77. G. Vitelli, *Papiri greci e latini* (1912–), I, 1307, col. 2, 2. Sometimes, especially during campaigns, sick or wounded soldiers were billeted with civilian households in towns: see, e.g., Harig 1971, 188ff.

78. *RIB* 139, 143–4, 146–7, 152, 156–60.

79. *CIL* III, 12336.

80. *De Med.* V, 19, 1B; V, 26, 23 f. For the formula and antiseptic quality see Majno 1975, 369.

6   Gods and their magic

1. For Galen's religious views see Kudlien 1981. Galen's medicine was predominantly secular, though on one occasion he let blood from his hand, apparently to good effect, after a dream instruction from Asklepios (XI 314K).

2. *Iliad* IV, 193; XI, 833.

3. Edelstein 1945, II, 228ff.

4. J. Toynbee, *Animals in Roman life and art* (London 1973), 223–6, Edelstein 1945, II, 227–30.

5. Pausanias, *Descrip. of Greece* II, xxviii, 1; Schouten 1967.

6. *IG* II², 4960.

7. Pausanias, *Descrip. of Greece* II, xxviii, 1; Pliny, *Nat. Hist.* XXIX, 22; Livy, Book XI, *periocha*.

8. For the use of analogy and pun decoding in the symbolic dreams see, e.g., Oberhelman 1981.

9. *Descrip. of Greece* II, xxvii, 3, trans. W. H. S. Jones; Herzog 1931, 6ff.; Majno 1975, 201ff.

10. Burford 1969.

11. Tomlinson 1983.

12. Pausanias, *Descrip. of Greece* II, xxvii, 1, trans. W. H. S. Jones.

13. *Ibid.* II, xxvii, 2.

14. Tomlinson 1983, 65–7.

15. Pausanias, *Descrip. of Greece* II, xxvii, 6, trans. W. H. S. Jones.

16. Travlos 1971, 127–37.

17. Roebuck 1951.

18. *Descrip. of Greece* II, iv, 5.

19. Roebuck 1951, 26.

20. Herzog and Schazmann 1932; Sherwin-White 1978.

21. Strabo, *Geographica* VIII, 6, 15; cf. also Pliny, *Nat. Hist.* XXIX, 1–2.

22. Edelstein 1945, II, 147; Behr 1968, 177ff; Kudlien 1981, 130; Oberhelman 1983; 1987.

23. *Hieroi Logoi* II, 7, trans. C. A. Behr.

24. Behr 1968, 27ff.

25. *Ibid.*, 31.

26. cf. Roebuck 1951, 156–7; Travlos 1971, pl. 184.

27. *Hieroi Logoi* II, 34–5, trans. C. A. Behr.

28. *Ibid.* IV, 16.

29. Galen, XVIIb 137K, trans. in Edelstein 1945, I, 202, no. 401.

30. Behr 1968, 166–7.

31. Krug 1985, figs 57–61.

32. *Ibid.*, fig. 65; Phillips 1973, pl. 7.

33. Roebuck 1951, 111–28.

34. *Ibid.*, pl. 40 no. 63.

35. Fenelli 1975.

36. *IG* II², 1532–9; W. H. D. Rouse, *Greek votive offerings* (Cambridge 1902).

37. Potter 1985.

38. Wells 1985, 41ff.

39. L. Vagnetti, *Il deposito votivo de Campetti a Veio* (Rome 1971).

40. See e.g. Celsus, *De Med.* IV, 2, 2. On the probable incidence of malaria see, e.g., E. Borza, 'Some observations on malaria and the ecology of central Macedonia in Antiquity', *American Journal of Ancient History* 4 (1979), 102–4.

41. Wells 1985, 43–4.

42. e.g. Pliny: W. H. S. Jones, *Pliny. Natural History* vol. VIII (London 1963), 577–83. Celsus: *De Med.* VI, 2–5. Note also *IG* IV², I, no. 121 in Edelstein 1945, I, 231 nos 6–7; and Galen: VII 706–732K, 'Galen on abnormal swellings', trans. by D. G. Lytton and L. M. Resuhr, *JHM* 33 (1978), 531–49.

43. *De Arch.* VIII, iii, 4–5, 17, trans. F. Grainger.

44. *Nat. Hist.* XXXI, iii–viii, trans. Rackham *et al.*

45. Seneca, *Epistulae Morales* LI.
46. Apollo: see J. J. Hatt, 'Apollon guérisseur en Gaule . . .', *in* Pelletier (ed.) 1985; Hochscheid: Dehn 1941, 104–11, pl. 14.
47. Aesculapius: see, e.g., E. Sikora, 'Le culte d'Esculape en Gaule' *in* Pelletier (ed.) 1985. Augst: F. Staehelin, *Die Schweiz in römischer Zeit* (Basel 1948), 538–41. Bath: Cunliffe 1984, 157–9.
48. Grenier 1960, 815–8; 666–8; 639–44.
49. Bernard and Vassal 1958; Martin 1965; Deyts 1983; Romeuf 1986.
50. Vatin 1969; 1972; Romeuf 1986.
51. e.g. Deyts 1983, no. 179, pl. LI.
52. e.g. *Ibid.*, no. 73, pl. XXII.
53. See, e.g., Celsus, *De Med.* VII, 18–24.
54. Bernard and Vassal 1958, 328–37.
55. Vatin 1969, 111, fig. 8; 1972, 40, pl. VI.
56. Cunliffe and Davenport 1985.
57. Cunliffe 1984, pl. 113d.
58. *Ibid.*, fig. 50.
59. Cunliffe and Davenport 1985, 182.
60. *Ibid.*, 130, 9A. I.
61. *Victoria County History: Somerset* 1906, 283, no. 46.
62. Wheeler 1932, 102, fig. 28, 6.
63. *RIB* 616, 617.
64. Wheeler 1932, 89, pl. XXVI, 121, 122.
65. *Ibid.*, 88ff., pl. XXV; pl. XXVI, 115–20; 101, pl. XXXIV.
66. e.g. Hochscheid: Dehn 1941, pl. 16 no. 10.
67. R. P. Wright, *Britannia* 16 (1985), 248–9.
68. Edelstein 1945, II, 256ff.
69. Eusebius Caesariensis, *De vita Constantini* III, 56.
70. Travlos 1971, 128.

7 Dying and death

1. *De Med.* IV, 32.
2. *Letters* 6, 4; 7, 21.
3. Pliny, *Nat. Hist.* XXV, vii, 24, trans. Rackham et al.
4. Pliny, *Nat. Hist.* XXV, vii, 23. See, especially, D. Gourevitch, 'Suicide among the sick in classical antiquity', *BHM* 43 (1969), 501–18.
5. Cunliffe 1969, 200.
6. *De Arch.* I, ii, 7.
7. *De Med.* I, 10, trans. W. G. Spencer.
8. Nutton 1983.
9. Wells 1964, 87; McNeill 1977, 116.
10. Republican epidemics: Livy, *History of Rome* XXXIX, 41; XL, 19, 6–8 and 36, 13–37, 7; XLI, 21, 5–10. Epidemic of AD 65: Suetonius, *Lives of the Caesars*, Nero 39, 1. Epidemic of AD 189: Dio Cassius, LXXII, 14, 3–4.
11. Birley 1966, 202–5.
12. Ammianus Marcellinus, 23, 6, 24.
13. Orosius, 7, 15, 5–6; 27, 7, trans. in Birley 1966, 202.
14. McNeill 1977, 116.
15. Gilliam 1961, 227–8.
16. Galen, *Methodus Medendi* XII; McNeill 1977, 117.
17. Procopius, *Persian Wars* II, 22, 6–39; Wells 1964, 89; Bratton 1981.
18. Procopius, *Persian Wars* II, 23, 1; McNeill 1977, 126–8. On ancient perceptions of food contamination as a cause of epidemic diseases see, e.g., E. Lieber, 'Galen on contaminated cereals as a cause of epidemics', *BHM* 44 (1970), 332ff.
19. Warwick 1968, 161; Wells 1982, 144.
20. G. Penso, *La médecine romaine: l'art d'Esculape dans la Rome antique* (Paris 1984), figs 137–41; Manchester 1983, 29.
21. Wells 1982, 152–60; 1964, 59–67.
22. Wells 1982, 153.
23. e.g. Celsus, *De Med.* IV, 29–31; V, 18, 32–6.
24. Aretaeus, *Chronic Diseases* II, 12.
25. Eisinger 1982, 279–302, esp. 284–8.
26. W. G. Spencer, *Celsus, De Medicina* vol. I (London 1935–8), 464.
27. Lucian, *The Cock* 23.
28. Celsus, *De Med.* IV, 31, trans. W. G. Spencer.
29. Elliot Smith and Dawson 1924.
30. Wells 1973, 399–400; 1982, 190–1.
31. Thucydides, II, 47–55; Wells 1964, 87–8; McNeill 1977, 105–6; Longrigg 1981.
32. Aretaeus: trans. in Wells 1964, 90. Hippocratic Corpus: *Epidemics* II, 36, 37; *Epidemics* V, 47, 74–6. See Majno 1975, 199–200.
33. Wells 1982, 181.
34. Warwick 1968, 151–2; Wells 1982, 181–3, Majno 1975, 197.
35. e.g. Hippocrates, *Epidemics* I, 3; VII, 7; VII, 49.
36. Caelius Aurelianus, *On Chronic Diseases* II, 197ff.; Grmek 1983, 283.
37. *CIG*, 3272; Wells 1964, 98–9, pl. 53.
38. *IG* IV², 122; Edelstein 1945, I, 227, 235–6, no. 33.
39. Celsus, *De Med.* III, 22, 8.
40. Manchester 1984, 163. Poundbury: Manchester 1984, 165. York: Warwick 1968, 161. Cirencester: Wells 1982, 181.
41. J. G. Andersen, *Studies in the mediaeval diagnosis of leprosy in Denmark* (Copenhagen 1969).
42. Manchester 1984, 168.
43. Pliny, *Nat. Hist.* XXVI, v. Cf. also Galen, 'On abnormal swellings', 14: VII 727–8K.
44. Møller-Christensen 1961; 1967; Manchester 1984, 167–8.
45. R. Reader 'New evidence for the antiquity of leprosy in early Britain', *Journal of Archaeological Science* I (1974), 205–7.
46. Grmek 1983, 297ff.; Manchester 1984, 172–3.
47. Manchester 1983, 45–9; Grmek 1983, 199–225.
48. Grmek 1983, 214–25.
49. A. Keaveney and J. Madden, *Hermes* 107 (1979), 499–500.
50. Grmek 1983, 208–10.
51. Some physicians were required to serve as forensic medical experts: see, e.g., D. W. Amundsen and G. B. Ferngren, 'The forensic role of physicians in Ptolemaic and Roman Egypt', *BHM* 52 (1978), 336–53.
52. Jones 1973, 1041.

Bibliography

In this select bibliography I have given preference generally to those works that are written in English and those that are most readily accessible.

Texts and translations

Anonymus Londinensis	*The medical writings of Anonymus Londinensis* W. H. S. Jones (Cambridge 1947)
Apicius	*The Roman cookery book: a critical translation of the art of cooking by Apicius* B. Flower and E. Rosenbaum (London 1958)
Aretaeus	*The extant works of Aretaeus the Cappadocian*, ed. and trans. by F. Adams (London 1856)
Aristides, *Hieroi Logoi*	*Aelius Aristides and the Sacred Tales* C. A. Behr (Amsterdam 1968)
Caelius Aurelianus	*Caelius Aurelianus On Acute Diseases and On Chronic Diseases*, ed. and trans. by I. E. Drabkin (Chicago 1950)
Cato, *De Agri Cultura*	*Marcus Porcius Cato On Agriculture*, trans. by W. D. Hooper and H. B. Ash. LCL (London 1967)
Celsus, *De Medicina*	*Celsus De Medicina*, trans. by W. G. Spencer. LCL, 3 vols (London 1935–8)
Dioscorides, *Materia Medica*	*Dioscorides Greek herbal*, trans. by J. Goodyer and ed. by R. T. Gunther (Oxford 1934)
Frontinus, *Aqueducts*	*Frontinus the Stratagems and the Aqueducts of Rome*, trans. by C. E. Bennett. LCL (London 1925)
Galen	*Claudii Galeni Opera omnia* Comprehensive Greek–Latin edition of Galen's works by C. G. Kühn 20 vols in 22. (Leipzig 1821–33; repr. Hildesheim 1964–5) This is abbreviated in the notes to K.
Galen	*Corpus medicorum Graecorum* Ediderunt Academiae Berolinensis Hauniensis Lipsiensis. (Various editors, Leipzig and Berlin 1914 ff). This edition is gradually superseding that of Kühn. English translations include: *Galen: On Prognosis*, trans. by V. Nutton, *CMG* v 8, 1 (Berlin 1979)
	Galen: On the Doctrines of Hippocrates and Plato, trans. by P. De Lacy, *CMG* v 4, 1, 2, 3 vols (Berlin 1978–84)
Galen	*Galen On Anatomical Procedures*, trans. by C. Singer (Oxford 1956)
Galen	*Galen On the Natural Faculties*, trans. by A. J. Brock. LCL (London 1916)
Galen	*Galen On the Usefulness of the Parts of the Body*, trans. by M. T. May, 2 vols (Ithaca, New York, 1968)
Galen	'Galen On Abnormal Swellings', trans. by D. G. Lytton and L. M. Resuhr, *JHM* 33 (1978), 531–49
Galen	'Galen On Tremor, Palpitation, Spasm, and Rigor', trans. by D. Sider and M. McVaugh, *Transactions and Studies of the College of Physicians of Philadelphia* new series 1, (1979), 183–210
Galen	*Galen On Respiration and the Arteries*, trans. by D. J. Furley and J. S. Wilkie (Princeton 1984)
Galen	*Galen: Three Treatises on the Nature of Science*, trans. by R. Walzer and M. Frede (Indianapolis 1985)
Greek Anthology	*The Greek anthology* vol. 4, trans. by W. R. Paton. LCL, 5 vols (London 1918)
Herodotus	*Herodotus*, trans. by A. D. Godley. LCL, 4 vols (London 1971)
Hippocrates	*Hippocrates*, trans. by W. H. S. Jones and E. T. Withington. LCL, 4 vols (London 1923–31)
Hippocrates	*The medical works of Hippocrates*, trans. by J. Chadwick and W. N. Mann (Oxford 1950)
Hippocrates	*Hippocratic writings*, trans. by J. Chadwick, W. N. Mann, I. M. Lonie and E. T. Withington. Ed. and introd. G. E. R. Lloyd (Harmondsworth 1978)
Homer, *Iliad*	*The Iliad*, trans. by A. T. Murray. LCL, 2 vols (London 1967)
Homer, *Odyssey*	*The Odyssey*, trans by A. T. Murray. LCL, 2 vols (London 1924)
Juvenal, Satires	*Juvenal and Persius*, trans. by G. G. Ramsay. LCL (London 1912)
Lucian	*Lucian, selected works*, trans. by B. P. Reardon (New York 1965)

Martial, *Epigrams*	*Martial Epigrams*, trans. by W. C. A. Ker. LCL, 2 vols (London 1968)
Paul	*The seven books of Paulus Aegineta*, trans. and commentary by F. Adams. 3 vols (London 1844–7)
Pausanias, *Description of Greece*	*Pausanias description of Greece*, trans. by W. H. S. Jones. LCL, 4 vols (London 1978)
Pliny, *Letters*	*The letters of the Younger Pliny*, trans. by B. Radice (Harmondsworth 1963)
Pliny, *Natural History*	*Pliny Natural History*, trans. by H. Rackham, W. H. S. Jones and D. E. Eichholz. LCL, 10 vols (London 1942–63).
Plutarch, *Parallel Lives*	*The Parallel Lives*, trans. by B. Perrin. LCL, 11 vols (London)
Scribonius Largus, *Compositiones*	*Scribonii Largi Compositiones*, ed. by S. Sconocchia (Leipzig 1983)
Seneca, *Epistulae Morales*	*Seneca Ad Lucilium Epistulae Morales*, trans. by R. M. Gummere. LCL, 3 vols (London 1917–25)
Soranus, *Gynaecology*	*Soranus' Gynecology*, trans. by O. Temkin (Baltimore 1956)
Tacitus, *Annals*	*Tacitus the Annals of Imperial Rome*, trans. by M. Grant (Harmondsworth 1971)
Vitruvius, *De Architectura*	*Vitruvius On Architecture*, ed. and trans. by F. Grainger. LCL, 2 vols (London 1970)

General works

ALLBUTT, T. C. 1921. *Greek medicine in Rome* (London, repr. New York 1970)

CASTIGLIONI, A. 1947. *A history of medicine* (London and New York)

EDELSTEIN, L. 1967. *Ancient medicine: selected papers*, eds O. and C. L. Temkin (Baltimore)

FRENCH, R. AND GREENAWAY, F. (EDS) 1986. *Science in the early Roman Empire: Pliny the Elder, his sources and influence* (London)

GARRISON, F. H. 1929. *An introduction to the history of medicine* (London)

GILLISPIE, C. C. (ED.) 1970–. *Dictionary of scientific biography* (New York)

HAMMOND, N. G. L. AND SCULLARD, H. H. 1970. *The Oxford classical dictionary* (Oxford)

HOLLÄNDER, E. 1912. *Plastik und Medizin* (Stuttgart)

JONES, A. H. M. 1973. *The later Roman empire 284–602* (Oxford)

KOELBING, H. M. 1977. *Arzt und Patient in der antiken Welt* (Zürich)

KOLLESCH, J. AND NICKEL, D. (TRANS. & ED.) 1979. *Antike Heilkunst: ausgewählte Texte aus dem medizinischen Schrifttum der Griechen und Römer* (Leipzig)

KRUG, A. 1985. *Heilkunst und Heilkult: Medizin in der Antike* (Munich)

LEITNER, H. 1973. *Bibliography to the ancient medical authors* (Bern)

LYONS, A. S. AND PETRUCELLI, R. J. 1978. *Medicine: an illustrated history* (New York)

MAJNO, G. 1975. *The healing hand: man and wound in the ancient world* (Cambridge, Massachusetts)

MEYER-STEINEG, T. AND SUDHOFF, K. 1921. *Geschichte der Medizin im Überblick mit Abbildungen* (Jena)

ROSTOVTZEFF, M. 1966. *The economic history of the Roman empire* (Oxford 2nd edn)

SCARBOROUGH, J. 1969. *Roman medicine* (London)

SCHOUTEN, J. 1967. *The rod and serpent of Asklepios: symbol of medicine* (London)

SIGERIST, H. E. 1961. *A history of medicine* vol. 2. (Oxford and New York)

SINGER, C. 1928. *A short history of medicine* (Oxford)

STILLWELL, R. (ED.) 1976. *The Princeton encyclopaedia of classical sites* (Princeton)

TEMKIN, O. 1977. *The double face of Janus and other essays in the history of medicine* (Baltimore and London)

UNDERWOOD, E. A. (ED.) 1953. *Science, medicine, and history* (London)

Specific topics

AMULREE, LORD 1973. 'Hygiene conditions in ancient Rome and modern London', *Med. Hist.* 17, 244–55

AMUNDSEN, D. W. 1974. 'Romanticizing the ancient medical profession: the characterization of the physician in the Graeco-Roman novel', *BHM* 48, 320–37

AMUNDSEN, D. W. 1977. 'The liability of the physician in classical Greek legal theory and practice', *JHM* 32, 172–203

AMUNDSEN, D. W. AND DIERS, C. J. 1970. 'The age of menopause in classical Greece and Rome', *Human Biology* 42 (1), 79–86

AMUNDSEN, D. W. AND FERNGREN, G. B. 1979. 'The forensic role of physicians in Roman law', *BHM* 53, 39–56

ANDRÉ, J. 1981. *L'alimentation et la cuisine à Rome* (Rome)

ANDRÉ, J. 1987. *Être médecin à Rome* (Paris)

APPELBOOM, T. (ED.) 1987. *Art, history and antiquity of rheumatic diseases* (Brussels)

ASHBY, T. 1935. *The aqueducts of ancient Rome* (Oxford)

BAADER, G. 1967. 'Spezialärzte in der Spätantike', *Medizinhistorisches Journal* 2, 231–8

BALLESTER, L. G. 1981. 'Galen as a medical practitioner: problems in diagnosis', *in* V. Nutton (ed.), *Galen: problems and prospects* (London)

BALSDON, J. P. V. D. 1962. *Roman women* (London)

BARROW, M. V. 1972. 'Portraits of Hippocrates', *Med. Hist.* 16, 85–8

BEHR, C. A. 1968. *Aelius Aristides and the Sacred Tales* (Amsterdam)

BERNARD, R. AND VASSAL, P. 1958. 'Étude médicale des *ex-voto* des sources de la Seine', *Revue archéologique de l'est et du centre-est* 9, 328–37

BIRLEY, A. 1966. *Marcus Aurelius* (London)

BISHOP, W. J. 1960. *The early history of surgery* (London)

BLAYNEY, J. 1986. 'Theories of conception in the ancient Roman World', *in* B. Rawson (ed.), *The family in ancient Rome: new perspectives* (New York) 230–36

BLIQUEZ, L. J. 1981. 'Greek and Roman medicine: the probing surgical tools of antiquity', *Archaeology* 34 (2), 10–17

BLIQUEZ, L. J. 1983. 'Classical prosthetics', *Archaeology* 36 (5), 25–9

BOON, G. C. 1983. 'Potters, oculists and eye-troubles', *Britannia* 14, 1–12

BOURKE, J. B. 1967. 'A review of the palaeopathology of the arthritic diseases', *in* D. Brothwell and A. T. Sandison (eds), *Diseases in antiquity* (Springfield, Illinois)

BOURKE, J. B. 1971. 'The palaeopathology of the vertebral column in ancient Egypt and Nubia', *Med. Hist.* 15, 363–75

BRADLEY, K. R. 1980. 'Sexual regulations in wet-nursing contracts from Roman Egypt', *Klio* 62 (2), 321–5

BRADLEY, K. R. 1986. 'Wet-nursing at Rome: a study in social relations', *in* B. Rawson, (ed.), *The family in ancient Rome: new perspectives* (New York) 201–29

BRAIN, P. 1982. 'The Hippocratic physician and his drugs', *Classical Philology* 78, 48–51

BRATTON, T. L. 1981. 'The identity of the plague of Justinian', *Transactions and Studies of the College of Physicians of Philadelphia* Series 5, vol. 3, 113–24 and 174–80

BROCKINGTON, C. F. 1975. 'The history of public health', *in* W. Hobson (ed.), *The theory and practice of public health* (London)

BROTHWELL, D. 1963. *Digging up bones* (London)

BROTHWELL, D. (ED.) 1968. *The skeletal biology of earlier human populations* (Oxford)

BROTHWELL, D. AND P. 1969. *Food in antiquity* (London)

BROTHWELL, D. AND HIGGS, E. (EDS) 1970. *Science in archaeology* (2nd edn, London)

BROTHWELL, D. AND SANDISON, A. T. (EDS) 1967. *Diseases in antiquity* (Springfield, Illinois)

BURFORD, A. 1969. *The Greek temple builders of Epidauros* (Liverpool)

CARCOPINO, J. 1941. *Daily life in ancient Rome* (1973 reprint, London)

CARRICK, P. 1985. *Medical ethics in antiquity: Phiolosphical perspectives on abortion and euthanasia* (Dordrecht)

CHADWICK, J. AND MANN. W. N. 1950. *The medical works of Hippocrates* (Oxford)

COCKBURN, A. 1963. *The evolution and eradication of infectious diseases* (Baltimore)

COCKBURN, T. A. 1971. 'Infectious diseases in ancient populations', *Current Anthropology* 12, 45–62

COCKBURN, A, AND E. (EDS) 1983. *Mummies, disease and ancient cultures* (Cambridge)

COHN-HAFT, L. 1956. *The public physicians of ancient Greece* (Northampton, Mass.)

COOKE, C. AND ROWBOTHAM, T. C. 1968. 'Dental report' *in* L. P. Wenham, *The Romano-British cemetery at Trentholme Drive, York* (London) 179–216

CUNLIFFE, B. 1969. *Roman Bath* (Oxford)

CUNLIFFE, B. 1980. 'The excavation of the Roman spring at Bath 1979', *Antiquaries Journal* 60, 187–206

CUNLIFFE, B. 1984. *Roman Bath discovered* (London)

CUNLIFFE, B. AND DAVENPORT, P. 1985. *The temple of Sulis Minerva at Bath vol. 1: the site* (Oxford)

DAVIES, R. W. 1969. 'The *medici* of the Roman armed forces', *Epigraphische Studien* 8, 83 ff.

DAVIES, R. W. 1970a. 'Some Roman medicine', *Med. Hist.* 14, 101–6

DAVIES, R. W. 1970b. 'The Roman military medical service', *Saalburg Jahrbuch* 27, 84–104

DAVIES, R. W. 1971. 'The Roman military diet', *Britannia* 2, 122–42

DAVIES, R. W. 1972. 'Some more military *medici*', *Epigraphische Studien* 9, 1 ff.

DAWSON, W. R. 1953. 'The Egyptian medical papyri' *in* E. A. Underwood (ed.), *Science, medicine and history* (London)

DECOUFLÉ, P. 1964. 'La notion d'*ex-voto* anatomique chez les etrusco-romains', *Collection Latomus* 72

DEHN, W. 1941. 'Ein Quellheiligtum des Apollo und der Sirona bei Hochscheid, Kr. Bernkastel', *Germania* 25, 104–11

DEYTS, S. 1983. *Les bois sculptés des sources de la Seine* (42nd supplement to *Gallia*, Paris)

DI BENEDETTO, V. 1986. *Il medico e la malattia: la scienza di Ippocrate* (Turin)

DICKISON, S. K. 1973. 'Abortion in antiquity', *Arethusa* 6, 159–66

DODDS, E. R. 1965. 'Man and the daemonic world', *in Pagan and Christian in an age of anxiety* (Cambridge)

DRABKIN, I. E. 1944. 'On medical education in Greece and Rome', *BHM* 15, 333–51

DRABKIN, I. E. 1951. 'Soranus and his system of medicine', *BHM* 25, 503–18

EDELSTEIN, E. J. AND L. 1945. *Asclepius: a collection and interpretation of the testimonies*, 2 vols (Baltimore)

EDELSTEIN, L. 1956. 'The professional ethics of the Greek physician', *BHM* 30, 391–419

EDELSTEIN, L. 1967. 'The dietetics of antiquity', *in Ancient medicine: selected papers* (Baltimore), 303–18

EISINGER, J. 1982. 'Lead and wine: Eberhard Gockel and the *colica Pictonum*', *Med. Hist.* 26, 279–302

ELLIOT SMITH, G. AND DAWSON, W. R. 1924. *Egyptian Mummies* (London)

ELLIOT SMITH, G. AND WOOD JONES, F. 1908. Anatomical report. *Archaeological survey of Nubia* Bulletin 1

ELLIOT SMITH, G. AND WOOD JONES, F. 1910. Report on the human remains. *Archaeological survey of Nubia* Bulletin 2

EMERY, G. T. 1963. 'Dental pathology and archaeology', *Antiquity* 37, 274–81

ENGELS, D. 1980. 'The problem of female infanticide in the Graeco-Roman world', *Classical Philology* 75, 112–20

ESCHEBACH, H. 1984. 'Die Ärzthäuser in Pompeji', *Antike Welt* Sonderheft 15

FENELLI, M. 1975. 'Contributo per lo studio del votivo anatomico: i votivi anatomici di Lavinio', *Archeologia Classica* 27, 206 ff.

FERGUSON, J. 1970. *The religions of the Roman empire* (London)

FERNGREN, G. B. 1985. 'Roman lay attitudes towards medical experimentation', *BHM* 59, 495–505

FESTUGIÈRE, A. J. 1954. 'Popular piety: Aelius Aristides and Asclepius', *in Personal religion among the Greeks* (Berkeley and Los Angeles)

FEUGÈRE, M., KÜNZL, E. AND WEISSER, U. 1985. 'Die Starnadeln von Montbellet (Saône-et-Loire). Ein Beitrag zur antiken und islamischen Augenheilkunde', *Jahrbuch des römisch-germanischen Zentralmuseums* 32, 436–508

FISCHER, K.-D. 1979. 'Zur Entwicklung des ärztlichen Standes im römischen Kaiserreich', *Medizinhistorisches Journal* 14, 165–75

FLOWER, B. AND ROSENBAUM, E. 1958. *The Roman cookery book: a critical translation of the art of cooking by Apicius* (London)

FONTANILLE, M-T. 1977. *Avortement et contraception dans la médecine gréco-romaine* (Paris)

FORBES, R. J. 1955a–c. *Studies in ancient technology* vols 1–3 (Leiden)

FORBES, R. J. 1966a–b. *Studies in ancient technology* vols 5–6 (2nd edn, Leiden)

FRASER, P. M. 1972. *Ptolemaic Alexandria*, 3 vols (Oxford): vol. 1, 336–376, 'Alexandrian Science: Medicine'.

FREDE, M. 1982. 'The method of the so-called Methodical School of medicine', *in* J. Barnes et al. (eds), *Science and speculation: studies in Hellenistic theory and practice* (Cambridge and Paris), 1–23

GARNSEY, P. AND WHITTAKER, C. R. (EDS) 1983. *Trade and famine in classical antiquity* (Cambridge)

GASK, G. E. AND TODD, J. 1953. 'The origin of hospitals', *in* A. E. Underwood (ed.), *Science, medicine and history* (London)

GHALIOUNGUI, P. 1963. *Magic and medical science in ancient Egypt* (London)

GHALIOUNGUI, P. 1973. *The house of life, per ankh: magic and medical science in ancient Egypt* (Amsterdam)

GHALIOUNGUI, P. 1983. *The physicians of Pharaonic Egypt* (Cairo)

GILLIAM, J. F. 1961. 'The plague under Marcus Aurelius', *American Journal of Philology* 73, 225–51

GOUREVITCH, D. 1984a. *Le triangle Hippocratique dans le monde gréco-romain: le malade, sa maladie et son médecin* (Rome)

GOUREVITCH, D. 1984b. *Le mal d'être femme: la femme et la médecine dans la Rome antique* (Paris)

GRENIER, A. 1960. *Manuel d'archéologie gallo-romaine, IV, 2: les monuments des eaux* (Paris)

GRENSEMANN, H. 1982. *Hippokratische Gynäkologie* (Wiesbaden)

GRMEK, M. D. (ED.) 1980. *Actes du Colloque hippocratique de Paris (4–9 Septembre 1978)* (Paris)

GRMEK, M. D. 1983. *Les maladies à l'aube de la civilisation occidentale* (Paris)

GUMMERUS, H. 1932. *Der Ärztestand im römischen Reiche nach den Inschriften* (Helsingfors)

GUNTHER, R. T. 1934. *The Greek herbal of Dioscorides* (Oxford)

HAMILTON, J. S. 1986. 'Scribonius Largus on the medical profession', *BHM* 60, 209–16

HANSON, A. E. 1985. 'Papyri of medical content', *Yale Classical Studies* 28, 25–48

HANSON, A. E. 1987. 'The eight months' child and the etiquette of birth: *obsit omen!*', *BHM* 61, 589–602

HARE, R. 1967. 'The antiquity of disease caused by bacteria and viruses. A review of the problem from a bacteriologist's point of view', *in* D. Brothwell and A. T. Sandison (eds) *Diseases in antiquity* (Springfield, Illinois)

HARIG, G. 1971. 'Zum Problem "Krankenhaus" in der Antike', *Klio* 53, 179–95

HARIG, G. 1983. 'Die philosophischen Grundlagen des medizinischen Systems des Asklepiades von Bithynien', *Philologus* 127, 43–60

HARIG, G. AND KOLLESCH, J. 1978. 'Der Hippokratische Eid: zur Entstehung der antiken medizinischen Deontologie', *Philologus* 122, 157–76

HARRIS, C. R. S. 1973. *The heart and the vascular system in ancient Greek medicine from Alcmaeon to Galen* (Oxford)

HARRIS, J. E. AND PONITZ, P. V. 1980. 'Dental health in ancient Egypt' *in* A. and E. Cockburn (eds) *Mummies, disease and ancient cultures* (Cambridge)

HARRIS, W. V. 1982. 'The theoretical possibility of extensive infanticide in the Graeco-Roman world', *Classical Quarterly* 32, 114–16

HART, G. D. (ED.) 1983. *Disease in ancient man: an international symposium* (Toronto)

HENIG, M. 1984. *Religion in Roman Britain* (London)

HERSCHEL, C. 1913. *The two books on the water supply of the city of Rome of Sextus Julius Frontinus* (New York)

HERZOG, R. 1931. 'Die Wunderheilungen von Epidauros', *Philologus* Suppl. 22, 3 (Leipzig)

HERZOG, R. AND SCHAZMANN, P. 1932. *Kos I: Asklepieion* (Berlin)

HOFFMANN-AXTHELM, W. 1981. *History of dentistry* (Chicago)

HOPKINS, K. 1966. 'Contraception in the Roman empire', *Comparative studies in society and history* 8, 124–51

HOWE, G. M. 1972. *Man, environment and disease in Britain: a medical geography of Britain through the ages* (Newton Abbot)

HURD-MEAD, K. C. 1938. *A history of women in medicine* (Haddam)

HUXLEY, H. H. 1957. 'Greek doctor and Roman patient', *Greece and Rome* 26, 132–8

JACKSON, R. 1986. 'A set of Roman medical instruments from Italy', *Britannia* 17, 119–67

JONES, W. H. S. 1946. *Philosophy and medicine in ancient Greece* (Baltimore: *BHM* supplement no. 8)

JONES, W. H. S. 1947. *The medical writings of Anonymus Londinensis* (Cambridge)

JOUANNA, J. 1974. *Hippocrate. Pour une archéologie de l'école de Cnide* (Paris)

KING, H. 1983. 'Bound to bleed: Artemis and Greek women', *in* A. Cameron and A. Kuhrt (eds), *Images of women in antiquity* (London), 109–27

KING, H. 1986. 'Agnodike and the profession of medicine', *Proceedings of the Cambridge Philological Society* 212, 53–77

KIRK, G. S. AND RAVEN, J. E. 1957. *The presocratic philosophers* (Cambridge)

KOELBING, H. M. 1977. *Arzt und Patient in der antiken Welt* (Zürich)

KOLLESCH, J. 1979. 'Ärztliche Ausbildung in der Antike', *Klio* 61 (2), 507–13

KUDLIEN, F. 1967. *Der Beginn des medizinischen Denkens bei den Griechen* (Zurich and Stuttgart)

KUDLIEN, F. 1968. *Die Sklaven in der griechischen Medizin der klassischen und hellenistischen Zeit* (Wiesbaden)

KUDLIEN, F. 1970. 'Medical ethics and popular ethics in Greece and Rome', *Clio Medica* 5, 91–121

KUDLIEN, F. 1976. 'Medicine as a "Liberal Art" and the question of the physician's income', *JHM* 31, 448–59

KUDLIEN, F. 1979. *Der griechische Arzt im Zeitalter des Hellenismus: seine Stellung in Staat und Gesellschaft* (Mainz)

KUDLIEN, F. 1981. 'Galen's religious belief' *in* V. Nutton (ed.), *Galen: problems and prospects* (London)

KUDLIEN, F. 1986. *Die Stellung des Arztes in der römischen Gesellschaft* (Stuttgart)

KÜNZL, E. 1982a. 'Ventosae cucurbitae romanae?', *Germania* 60, 513–32

KÜNZL, E. 1982b. 'Medizinische Instrumente aus Sepulkralfunden der römischen Kaiserzeit', *Bonner Jahrbücher* 182, 1–137

KÜNZL, E. 1983. 'Eine Spezialität römischer Chirurgen: die Lithotomie', *Archäologisches Korrespondenzblatt* 13, 487–93

KÜNZL, E. 1984. 'Einige Bemerkungen zu den Herstellern der römischen medizinischen Instrumente', *Alba Regia* 21, 59–65

KÜNZL, E. 1986. 'Operationsräume in römischen Thermen', *Bonner Jahrbücher* 186, 491–509

LEFKOWITZ, M. R. AND FANT, M. B. 1982. *Women's life in Greece and Rome* (London)

LEWIS, N. 1976. *The interpretation of dreams and portents* (Toronto)

LLOYD, G. E. R. 1970. *Early Greek science: Thales to Aristotle* (London)

LLOYD, G. E. R. 1973. 'Hellenistic biology and medicine', chapter 6 of *Greek science after Aristotle* (London)

LLOYD, G. E. R. 1975a. 'Alcmaeon and the early history of dissection'. *Sudhoffs Archiv* 59, 113 ff.

LLOYD, G. E. R. 1975b. 'A note on Erasistratus of Ceos', *Journal of Hellenic Studies* 95, 172–5

LLOYD, G. E. R. 1975c. 'The Hippocratic question', *Classical Quarterly* 25, 171–92

LLOYD, G. E. R. (ED.) 1978. *Hippocratic Writings* (Harmondsworth)

LLOYD, G. E. R. 1979. *Magic, reason and experience: studies in the origins and development of Greek science* (Cambridge)

LLOYD, G. E. R. 1983. 'The critique of traditional ideas in Soranus' Gynaecology', *in Science, folklore and ideology: studies in the life sciences in ancient Greece* (Cambridge)

LONGFIELD-JONES, G. M. 1986. 'A Graeco-Roman speculum in the Wellcome Museum', *Med. Hist.* 30, 81–9

LONGRIGG, J. 1981. 'Superlative achievement and comparative neglect: Alexandrian medical science and modern historical research', *History of Science* 19, 155–200

LONIE, I. M. 1977. 'A structural pattern in Greek dietetics and the early history of Greek medicine', *Med. Hist.* 21, 235–60

LONIE, I. M. 1978. 'Cos versus Cnidus and the historians', *History of Science* 16, 42–75 and 77–92

MACDOUGALL, E. B. AND JASHEMSKI, W. F. (EDS) 1981. *Ancient Roman gardens* (Dumbarton Oaks, Washington)

MAJNO, G. 1975. *The healing hand: man and wound in the ancient world* (Cambridge, Massachusetts)

MANCHESTER, K. 1983. *The archaeology of disease* (Bradford)

MANCHESTER, K. 1984. 'Tuberculosis and leprosy in antiquity: an interpretation', *Med. Hist.* 28, 162–73

MANULI, P. AND VEGETTI, M. 1977. *Cuore, sangue e cervello: biologia e antropologia nel pensiero antico* (Milan)

MARTIN, R. 1965. 'Wooden figures from the source of the Seine', *Antiquity* 39, 247–52

MCKAY, A. G. 1975. *Houses, villas and palaces in the Roman world* (London)

MCNEILL, W. H. 1977. *Plagues and peoples* (Oxford)

MEYER-STEINEG, T. 1912. 'Chirurgische Instrumente des Altertums', *Jenaer medizin-historische Beiträge* 1, 1 ff.

MICHLER, M. 1968. *Die alexandrinischen Chirurgen* (Wiesbaden)

MILLER, T. S. 1985. *The birth of the hospital in the Byzantine empire* (Baltimore and London)

MILNE, J. S. 1907. *Surgical instruments in Greek and Roman times* (Oxford; reprinted Chicago 1970)

MØLLER-CHRISTENSEN, V. 1938. *The history of the forceps* (Copenhagen and London)

MØLLER-CHRISTENSEN, V. 1961. *Bone changes in leprosy* (Bristol)

MØLLER-CHRISTENSEN, V. 1967. 'Evidence of leprosy in earlier peoples' *in* D. Brothwell and A. T. Sandison (eds), *Diseases in antiquity* (Springfield, Illinois)

MØLLER-CHRISTENSEN, V. 1973. 'Osteo-archaeology as a medico-historical auxiliary science', *Med. Hist.* 17, 411–18

MORAUX, P. 1985. *Galien de Pergame. Souvenirs d'un médecin* (Paris)

MORSE, D. 1967. 'Tuberculosis', *in* D. Brothwell and A. T. Sandison (eds), *Diseases in antiquity* (Springfield, Illinois)

MUDRY, P. 1985. 'Médecins et spécialistes. Le problème de l'unité de la médecine à Rome au premier siècle ap. J.-C.', *Gesnerus* 42, 329–36

NICKEL, D. 1979. 'Berufsvorstellungen über weibliche Medizinalpersonen in der Antike', *Klio* 61 (2), 515–18

NIELSEN, H. 1974. *Ancient ophthalmological agents* (Odense)

NUTTON, V. 1969. 'Medicine and the Roman army: a further reconsideration', *Med. Hist.* 13, 260–70

NUTTON, V. 1971. 'Two notes on immunities', *Journal of Roman Studies* 61, 52–63

NUTTON, V. 1972. 'Roman oculists', *Epigraphica* 34, 16–29

NUTTON, V. 1973. 'The chronology of Galen's early career', *Classical Quarterly* 23, 158–71

NUTTON, V. 1977. '*Archiatri* and the medical profession in antiquity', *Papers of the British School at Rome* 45, 191–226

NUTTON, V. 1981a. 'Continuity or rediscovery? The city physician in classical antiquity and mediaeval Italy', in A. W. Russell (ed.), *The town and state physician in Europe, from the Middle ages to the Enlightenment* (Wolfenbüttel) 9–46

NUTTON, V. (ED.) 1981b. *Galen: problems and prospects* (London)

NUTTON, V. 1983. 'The seeds of disease: an explanation of contagion and infection from the Greeks to the Renaissance'. *Med. Hist.* 27, 1–34

NUTTON, V. 1984. 'Galen in the eyes of his contemporaries', *BHM* 58, 315–24

NUTTON, V. 1985a. 'The drug trade in antiquity', *Journal of the Royal Society of Medicine* 78, 138–45

NUTTON, V. 1985b. 'Murders and miracles, lay attitudes towards medicine in classical antiquity', in R. S. Porter (ed.), *Patients and practitioners: lay perceptions of medicine in pre-industrial society* (Cambridge)

NUTTON, V. 1986. 'The perils of patriotism: Pliny and Roman medicine', in R. French and F. Greenaway (eds), *Science in the early Roman empire* (London)

OBERHELMAN, S. M. 1981. 'The interpretation of prescriptive dreams in ancient Greek medicine', *JHM* 36, 416–24

OBERHELMAN, S. M. 1983. 'Galen, *On Diagnosis from Dreams*', *JHM* 38, 36–47

OBERHELMAN, S. M. 1987. 'The diagnostic dream in ancient medical theory and practice', *BHM* 61, 47–60

ORTNER, D. J. AND PUTSCHAR, W. G. J. 1984. *Identification of pathological conditions in human skeletal remains* (Washington)

PATRICK, A. 1967. 'Disease in antiquity: ancient Greece and Rome', in D. Brothwell and A. T. Sandison (eds), *Diseases in antiquity* (Springfield, Illinois)

PEARCY, L. T. 1985. 'Galen's Pergamum', *Archaeology* 38 (6), 33–9

PELLETIER, A. (ED.) 1985. *La médecine en Gaule: villes d'eaux, sanctuaires des eaux* (Paris)

PENELLA, R. J. AND HALL, T. S. 1973. 'Galen's "On the Best Constitution of our Body". Introduction, translation, and notes', *BHM* 47, 282–96

VON PETRIKOVITS, H. 1975. *Die Innenbauten römischer Legionslager während der Prinzipatszeit* (Opladen)

PHILLIPS, E. D. 1973. *Greek medicine* (London)

PHILLIPS, J. H. 1980. 'The emergence of the Greek medical profession in the Roman Republic', *Transactions and Studies of the College of Physicians of Philadelphia* new series 2, 267–75

POMEROY, S. B. 1983. 'Infanticide in Hellenistic Greece', in A. Cameron and A. Kuhrt (eds), *Images of women in antiquity* (London), 207–22

POTTER, P. 1976. 'Herophilus of Chalcedon: an assessment of his place in the history of anatomy', *BHM* 50, 45–60

POTTER, T. W. 1985. 'A Republican healing sanctuary at Ponte di Nona near Rome and the classical tradition of votive medicine', *Journal of the British Archaeological Association* 138, 23–47

RANKE, H. 1941. *Medicine and surgery in ancient Egypt* (Philadelphia)

REECE, R. 1982. 'Bones, bodies and dis-ease', *Oxford Journal of Archaeology* 1 (3), 347–58

RÉMY, B. 1984. 'Les inscriptions de médecins en Gaule', *Gallia* 42, 115–52

RENFREW, J. 1985. *Food and cooking in Roman Britain* (London)

RICCI, J. V. 1949. *The development of gynaecological surgery and instruments* (Philadelphia)

RIDDLE, J. M. 1985. *Dioscorides on pharmacy and medicine* (Austin, Texas)

ROEBUCK, C. 1951. 'The Asklepieion and Lerna', *Corinth* 14 (Princeton)

ROMEUF, A-M. 1986. '*Ex-voto* en bois de Chamalières (Puy-de-Dôme) et des sources de la Seine. Essai de comparaison', *Gallia* 44, 65–89

ROUSSELLE, R. 1985. 'Healing cults in antiquity: the dream cures of Asclepius of Epidaurus', *Journal of Psychohistory* 12, 339–51

SANDISON, A. T. 1968. 'Pathological changes in the skeletons of earlier populations due to acquired disease and difficulties in their interpretation', in D. Brothwell (ed.), *The skeletal biology of earlier human populations* (Oxford)

SANDISON, A. T. 1980. 'Diseases in ancient Egypt', in A. and E. Cockburn (eds), *Mummies, disease and ancient cultures* (Cambridge)

SARTON, G. 1954. *Galen of Pergamon* (Kansas)

SAUNDERS, J. B. DE C. M. 1963. *The transition from ancient Egyptian to Greek medicine* (Lawrence, Kansas)

SCARBOROUGH, J. 1975. 'The drug lore of Asclepiades of Bithynia', *Pharmacy in History* 17, 43–57

SCARBOROUGH, J. 1976. 'Celsus on human vivisection at ptolemaic Alexandria', *Clio Medica* 11, 25–38

SCARBOROUGH, J. 1981. 'The Galenic question', *Sudhoffs Archiv* 65, 1–31

SCARBOROUGH, J. 1982. 'Roman pharmacy and the eastern drug trade', *Pharmacy in History* 24, 135–43

SCARBOROUGH, J. 1984. 'The myth of lead poisoning among the Romans: an essay review', *JHM* 39, 469–75

SCARBOROUGH, J. 1985a. 'Erasistratus: student of Theophrastus?', *BHM* 59, 515–17

SCARBOROUGH, J. 1985b. *Pharmacy's ancient heritage: Theophrastus, Nicander, and Dioscorides* (Lexington, Kentucky)

SCARBOROUGH, J. 1986. 'Pharmacy in Pliny's Natural History: some observations on substances and sources' in R. French and F. Greenaway (eds), *Science in the early Roman empire* (London)

SCARBOROUGH, J. 1987. 'Texts and sources in ancient pharmacy', *Pharmacy in History* 29, 81–4 and 133–9

SCARBOROUGH, J. AND NUTTON, V. 1982. 'The *Preface* of Dioscorides' *Materia Medica*: introduction, translation, and commentary', *Transactions and Studies of the College of Physicians of Philadelphia* new series 4, 187–227

SCHULTZE, R. 1934. 'Die römischen Legionslazarette in Vetera und anderen Legionslagern', *Bonner Jahrbücher* 139, 54–63

SHAW, B. D. 1987. 'The age of Roman girls at marriage: some reconsiderations', *Journal of Roman Studies* 77, 30–46

SHERWIN-WHITE, S. 1978. *Ancient Cos. An historical study from the Dorian settlement to the imperial period* (Göttingen)

SHORTER, E. 1983. *A history of women's bodies* (London)

SIMON, B. 1978. *Mind and madness in ancient Greece: the classical roots of modern psychiatry* (Ithaca and London)

SMITH, W. D. 1973. 'Galen on Coans versus Cnidians', *BHM* 47, 569–85

SMITH, W. D. 1979. *The Hippocratic tradition* (New York and London)

SMITH, W. D. 1982. 'Erasistratus's dietetic medicine' *BHM* 56, 398–409

VON STADEN, H. 1975. 'Experiment and experience in Hellenistic medicine', *Bulletin of the Institute of Classical Studies* 22, 178–99

VON STADEN, H. 1988. *Herophilus: the art of medicine in early Alexandria* (Cambridge)

STEINBOCK, R. T. 1976. *Palaeopathological diagnosis and interpretation* (Illinois)

STEPHENS, G. R. 1984/5. 'Aqueduct delivery and water consumption in Roman Britain', *Bulletin of the Institute of Archaeology, University of London* 21/22, 111–17

STEPHENS, G. R. 1985. 'Civic aqueducts in Britain', *Britannia* 16, 197–208

SUDHOFF, K. 1964. *Geschichte der Zahnheilkunde* (Hildesheim)

TABANELLI, M. 1958. *Lo strumento chirurgico e la sua storia* (Milan)

TABANELLI, M. 1962. *Gli ex-voto poliviscerali etruschi e romani* (Florence)

TABANELLI, M. 1963. *La medicina nel mondo degli Etruschi* (Florence)

TEMKIN, O. 1956. *Soranus' Gynecology* (Baltimore)

TEMKIN, O. 1973. *Galenism* (New York)

TEMKIN, O. 1979. 'Medical ethics and honoraria in Late Antiquity; *in* C. E. Rosenberg (ed.), *Healing and History: essays for George Rosen* (New York) 6–26

THIVEL, A. 1981. *Cnide et Cos?: essai sur les doctrines médicales dans la collection Hippocratique* (Paris)

TOLEDO-PEREYRA, L. H. 1973. 'Galen's contribution to the history of surgery', *JHM* 28, 357–75

TOMLINSON, R. A. 1969. 'Two buildings in sanctuaries of Asklepios', *Journal of Hellenic Studies* 89, 106–17

TOMLINSON, R. A. 1983. *Epidauros* (London)

TRAVLOS, J. 1971. *Pictorial dictionary of ancient Athens* Asklepieion 127–37 (London)

TZAVELLA-EVJEN, H. 1983. 'Homeric medicine' *in* R. Högg (ed.), *The Greek renaissance of the eighth century BC* (Stockholm) 185–8

VATIN, C. 1969. '*Ex-voto* de bois gallo-romains à Chamalières', *Revue Archéologique* 1, 103–14

VATIN, C. 1972. 'Wooden sculpture from Gallo-Roman Auvergne', *Antiquity* 46, 39–42

VOINOT, J. 1984. 'Inventaire des cachets d'oculistes gallo-romains', *Conférences Lyonnaises d'ophtalmologie* 150 (1981–2) 1–578

WALDRON, H. A. 1973. 'Lead poisoning in the ancient world', *Med. Hist.* 17, 391–9

WANGENSTEEN, O. H. AND S. D. 1978. *The rise of surgery* (Folkestone)

WARREN, C. P. W. 1970. 'Some aspects of medicine in the Greek Bronze Age', *Med. Hist.* 14, 364–77

WARWICK, R. 1968. 'The skeletal remains' *in* L. P. Wenham, *The Romano-British cemetery at Trentholme Drive, York* (London)

WATTS, W. J. 1973. 'Ovid, the law and Roman society on abortion', *Acta classica* 16, 89–101

WELLS, C. 1964. *Bones, bodies and disease* (London)

WELLS, C. 1967a. 'A Roman surgical instrument from Norfolk'. *Antiquity* 41, 139–41

WELLS, C. 1967b. 'Pseudopathology' *in* D. Brothwell and A. T. Sandison (eds), *Diseases in antiquity* (Springfield, Illinois)

WELLS, C. 1973. 'A palaeopathological rarity in a skeleton of Roman date', *Med. Hist.* 17, 399–400

WELLS, C. 1974. 'Osteochondritis dissecans in ancient British skeletal material', *Med. Hist.* 18, 365–9

WELLS, C. 1975. 'Ancient obstetric hazards and female mortality', *Bulletin of the New York Academy of Medicine* 51, 1235–49

WELLS, C. 1976. 'Romano-British pathology', *Antiquity* 50, 53–5

WELLS, C. 1982. 'The human burials' *in* A. McWhirr, L. Viner and C. Wells *Romano-British cemeteries at Cirencester* (Cirencester)

WELLS, C. 1985. 'A medical interpretation of the votive terracottas' *in* Potter 1985, 41–4

WHEELER, R. E. M. AND T. V. 1932. *Report on the excavation of the prehistoric, Roman, and post-Roman site in Lydney Park, Gloucestershire* (Oxford)

WHITE, K. D. 1970. *Roman farming* (London)

WHITE, K. D. 1984. *Greek and Roman technology* (London)

WILMANNS, J. C. 1987. 'Zur Rangordnung der römischen Militärärzte während der mittleren Kaiserzeit', *Zeitschrift für Papyrologie und Epigraphik* 69, 177–89

WOOD JONES, F. 1908. The pathological report. *Archaeological survey of Nubia* Bulletin 2

WROTH, W. 1882. 'Telesphorus', *Journal of Hellenic Studies* 3, 283–300

ZIMMERMAN, M. R. AND KELLEY, M. A. 1982. *Atlas of human palaeopathology* (New York)

ŽIVANOVIĆ, S. 1982. *Ancient diseases: the elements of palaeopathology* (London)

Index